NURSING PROCESS

Application of theories, frameworks, and models

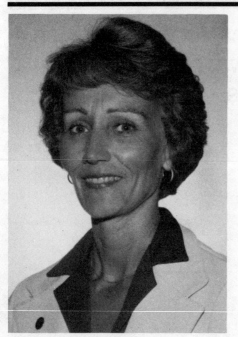

Janet W. Griffith, R.N., Ph.D., is an Associate Professor in the Graduate Pediatric and Women's Health Department at Indiana University School of Nursing. She has taught the nursing process and application of nursing models and frameworks to nursing faculty and students since the early 1970s. Currently, Dr. Griffith is teaching graduate nursing students to analyze and apply nursing theories in the nursing process.

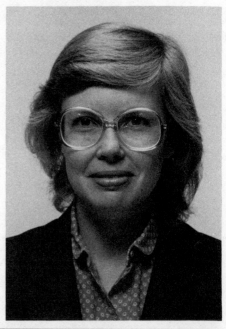

Paula J. Christensen, R.N., M.S., is a clinical nurse specialist in psychiatric/mental health at SwedishAmerican Hospital, Rockford, Illinois. She has experience teaching the nursing process and nursing and behavioral theories in undergraduate nursing education. Her current practice includes working with nurses to enhance the theoretical and clinical application of the nursing process.

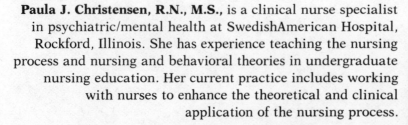

NURSING PROCESS

Application of theories, frameworks, and models

Edited by **JANET W. GRIFFITH, R.N., Ph.D.**

Associate Professor,
Graduate Pediatric and Women's Health Department,
Indiana University School of Nursing,
Indianapolis, Indiana

PAULA J. CHRISTENSEN, R.N., M.S.

Clinical Nurse Specialist,
Psychiatric/Mental Health,
SwedishAmerican Hospital,
Rockford, Illinois

The C. V. Mosby Company

ST. LOUIS • TORONTO • LONDON   1982

MOSBY

A TRADITION OF PUBLISHING EXCELLENCE

Editor: Pamela L. Swearingen
Assistant editor: Bess Arends
Book design: Kay Kramer
Cover design: Diane Beasley
Production: Susan Trail

The C.V. Mosby Company
11830 Westline Industrial Drive, St. Louis, Missouri 63141

Library of Congress Cataloging in Publication Data

Main entry under title:

Nursing process.

  Bibliography: p.
  Includes index.
  1. Nursing. 2. Nursing—Philosophy. I. Griffith,
Janet W. II. Christensen, Paula J. [DNLM:
1. Nursing process. WY 100 N9759]
RT42.N87   610.73   81-14191
ISBN 0-8016-1984-X   AACR2

GW/VH/VH 9 8 7 6 5 4 3 2   03/D/350

CONTRIBUTORS

Phyllis Baker Andrews
R.N., M.S.N.

Assistant Professor, Miami University, Oxford, Ohio

Paula J. Christensen
R.N., M.S.

Clinical Nurse Specialist, Psychiatric/Mental Health, SwedishAmerican Hospital, Rockford, Illinois

Joanne Renaud Cross
R.N., M.S.N.

Assistant Professor, Wright State University School of Nursing, Dayton, Ohio

Linda L. Delaney
R.N., M.S.

Oncology Clinical Specialist, Veteran's Administration Medical Center, Dayton, Ohio

Janet W. Griffith
R.N., Ph.D.

Associate Professor, Graduate Pediatric and Women's Health Department, Indiana University School of Nursing, Indianapolis, Indiana

Bonnie L. Sommerville
R.N., M.S.

Assistant Director of Staff Development, The Children's Medical Center, Dayton, Ohio

Grace Murabito Thomas
R.N., M.S.

Assistant Professor, Wright State University School of Nursing, Dayton, Ohio

The inception and initial planning for this book were completed when all the writers were on the faculty of Wright State University in January 1980.

This book is dedicated to all nurses and students of nursing
who aspire to practice professional nursing with
individual, family, and community clients

PREFACE

Dynamic changes have occurred in nursing practice over the last two decades. One major change is more rigorous application of the scientific process, which involves thorough and systematic investigation of a problem within a defined theoretical framework. Nursing is moving toward more rigorous application of scientific methods through refinement of the nursing process. The standards of nursing practice demonstrate the profession's commitment to the scientific approach in the nursing process. Nurses have developed systematic assessment tools, diagnostic categories, and improved implementation strategies. Gradually nurses are learning to apply theoretical frameworks to the nursing process. These theoretical approaches provide the base for application of the scientific process. Theories, frameworks, and conceptual models direct the focus of the nursing process and guide selection of implementation strategies.

This book is written primarily for professional student nurses, practitioners, and educators to enhance their knowledge and application of the contemporary nursing process. The contemporary approach uses eclectic theoretical frameworks and models as the basis for the nursing process. The basic components of the nursing process—assessing, analyzing and diagnosing, planning, implementing, and evaluating—are described in this book. These same components were identified by the National Council of State Boards of Nursing, Inc., for the revised State Board Examination.

This book describes how theoretical approaches are applied in each component of the nursing process. This is accomplished in three ways. First, the rationale and method of applying theoretical approaches are described. Second, each component of the nursing process is explained in detail, and the application of these approaches is demonstrated. Third, application of the nursing process to individual, family, and community clients is illustrated through the use of theoretical approaches.

Highlights of this book include a brief description of numerous frameworks and models from nursing and the behavioral sciences. These eclectic theoretical approaches are applied to individual, family, and community clients across all clinical areas. The complex process of analysis and synthesis, along with diagnosis, is explained in detail. Also, guidelines for applying the nursing process are a unique feature in the component chapters.

There are three sections in this book. Section I begins with a discussion of the relevance of a theoretical approach as the basis for professional nursing practice. The historical evolution of the nursing process and theory development is presented, and several nursing and behavioral theoretical frameworks and conceptual models are described. The explanations of these frameworks are the bases for understanding their application in subsequent chapters.

Section II describes in detail each component of the nursing process. It shows how to apply different frameworks and models and provides guidelines for applying each one. Examples are shown for applying each component to the individual, family, and community.

Section III is composed of case studies for an individual, a family, and a community. Each case study is critiqued to show how the guidelines and theoretical approaches are incorporated in the process.

We recommend that the reader begin with Chapter 1 and proceed in sequence through Chapter 11, since the book presents a continuum. Each chapter provides the basis for the next chapter. The first 11 chapters are the foundation for understanding the case studies in Section III. Appendix C contains additional summaries of theoretical frameworks and models not included in Chapter 2. A glossary and a complete list of the guidelines from each chapter are also in the appendixes.

We wish to express our extreme gratitude to the contributing writers for their diligent work. Their cooperation, support, and continued effort over the year are greatly appreciated. We also wish to thank our families and friends, especially Michelle Griffith and Roger Benedict, for their encouragement and support in writing this book. Appreciation is also given to Mary Anne Berry, the efficient typist whose assistance was invaluable. Last, we are indebted to The C.V. Mosby Company for their recognition and financial support of this contribution to the nursing profession.

Janet W. Griffith
Paula J. Christensen

CONTENTS

I

THEORY-BASED NURSING PRACTICE

Relevance of THEORETICAL APPROACHES in nursing practice

JANET W. GRIFFITH

Nursing is based on the integration and application of knowledge from the natural, behavioral, and humanistic sciences. This knowledge base rapidly changes and expands as new theories and research provide more information. Our knowledge and values about life, people, and events influence the way we perceive and understand the world around us. Some people perceive life and events as isolated, unrelated facts; this fragmented perception limits their perspective. Others, who perceive events from a broad, comprehensive viewpoint, are able to relate them to other events. The latter approach is more abstract and helps us organize facts and isolated events within frameworks. This approach helps nurses understand a client's complex problems and apply their broad knowledge base.

Nurses use theoretical frameworks and conceptual models, such as Maslow's hierarchy of needs[13] or Erikson's developmental stages,[5] to establish a frame of reference for understanding clients and their environments. These frameworks guide the way we observe and classify people and situations. As nurses, we use these frameworks or theoretical approaches as our frame of reference in each component of the nursing process.

Nursing practice has progressed from using particular examples of scientific rationale, such as aseptic technique and learning principles, to full application of the scientific approach in the nursing process. The scientific approach, which is used by all professional disciplines, involves rigorous investigation of a problem within a defined theoretical framework. Today professional nurses are using theoretical frameworks and conceptual models to organize knowledge, understand the client's health status, and guide their nursing practice. This theoretical approach assists nurses in interpreting the client's health and determining appropriate nursing strategies.

This chapter begins with a brief historical overview of nursing and the nursing process. The writers' philosophy of nursing is described and terms such as theories, frameworks, and models are defined. Hereafter the term "approach" includes theories, frameworks, and models, unless one is specified. There is a discussion of nursing frameworks and models and their application to practice. In this book the term "client" refers to the individual, family, or community, unless specifically stated.

HISTORICAL PERSPECTIVES: NURSING AND THE NURSING PROCESS

In the past, nursing was described in functional terms: the activities nurses performed. Beginning in the 1960s, the interpersonal, intellectual, and scientific aspects of nursing were emphasized by the profession. The interpersonal aspects of the client-nurse relationship were addressed by Ida Jean Orlando.[17] She also stressed the need for deliberative rather than intuitive nursing actions. Lois Knowles[12] incorporated the scientific approach by describing nursing as involving discovery, delving, doing, and discrimination. With continued focus on the scientific approach, nursing leaders explained how to apply this approach in the nursing process. In 1966 Kelly[10] described available data for nursing assessment as the client's physical signs and symptoms, the medical history and diagnosis, the social history and cultural background, and the physical or psychological factors in the environment. Dorothy Johnson[8] stressed the importance of systematically collecting data and rigorously analyzing it. Nursing diagnosis was defined at that time as determining the cause and alleviation of a symptom.[10]

In 1967 Yura and Walsh[25] wrote the first comprehensive book describing four components of the nursing process. These authors emphasized the intellectual, interpersonal, and technical skills of nursing practice. By the 1970s the profession viewed nursing as a scientific discipline oriented toward a theoretically based practice that focused on the client. The steps of the nursing process were legitimized in 1973, when the American Nurses' Association[2] wrote the Standards of Nursing Practice. Thereafter, several states initiated revisions of their nurse practice acts to reflect this broader scope of nursing practice. Recently the state board examinations were revised to test knowledge of assessing, analyzing, planning, implementing and evaluating—the five major components of the nursing process. These components are illustrated in Fig. 1, which depicts the sequence of the steps and the evaluative feedback process. The components of the nursing process are as follows:

1. Nursing assessment
   a. Data collection
2. Analysis/synthesis of data
   a. Nursing diagnosis
3. Nursing plans
   a. Goals and objectives
   b. Plans for implementation
   c. Scientific rationale
4. Nursing implementation
5. Evaluation

In nursing practice, nurses' roles are independent, interdependent, and dependent. Some independent actions are assessing, analyzing and diagnosing, planning, implementing, and evaluating. Interdependent activities involve coordinating and planning with other health team members. Dependent activities include implementing the physician's orders to administer medications or treatments. The nursing process enhances each of the three roles for the client's benefit.

The nursing process is a means for nurses to demonstrate accountability and responsibility to clients. As health care costs increase, both consumers and administrators of health care agencies are concerned about cost effec-

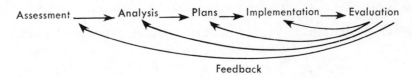

Fig. 1. An interactional feedback model depicting components in the nursing process.

tiveness and accountability. Service providers, including nurses, are watched by those paying for their services, namely consumers and the government, to determine the worth of their services. Nurses are expected to be accountable for their actions and to evaluate the effectiveness of their care. Evaluation is a way to demonstrate accountability and responsibility for one's actions to the consumer and to the health care agency. The nursing process is one tool to evaluate the effectiveness of nursing care and to demonstrate nurses' accountability.

PHILOSOPHY OF NURSING

Our description of the nursing process is influenced by our beliefs about individuals, society, health, and nursing. Individuals are complex biopsychosocial, cultural, and spiritual beings whose behavior patterns develop from genetic inheritance and interaction with their environment. Individuals act and react to continuous changes and forces in their life experiences as they strive toward self-actualization.

Society is composed of individuals, groups, families, and communities with common goals and values. Society encompasses the social, economic, political, and environmental forces and changes during reciprocal interactions and relationships.

Health is viewed as changing biopsychosocial and spiritual levels of wellness and illness. It is influenced by and encompasses the individual's genetic inheritance, capabilities, life experiences, and interaction with societal and environmental forces and changes.

Nursing is an applied science that employs intellectual, interpersonal, and technical skills throughout the nursing process to assist clients in achieving maximum health potential. Nurses use theoretical approaches to guide and support each component of the nursing process. The nurse functions as a health team member through independent, interdependent and dependent roles within the health care system, serving as the client's advocate and assuming responsibility and accountability to the client. The client-nurse relationship is interdependent, based on personal perceptions, values, and goals. Clients are active participants in each step of the nursing process through mutual decision making.

DEFINITION OF TERMS

The terms "theory," "theoretical framework," and "conceptual model" are frequently used indiscriminately and interchangeably in nursing and in other disciplines. These terms have been defined differently by various writers, and this has led to a great deal of confusion. In this text these terms are defined as follows.

Concepts and principles

A concept is an abstraction that conveys general notions, thoughts, or ideas. Concepts are names, labels, or categories for objects, persons, or events. They have varying degrees of abstraction; some terms, such as anxiety or pain, are more abstract than concepts such as medication or procedure. All concepts are intangible, descriptive terms that individuals interpret according to their impressions and experiences. Concepts must be specifically defined, since people have different meanings for them. Alone, they are useless. In a conceptual framework, the meaning and relationship of concepts determine their applicability to practice. Concepts used in nursing include health and illness, stress and adaptation, family and community, environment and society, and nursing care plans and evaluation.

Principles are guiding rules or laws that have been supported over time and proven through research. They are more exact, proven theories that are predictive. Principles define the relationship between two or more concepts and form the rule for generalizations; they are used to explain actions or provide rationale for behaviors. Examples of principles commonly applied in nursing are those of aseptic technique and of learning. Principles are typically cited as scientific rationale to explain or justify specific nursing strategies.

Conceptual models

A conceptual model is a group of concepts, ideas, or theories that are interrelated, but in which the relationship is not clearly defined. It is an abstract representation of reality that cannot be tested. A conceptual model is not a theory, because it does not describe the interrelationships among the concepts, nor does it explain how or why the phenomena occur.

Examples that may be considered conceptual models in nursing are Imogene King's model of nursing,[11] Dorothy Orem's self-care nursing model,[16] and Dorothy Johnson's behavioral system model for nursing.[9] The nursing process may also be considered a model because it resembles systems theory.

Theoretical frameworks

Theoretical frameworks are related concepts that specifically describe or explain phenomena. Since they are broader than theories, they are difficult to prove. The interrelationships among the concepts may be loosely or specifically described. The concepts are derived from scientifically supported generalizations and research. Frameworks are not amenable to testing.

Some nurses believe that Abraham Maslow's hierarchy of needs[13] is an example of a nonnursing theoretical framework. Sr. Callista Roy's adaptation model[20] and Martha E. Rogers' science of unitary man[19] may be considered theoretical frameworks in nursing. The basic difference between theories and theoretical frameworks is that only theories are amenable to testing.

Theory

A theory is a scientifically supported statement that describes, explains, or predicts the interrelationships among concepts. The concepts and theoretical statements are interrelated and are amenable to testing. Different definitions and levels of theory are described in the literature.* Some authors classify theories as descriptive, exploratory, and predictive.[23] Descriptive theory, the lowest level, identifies major elements or events of phenomena and their relationships, but does not explain how or why they are related. Explanatory theory attempts to explain causal relationships among the concepts. Predictive theory consistently predicts future outcomes. It is the most desirable level but is difficult to test and prove.

There is no consensus among the disciplines as to what a theory is; however, the following examples may be considered theories. Erik Erikson's developmental model[5] is often treated as a descriptive theory. An example of an explanatory theory is general systems theory, developed by von Bertalanffy.[24] Selye's theory of stress and the general adaptation syndrome[22] may be considered a predictive theory, since it has been repeatedly tested and supported. In the social sciences, including nursing, it is generally accepted that predictive theories are being pursued but presently do not exist.

NURSING FRAMEWORKS AND MODELS

Since the 1960s there has been a growing interest in developing nursing theories. This interest emerged from the desire to clarify the nature of nursing. Margaret Newman described three general approaches that nurses use to develop nursing theory.[14] One approach is to borrow theory from other disciplines and integrate it into a science of nursing. An example of this approach is the use of systems theory as seen in Johnson's behavioral system model for nursing.[9] A second approach is to analyze nursing practice situations for the theoretical underpinnings. Orem's self-care nursing model[16] is representative of this approach. The third approach is to develop a conceptual model from which theories can be derived. This is the aim of nursing theorists, but presently nursing frameworks and models reflect a synthesis of the first two approaches. They combine scientific theories with analyses from nursing practice. Nursing approaches describe the relationships of the client and nurse with health and the environment. They focus on the interactions between the client and nurse by describing the nursing activities or the relationship between the client and nurse.

There are different opinions as to whether nursing frameworks and models meet the criteria of *theory* in the rigid sense. Most nursing theorists prefer to call their work *models*, because they do not meet the narrow criteria of theory.[18] However, two writers believe that some nursing models meet the criteria of descriptive theory.[6] Nursing educators also frequently refer to nursing theories as a way of collectively describing nursing frameworks and models.

---

*References 3, 4, 7, 15, 23.

In the future, nursing theories must clearly differentiate activities that are unique to nursing. Nursing must distinguish either a separate body of knowledge or a distinct manner of applying shared knowledge. Future nursing theories will strive to describe, explain, and predict nursing actions that facilitate the prevention of illness, and the maintenance and promotion of a client's maximum health potential.

APPLICATION TO NURSING PRACTICE

Historically, nursing used rational approaches and a scientific base to explain nursing practice. Professionals in all disciplines, including nurses, use the scientific process with theoretical frameworks to collect information, seek new knowledge, and direct their actions. The nursing process is an adaptation of scientific approach to nursing practice. Recently, nurses are using theoretical frameworks and conceptual models to guide and support the nursing process. The scientific approach, with a theoretical base, provides a method and focus for data collection, analysis of client health patterns, and diagnosis of client concerns or problems. The theoretical base also guides selection of nursing implementation strategies.

Scientific theories, theoretical frameworks, and conceptual models are systematically applied in each step of the nursing process. Nurses must understand specific aspects of each theoretical approach for effective use in the nursing process. For each theoretical approach the nurse must understand the underlying assumptions, the definition of each concept, and the interrelationships of the concepts. Misunderstanding these aspects may lead the nurse to apply an inappropriate model or framework to a client's situation.

In choosing the most appropriate approach, the nurse considers the client's health status and comprehensive situation along with the above aspects of each approach. Selection of a specific framework or model is based on the following considerations recommended by Hardy[7]:

1. Which theory deals most adequately with the variables of concern to the health professional? The key point is to identify the "variables of concern" in the client's situation that most closely fit a theoretical approach. For example, Aquilera's crisis theory[1] would be appropriate for a rape victim, while a family developmental framework is more appropriate for an expectant couple.

2. Which variables or concepts of the theory can be altered or modified to improve the client's health status and situation? The key point is to identify theoretical frameworks that focus on improving the client's health status. For example, the family with dysfunctional communication can be assisted using Virginia Satir's family model,[21] which addresses family communication. Erikson's developmental model[5] is useful with children exhibiting psychosocial behavioral problems, since the concepts address these behaviors.

3. Is the change in the client's health status significant enough to develop a plan of action based on the theory? In other words, does the theory support the main focus of change and direct the course of nursing strategies? For example, Roy's adaptation model[20] guides various strategies for helping clients adapt to physiological alterations. Systems theory[24] can be used to

implement change in a community. The selection and application of the most appropriate theory, framework, or model facilitates rational decision making in each component of the nursing process.

Since individual, family, and community clients each present unique health situations, the nurse needs to have a broad knowledge of different theoretical approaches to select the most appropriate one. The nurse initiates the selection process by collecting basic information about the client. Next, the nurse determines the appropriate theoretical approach to guide further data collection and analysis of the client's behaviors. Selection of the most appropriate theoretical model is based on the nurse's knowledge of the client's situation and consideration of which model addresses the client's health concerns that can be significantly altered through nursing implementation strategies.

SUMMARY

Professional nursing has evolved from application of scientific principles to a discipline that applies theories, frameworks, models, and principles to practice. Theories describe, explain, and predict the interrelationships among concepts. Theoretical frameworks are broader than theories, less precisely defined, and show interrelationships among concepts. Conceptual models are composed of related concepts, but the precise relationships are undefined. Neither frameworks nor conceptual models are amenable to testing or proving. Concepts are abstract mental formulations for objects, ideas, persons, or events, which vary in concreteness. Principles are guiding rules or laws that have been supported over time.

Together, theories, frameworks, models, and principles serve to identify and classify phenomena. They are used throughout the nursing process to guide assessment, organize the data for analysis, and direct nursing implementation. Theoretical approaches are the means to justify each step in the nursing process and demonstrate the nurse's accountability to the client.

REFERENCES

1 Aguilera, D.C., and Messick, J.M.: Crisis intervention: theory and methodology, ed. 4, St. Louis, 1982, The C.V. Mosby Co.

2 American Nurses' Association: Standards of nursing practice, Kansas City, 1973, The Association.

3 Dickoff, J., James, P., and Weidenbach, E.: Theory in a practice discipline. I. Practice oriented theory, Nurs. Res. **17:**415, 1968.

4 Dickoff, J., and James, P.: Theory development in nursing. In Verhonick, P.J., editor: Nursing research 1, Boston, 1975, Little, Brown & Co.

5 Erikson, E.: Childhood and society, ed. 2, New York, 1963, W.W. Norton & Co., Inc.

6 Flaskerud, J.H., and Halloran, E.J.: Areas of agreement in nursing theory development, Adv. Nurs. Sci. **3:**1, Oct. 1980.

7 Hardy, M.E., and Conway, M.E.: Role theory: perspectives for health professionals, New York, 1978, Appleton-Century-Crofts.

8 Johnson, D.: Professional practice in nursing. In

The shifting scene: directions for practice, NLN Pub. No. 15-1252, New York, 1967, National League for Nursing.

9 Johnson, D.E.: The behavioral system model for nursing. In Reihl, J.P., and Roy, Sr.C., editors: Conceptual models for nursing practice, ed. 2, New York, 1980, Appleton-Century-Crofts.

10 Kelly, K.: Clinical inference in nursing, Nurs. Res. **15:**23, 1966.

11 King, I.M.: Toward a theory of nursing, New York, 1971, John Wiley & Sons, Inc.

12 Knowles, L.N.: Decision making in nursing: a necessity for doing, ANA Clinical Sessions 1966, New York, 1967, Appleton-Century-Crofts.

13 Maslow, A.: Motivation and personality, ed. 2, New York, 1970, Harper & Row, Publishers, Inc.

14 Newman, M.A.: Nursing's theoretical evolution, Nurs. Outlook **20:**449, 1972.

15 Newman, M.A.: Theory development in nursing, Philadelphia, 1979, F.A. Davis Co.

16 Orem, D.E.: Nursing: concepts of practice, New York, 1980, McGraw-Hill Book Co.

17 Orlando, I.J.: The dynamic nurse-patient relationship: function, process and principles, New York, 1961, G.P. Putnam's Sons.

18 Reihl, J.P., and Roy, Sr.C.: Conceptual models for nursing practice, ed. 2, New York, 1980, Appleton-Century-Crofts.

19 Rogers, M.E.: An introduction to the theoretical basis of nursing, Philadelphia, 1970, F.A. Davis Co.

20 Roy, Sr.C.: Introduction to nursing: an adaptation model, Englewood Cliffs, N.J., 1976, Prentice-Hall, Inc.

21 Satir, V.: Peoplemaking, Palo Alto, Cal., 1972, Science and Behavior Books, Inc.

22 Selye, H.: The stress of life, New York, 1956, McGraw-Hill Book Co.

23 Stevens, B.J.: Nursing theory: analysis, application, evaluation, Boston, 1979, Little, Brown & Co.

24 von Bertalanffy, L.: General systems theory: foundations, development, and application, New York, 1968, George Braziller, Inc.

25 Yura, H., and Walsh, M.B.: The nursing process: assessing, planning, implementing, evaluating, New York, 1967, Appleton-Century-Crofts.

BIBLIOGRAPHY

Byrne, M.L., and Thompson, L.F.: Key concepts for the study and practice of nursing, ed. 2, St. Louis, 1978, The C.V. Mosby Co.

Carrieri, V., and Sitzman, J.: Components of the nursing process, Nurs. Clin. North Am. **6:**115, 1971.

Ellis, R.: Characteristics of significant theories, Nurs. Res. **17:**217, 1968.

Fredette, S.: The art of applying theory to practice, Am. J. Nurs. **74:**865, 1974.

Hardy, M.E.: Theoretical foundations for nursing, New York, 1973, MMS Information Corporation.

Hardy, M.E.: Theories: components, development, evaluation, Nurs. Res. **23:**100, 1974.

Harris, R.B.: A strong vote for nursing process, Am. J. Nurs. **79:**1999, 1979.

Jacox, A.: Theory construction in nursing: an overview, Nurs. Res. **23:**4, 1974.

La Monica, E.L.: The nursing process: a humanistic approach, Reading, Mass., 1979, Addison-Wesley Publishing Co., Inc.

Marriner, A.: The nursing process: a scientific approach to nursing care, St. Louis, 1975, The C.V. Mosby Co.

Mitchell, P.H.: Concepts basic to nursing, ed. 2, New York, 1977, McGraw-Hill Book Co.

Murray, R., and Zentner, J.: Nursing concepts for health promotion, ed. 2, Englewood Cliffs, N.J., 1979, Prentice-Hall, Inc.

Nursing Theories Conference Group: Nursing theories: the base for professional nursing practice, Englewood Cliffs, N.J., 1980, Prentice-Hall, Inc.

Putt, A.M.: General systems theory applied to nursing, Boston, 1978, Little, Brown & Co.

Reilly, D.E.: Why a conceptual framework? Nurs. Outlook **23:**566, 1975.

Yura, H., and Walsh, M.B. The nursing process: assessing, planning, implementing, evaluating, ed. 3, New York, 1978, Appleton-Century-Crofts.

Overview of selected
THEORETICAL APPROACHES

JANET W. GRIFFITH

This chapter presents an overview of selected nursing and behavioral theories, frameworks, models, and principles. These approaches are commonly used in the nursing process. The basic structure and essence of each approach are described; a skeletal picture of the concepts is presented. The purpose of presenting these approaches is to give the reader a background knowledge to understand their application in the ensuing chapters. Readers are strongly encouraged to review the literature on each theoretical approach before using it in the nursing process.

There are two main sections in this chapter. The first section describes five nursing frameworks and models; the second discusses frameworks, models, and principles from other disciplines. The theoretical approaches selected for this chapter are in no way inclusive; many other approaches are both available and relevant in nursing practice. Appendix C also contains other nursing and behavioral approaches. They serve as a reference for this book and as a guide in applying the nursing process.

NURSING FRAMEWORKS AND MODELS
King's conceptual framework

In 1971 Imogene King[2] described a framework of concepts she views as essential to nursing. These concepts were drawn from behavioral science theories and from her philosophy of nursing. Man is the focus of this framework, which also includes concepts of perception, interpersonal relationships, social systems, and health. King interrelates these concepts by stating, "Man functions in social systems through interpersonal relationships in terms of his perceptions which influence his life and his health."[2] A description of each concept follows.

Man, the focus, is considered in three dimensions. First, man is a *reacting being*, who is aware of events in the environment. He responds biopsychosocially as a whole. Second, man is *time oriented*. He can recall past events, which influence present and future decisions and goals. Man's time orientation influences present reactions. Last, man is a *social being*. He constantly interacts with others and the environment. Through interactions and communication, man exchanges thoughts and feelings, information, and energy. This facilitates his functioning and adaptation.

Social systems defined by King are as follows:

> Groups of individuals join together in a network or system of social relationships to achieve common goals developed about a system of values with an organized set of practices and the methods to regulate practices and administer the rules. The members of the groups interact according to standards or norms based on a set of roles and status.*

Common social systems include the family, church, school, community, hospitals, governmental agencies, and social groups. Each social system develops values according to its membership. These values influence the groups' interaction and practices. The values, beliefs, and attitudes may become norms, standards, or rules that guide acceptable behavior of the members. These behaviors influence the role, status, and authority of the members.

Interpersonal relationships develop as individuals continually interact with others. King defines interpersonal relationships as "the interaction of two or more individuals in . . . time for some purpose or goal."[2] They involve forms of communication based on perception, judgment, action, reaction, interaction, transaction, and feedback. An individual's expectations, goals, needs, values, and exchange of energy influence behavior and interpersonal relationships.

Perception refers to the way an individual interprets reality. The meaning an individual gives to events directly influences the individual's response to the environment. The five senses are used in perception. An individual interprets the way he sees himself functioning, feedback from others, and the events going on around him.

Health is defined as "a dynamic state in the life cycle of an organism that implies continuous adaptation to stresses in the internal and external environment through optimum use of one's resources to achieve maximum potential for daily living."[2] Continual changes in biopsychosocial areas occur through environmental change and demands. Stress and adaptive responses may also occur in each of these areas.

In summary, King views nursing as assisting man through interpersonal relationships in meeting his basic needs throughout the life cycle. Man's perceptions influence his interactions in social systems and his health. Nurses function in social systems to promote man's optimum health. King's framework is applicable to individuals and families in the nursing process. It is an excellent assessment tool and can guide the analysis, diagnosis, and planning strategies.

Levine's conservation principles of nursing

Myra Levine's beliefs about nursing[3] reflect an integration of scientific and behavioral theories and concepts. This holistic approach recognizes the integrated process by which clients adapt to internal and external environmental factors.

According to Levine, nursing involves human interactions, recognizes that people are dependent on their relationships with others, and supports or promotes the client's adjustment through intervention. Nurse-client inter-

---

*From King, I.M.: Toward a theory for nursing, New York, 1971, John Wiley & Sons, Inc.

actions are based on the *conditions* in which the client enters the system, the *functions* of the nurse in the setting, and the *responsibilities* of the nurse in that setting. The nurse actively participates in the client's environment to facilitate adaptation through supportive or therapeutic interventions. *Supportive* interventions include maintaining the client's present state of health or decreasing deterioration. *Therapeutic* interventions favorably influence health to promote or optimize the client's well-being.

By viewing the client holistically, the nurse incorporates principles of conservation of energy and structural, personal, and social integrity in nursing interventions. Levine believes that nursing interventions are directed toward conservation or "keeping together" each of these aspects to maintain the client's balance of unity and integrity. Based on scientific knowledge and skill, nursing intervention requires active client participation in the plan of care within safe limits of the individual's ability to participate. Through supportive and therapeutic interventions, the nurse applies Levine's four principles of conservation to maintain and promote the client's unity and integrity.[3,4]

1. *Conservation of energy* refers to maintaining the ability to do the work required to preserve balance in the system. It is essential to have a balance of energy intake and output to maintain integrity. Energy forms include food, activity, and rest to promote healing, restore structural integrity, and prevent fatigue.

2. *Conservation of structural integrity* refers to preventing disease and promoting, maintaining, or restoring the physical structure and functioning of the body.

3. *Conservation of personal integrity* refers to preserving the client's right to privacy, dignity, and honesty. Each client's sense of self-worth, uniqueness, and identity should be supported during nurse-client interactions and interventions.

4. *Conservation of social integrity* refers to recognizing each client as a social being involved in dependent relationships with others. The client's significant others should be respected and involved with the client and with the plan of care.

Levine's principles serve as a useful framework to guide the nursing assessment, analysis/synthesis, and planning components of the nursing process. They may be used effectively with individuals or families. Levine's views of nursing are applicable as the scientific rationale to support nursing plans.

Orem's self-care nursing model

Dorothy Orem's model[5] focuses on the art and practice of nursing. Nursing is described as providing assistance with self-care activities when the individual is unable to perform those activities. Self-care activities are those personal tasks the individual personally initiates and performs to maintain life, health, and well-being. Self-care activities contribute to the maintenance and promotion of structural integrity, functioning, and development.

Orem identifies three requisites for self-care: universal, developmental, and health deviation.[6] These requisites represent the individual's purpose for self-care.

Universal requisites are those demands and actions necessary to meet the basic needs in daily living. They are common to everyone throughout the life cycle and are adjusted for age, developmental stage, environment, and other factors. They are associated with maintaining life processes, structural integrity, and functioning.

Orem identifies eight universal self-care requisites: maintenance of sufficient air, water, and food; balance between activity and rest; balance between solitude and social interaction; provision of care associated with elimination processes and excrements; prevention of hazards to human life, functioning, and well-being; and promotion of human functioning and development within social groups.

Developmental self-care requisites are associated with developmental processes and conditions occurring during the life cycle. There are two categories of developmental self-care. The first is maintaining conditions that support life processes and promote development. The second is the prevention of harmful effects on human development and the provision of care to overcome these effects.

Health-deviation self-care requisites are associated with individuals who are ill, injured, or have a pathological condition and are receiving medical care. Orem identified six requisites for individuals with health deviations. These requisites include (1) seeking and securing appropriate medical assistance; (2) recognizing and taking care of these conditions; (3) implementing prescribed diagnostic, therapeutic, and rehabilitative measures; (4) recognizing and regulating the effects of treatment; (5) modifying the self-concept and acceptance of the condition; and (6) learning to live with the condition in a life-style that promotes continued development.

Orem describes three types of nursing care that support the three primary self-care requisites.[5] The first is the supportive-educative approach for the client who is able to and should learn self-care activities. This approach facilitates universal self-care through support, teaching, guidance, and environmental change. The second approach, partly compensatory, assists clients who are unable to perform some self-care activities. The nurse augments developmental self-care requisites by assisting the client with these activities. Last, the wholly compensatory approach of nursing care is provided to incapacitated clients. The nurse performs all self-care activities for the client. Frequently, the types of nursing care overlap in assisting individual clients.

In summary, Orem's model describes three broad requisites for self-care: universal, developmental, and health deviation. She also identifies three nursing approaches that assist clients in meeting their self-care needs. In working with clients the nurse assists clients in meeting requisites in each area through the use of one or more nursing care approaches. Orem's model can be applied to individuals or families in the assessment and analysis components of the nursing process. The different nursing approaches are excellent guides for implementation plans.

Peplau's interpersonal model

In 1952 Hildegard Peplau[8] described nursing as a therapeutic interpersonal relationship. This relationship facilitates the growth and development of both client and nurse. It helps the client progress toward constructive, productive, and creative living. Nurses help clients (1) examine their interpersonal relationships, felt needs, and problems; and (2) define, understand, and productively resolve them. During the relationship, the attitudes toward the client and the relationship are also examined by the nurse. This helps the nurse understand the interpersonal dynamics and develop therapeutic use of self. The nurse uses communication techniques, unconditional acceptance, and empathy. These skills promote a trusting nurse-client relationship and promote self-reliance and independent decision making. Peplau describes four phases in a goal-directed interpersonal relationship: orientation, identification, exploitation, and resolution.

Orientation refers to the initiation of the relationship when the client recognizes a felt need or difficulty and seeks professional assistance. Upon mutual agreement, the nurse defines the nature of the reciprocal relationship and its purposes. The nurse explains that the collaborative role is to identify, examine, and find ways to resolve the client's problem.

Identification begins the working phase. The nurse-client relationship develops and strengthens as initial attitudes of the client and nurse are explored. Their perceptions and expectations of each other are clarified. A trusting relationship may develop if they openly share their thoughts and feelings. During this phase, they work to identify the client's problems or difficulties.

Exploitation refers to the discussion of solutions after mutual identification and understanding of the client's problems. The client's roles and responsibilities in resolving the problem are clarified. The client gradually assumes responsibility for control of the problem and decision making. There is progressive independence and self-reliance. During this phase, the client may test the relationship and experience dependent and independent feelings, which need to be discussed.

Resolution refers to the final phase, as the client and nurse collaborate to resolve the problem; they also must work through their psychological dependency needs. They should discuss termination before the last meeting, because this prepares them for the final separation. Successful resolution occurs when both of them summarize the relationship, its meaning, and accomplishments. This promotes the growth and maturity of both individuals.

In summary, Peplau's model describes nursing as a therapeutic, growth-producing relationship. It proceeds through four phases: orientation, identification, exploitation, and resolution. The nurse and client explore their relationship, the client's problems, and potential solutions. This model is a useful guide to plan implementation strategies or to cite as scientific rationale. It also may serve as a supporting approach to assess and analyze the nurse-client relationships. It can be applied to both individual and family clients.

Roy's adaptation model

Sister Callista Roy's model[11] reflects the general systems theory approach. It explains how an individual interacts with and adapts to the environment. The model is based on assumptions that individuals are biopsychosocial beings interacting with a dynamic environment. This interaction requires use of adaptive mechanisms to conserve energy and maintain equilibrium.

In Roy's model, nursing assists the client in adapting in four modes. Adaptation is the process of responding to and satisfactorily coping with environmental changes. Problems occur through failure of coping mechanisms. The four modes are basic physiological needs, self-concept, role mastery or function, and interdependence.

There are seven areas of *basic physiological needs*. First, exercise and rest are needed. Excesses or deficits in this area could produce immobility, hyperactivity, fatigue, or insomnia. The second need is nutrition. Potential problems include malnutrition, nausea, and vomiting. Elimination needs are third. Problems may result in retention, hyperexcretion, constipation, diarrhea, and incontinence. Fourth are fluid and electrolytes. Excesses or deficits may cause dehydration, edema, and electrolyte imbalance. The fifth need, oxygen, if unmet may lead to ischemia or fatigue. Circulation needs are sixth, and problems include shock or overload. Last is regulation of temperature, senses, and the endocrine system. Problems in these areas may cause fever or hypothermia, sensory deprivation or overload, and endocrine imbalance.

Self-concept has three parts: physical, personal, and interpersonal. The physical self includes body images and sensations. The personal self consists of moral and ethical issues, consistency of self-behavior with values, and one's self-ideal and expected behaviors. The interpersonal self-concept is the individual's perception of one's interactions with others.

Role mastery includes both instrumental and expressive aspects of the individual's position in society. Problems that may occur in this mode are role conflict and role failure.

Interdependence is the ability to achieve a comfortable balance between dependence and independence. Problems in this mode may result in alienation, rejection, aggression, hostility, loneliness, dominance, and exhibition.

Roy's model also includes the regulator and cognator subsystems. The regulator subsystem reacts to internal and external physical stimuli. The cognator subsystem adapts to internal and external psychosocial stimuli. These stimuli are received through perception, learning, judgment, and emotion. The client develops maladaptive behaviors when the cognator or regulator subsystem is ineffective.

There are three sources of stimuli: focal, contextual, and residual.[10] Focal stimuli are related to environmental changes. Contextual stimuli are from all other internal and external sources that influence the situation. Residual stimuli are the personal characteristics of the individual that are relevant to the situation.[10]

In summary, the purpose of nursing, according to Roy, is to change the stimuli to promote the client's adaptation. The nurse examines the client's four modes to identify problems. Next, the nurse identifies and alters the stimuli that produced the maladaptation. When the stimuli are altered, the client's regulator and cognator subsystems may resume effective adaptive behaviors. Roy's model includes biopsychosocial areas and is broad enough to use with individuals or families in the nursing process. It is an excellent tool for assessing and analyzing clients' health patterns. When nursing implementation strategies are directed at changing sources of stimuli, Roy's model is a useful guide.

DIVERSE FRAMEWORKS, MODELS, AND PRINCIPLES
Duvall's family developmental framework

Evelyn Duvall's family developmental framework[1] provides a guide to examine and analyze the basic changes and developmental tasks common to most families during their life cycle. Although each family has unique characteristics, normative patterns of sequential development have been described by Duvall. These stages and developmental tasks illustrate common family behaviors that may be expected at specific times in the family life cycle. The stages of family development are marked by the age of the oldest child, although there is some overlapping of stages when there are several children in the family.

Stage I *(beginning families)* begins with the married couple as they establish a mutually satisfying relationship. The couple's tasks center on forming an intimate relationship and balance in their lives together, family planning, and establishing a harmonious relationship with in-laws and new friends. Adjusting to pregnancy and planning for parenthood are also critical tasks during this stage.

Stage II *(early childbearing)* begins when the first child is between birth and 30 months; at this time the family tasks involve adjusting to the critical needs and demands of an infant while continuing to establish a satisfying home environment. Changes in roles and responsibilities with parenthood are critical tasks.

Stage III *(families with preschoolers)* begins as the parents adapt to the challenging needs and interests of the preschool child in a way to promote the child's growth. In adapting to the preschooler's needs, the parents may find their energy and privacy reduced. With the addition of another infant, parents may experience increased child-rearing responsibilities and the need for more living space in the home and for more personal time to maintain intimacy and communication between the parents.

Stage IV *(families with schoolchildren)* begins as the oldest child enters school; the family tasks revolve around adjusting to community activities involving the child, encouraging the child's educational achievement, and maintaining a satisfying marital relationship. Critical tasks include balancing time and energy to meet the demands of work, the children's needs and activities, adult social interests, and the requirements of open communication and harmony in the marital and in-law relationships.

Stage V *(families with teenagers)* begins when the oldest child becomes a teenager; a gradual emancipation commences as the child develops increasing independence and autonomy. Families with teenagers must adapt to balancing freedom for growth with meeting family responsibilities. Critical tasks during this period are maintaining open communication between parents and teenagers, continuing intimacy in the marital relationship, and establishing outside interests and careers as teenagers leave the home.

Stage VI *(launching center families)* begins when the first child leaves the home and lasts until the last child has left. Parents must both prepare their children to live independently and accept the departure of the children. After the children have left, the parents must reorganize to reestablish the family unit. Husband and wife roles and responsibilities will shift during this period as a wife may return to work. With the birth of grandchildren, the parental roles and self-images require some family accommodation.

Stage VII *(middle-aged families)* begins once the children have left the home, when middle-aged parents have more time and freedom to cultivate their social and leisure interests. This may also be a period for rebuilding the marriage and maintaining satisfying relationships both with aging parents and with the children and their families. Planning for retirement while maintaining physical and emotional health and careers are major family concerns.

Stage VIII *(aging families)* begins with the retirement of one or both spouses and continues until the deaths of both marital partners. Critical tasks focus on finding sufficient energy and motivation to seek and engage in pleasurable leisure activities within financial and health limitations. Major tasks are adjusting to retirement with changing life-styles and accepting the deaths of friends and spouse. Within this period the family may also close the home and move into a retirement community, thus having to establish new ties with friends in a new community and to find new leisure activities.

Within each of the successive stages of family development, Duvall identified eight basic tasks that lead to successful family life within society. These tasks promote family adjustment and adaptation of the individual members. When families fail to accomplish these tasks, the family collectively or its members individually may experience unhappiness, societal disapproval, and difficulty in achieving harmony and self-actualization. The family tasks involve responsibilities to satisfy the biological, cultural, and personal needs and aspirations of the members at each stage of family development. These eight basic tasks include:

1. *Physical maintenance:* The family is responsible for providing shelter, appropriate clothing, and sufficient nourishing food, along with adequate health care.

2. *Allocation of resources:* Resources include finances, personal time, energy, and relationships. Family members' needs are met through division of costs and labor to provide material goods, space, and facilities, and through interpersonal relations to share authority, respect, and affection.

3. *Division of labor:* Family members decide who will assume what responsibilities, such as providing income, managing the household tasks, maintaining the home and car, caring for young, old, or incapacited family members, and other designated tasks.

4. *Socialization of family members:* The family assumes responsibility for guiding development of mature and acceptable patterns of socially acceptable behavior in eating, elimination, sleeping, sexuality, aggression, and interaction with others.

5. *Reproduction, recruitment, and release of family members:* Childbearing, adoption, and rearing children are family responsibilities, along with incorporating new members through marriage. Policies are established for including others in the family, such as in-laws, relatives, step-parents, guests, and friends.

6. *Maintenance of order:* Order is maintained by the communication of acceptable behavior. The types and intensity of interactions, patterns of affection, and sexual expression are sanctioned by parental behavior to ensure acceptance in society.

7. *Placement of members in the larger society:* Family members establish roots in society through relationships in the church, school, political and economic system, and other organizations. The family also assumes responsibility for protecting family members from undesirable outside influences and may prohibit membership in objectionable groups.

8. *Maintenance of motivation and morale:* Family members reward each other for their achievements and provide for an individual's needs of acceptance, encouragement, and affection. The family develops a philosophy of life and sense of family unity and loyalty, thereby enabling members to adapt to both personal and family crises.

Duvall's framework is an excellent guide for assessing, analyzing, and planning in a family nursing process. The nurse must first determine the family's stage of development, then examine the tasks that are appropriate for the respective stage. Since physiological aspects are not addressed in this framework, they should be added for a comprehensive approach to the family.

Otto's framework of family strengths

Based on his research with numerous families, Herbert Otto[7] developed a tool for assessing families. Family strengths are defined as "those factors or forces that contribute to family unity and solidarity and that foster the development of the potentials inherent within the family."[7] Family strengths can be identified by the factors in Otto's framework.

Physical, emotional, and spiritual needs. The family's ability to provide the physical needs of food and shelter is considered a strength. This also includes space management for adequate living and play areas and sufficient privacy of members. Physical needs encompass providing good health and nutritionally balanced meals, along with the pleasure inherent in planning, preparing, and eating meals together.

Emotional needs are reflected in family members' sensitivity to each other's needs and the ability to express affection, warmth, caring, love, and understanding. Healthy families are able to give and receive love and affection from relatives, and the parents find sufficient satisfaction in sexual relations.

Family spiritual strengths include sharing basic beliefs and spiritual or religious values with members. Membership in church or related organizations is another strength, along with providing an atmosphere of honesty and integrity. Values and principles are demonstrated in daily life and in interpersonal relationships.

Child-rearing practices and discipline. Parents respect each other's views and decisions on child-rearing practices in healthy families. They share joint responsibility in child rearing and they foster self-discipline in the children.

Communication. The ability of family members to express a variety of feelings and emotions and to articulate ideas, concepts, beliefs, and values is considered a strength. There is an atmosphere of openness and freedom to share any matter of concern. Communication is a two-way process, involving sensitive listening and verbal expression. Open communication that leads to consensual decision making is considered a family strength.

Support, security, and encouragement. Family members share a sense of security—a belief that the family supports and encourages them. Members find "genuine and realistic commendation, praise, and recognition . . . for specific effort or achievement."[7] There is a sense of balance to family activities, and humor is seen as a family resource.

Growth-producing relationships and experiences within and without the family. Family members relate to each other and outsiders in ways that facilitate growth and maturation. They build, maintain, and develop friendships and relationships in the neighborhood, school, and vocational environments. Members have sufficient friends and continue making new friends. Involvement in varied activities and relationships that enrich their lives is considered a strength.

Responsible community relationships. Family strengths include assuming responsibility for leadership in local, school, social, cultural, or political organizations. Family members share opinions, beliefs, and concerns about local, regional, and national interests. Diversity of opinions is respected and considered a strength.

Growing with and through children. When parental relationships with children are used for personal growth and "actualization of personal potential," it is considered a family strength. Parents recognize that their children facilitate the parents' growth. The qualities of spontaneity, emotional honesty, and open communication are fostered to promote the growth of both parents and children.

Self-help and accepting help. The family demonstrates strength by taking the initiative and responsibility to help itself. If outside assistance is needed, the family seeks and accepts help from others.

Flexibility of family functions and roles. Family members are able to assume each other's roles and functions as necessary. Role interchange may occur between parents, or among parents and children.

Mutual respect for individuality. Family members recognize, respect, and treat each other as unique individuals.

Crisis as a means of growth. Crises or traumatic experiences are used constructively by the family. It grows in unity and understanding as a result of these experiences.

Family unity, loyalty, and intrafamily cooperation. The family shares traditions and rituals, along with "maintaining close, productive and growthful relationships"[7] with extended family members.

Flexibility of family strengths. Family members show the ability to be flexible and to adjust to different situations. Members can adapt to changes within the family and also to events outside the family.

In summary, Otto's framework addresses various areas of family strengths. It incorporates the interactional components along with basic needs, relationships outside the family, and growth-producing experiences. It is a useful guide to assess and analyze family strengths and identify areas needing improvement in the family nursing process.

**Satir's family
interactional model**

Virginia Satir[12] believes that the family's interactional health depends on its ability to share and understand the members feelings, needs, and behavior patterns. She thinks that healthy, nurturing families help their members know themselves through communication of everyday events. This communication promotes each individual's self-confidence and self-worth. Satir views the healthy family as hopeful, trusting of others, and curious about what society has to offer. The family operates on a growth-producing, reality-oriented basis. This promotes intimacy among its members. Family rules about money, chores, and power are explicit and understood by everyone. Also, the healthy family establishes links with society. These links are established through membership in various groups.

Satir's model of the healthy family consists of four concepts: self-worth, communication, rules, and links to society.

Each member and the family unit demonstrate feelings of high esteem and *self-worth*. These attitudes are conveyed by behaviors showing integrity, honesty, responsibility, compassion, and love. These attitudes flow outward from each individual, and a sense of trust radiates from all members. They accept their own strengths and inadequacies as well as those of others. Without self-worth, family members build walls of distrust, isolation, and loneliness. They fear others will cheat them, use them, or step on them. This leads to unhealthy family interaction.

Communication directly influences the relationship among family members. Patterns of communication include body movements, posture, tone of voice, and what is spoken. In healthy families, communication is open, direct, clear, and honest. The members are receptive and encourage open, honest sharing of feelings and needs. They value what others have to say, supporting each member's attempts in both verbal and physical communication. Unhealthy families block communication among members; they may give ambiguous messages or not listen at all. This leads to distrust and low self-worth among the family members.

Each family has a set of *rules* it lives by. These rules may be explicit or implicit. Most families assume that everyone knows and understands the rules, but this is not always true. Families have rules about money, responsibilities, activities, special privileges, privacy, sexual expression, language, territoriality, and authority. In many situations, rules define what actions are appropriate; they may also guide how feelings are expressed and may help achieve goals or impede goal achievement. Some rules may be outdated, unfair, unclear, or inappropriate. In healthy families the rules are known to all members, allow for freedom, and encourage discussion among the members. Unhealthy families may have implicit rules that restrict family members. These rules may be inflexible and inhibit the growth of the members.

The family unit and individual members have *links to society* through organizations and friends. The organizational links include schools, church, political groups, recreational groups, and clubs. Links with friends are usually formed through common interests. These links are a way the family and its members keep actively involved in the community and relate to the world around them. Healthy families have many links with society, believing society has much to offer and trusting their selection of groups to be a positive influence and interaction. They believe society offers opportunities for choices and change, growth, and development. These opportunities are welcomed, desirable, and normal. Unhealthy families view society with distrust and fear exposure to others' values. They avoid involvement in organizations, preferring to remain isolated. They do not welcome experiences outside the family.

In summary, Satir's family model depicts the healthy family as promoting self-worth among its members. Self-worth is encouraged through attitudes of acceptance, open communication, flexible rules, and trusting in each other and in society. These attitudes promote individuals' self-confidence, concern for others, and trust in interactions with others. Satir's model is useful in all components of the nursing process with a family. Since Satir does not include physical health, this aspect must be added in nursing assessment, analysis, and planning.

General systems theory

General systems theory serves as a model for viewing man as interacting with the environment. One of the first theorists to develop systems theory was Ludwig von Bertalanffy,[13] who synthesized the following abstract laws in systems theory development: (1) systems are organized complexities in which behavior is determined by interaction among various components; (2) no system repeats its interaction, but continuous interaction among variables produces uniquely dynamic situations infinitely; (3) evolution proceeds from a less to a more differentiated state; dynamic interaction between individuals and the environment results in increasing complexity for both; (4) there are regular changes in the evolution of all systems as they move toward higher states of order, differentiation, and probability; (5) people are living, open (metabolizing) systems, exhibiting self-differentiation, providing energy, and having a stored information system (genetic code) to steer the process.

A *system* consists of a set of interacting components within a boundary that filters the type and rate of exchange with the environment. Systems are composed of both structural and functional components. Structure refers to the arrangements of the parts at a given time, while function is the process of continuous change in the system as matter, energy, and information are exchanged with the environment.

All living systems are *open*, in that there is continual exchange of matter, energy, or information. In open systems there are varying degrees of interaction with the environment from which the system receives input and gives back output in the form of matter, energy, and information. Theoretically, no closed systems exist, as they would be totally isolated from interacting with the environment.

The universe consists of a *hierarchy of systems* (numerous suprasystems, systems, and subsystems), and each system may be viewed as having one or more suprasystems and subsystems. For example, the individual as a system belongs to suprasystems in a family, community, and region. An individual's subsystems are composed of organ systems, or biopsychosocial components.

Each system has discrete, definable *boundaries* that filter and regulate the flow of input and output exchange with the environment. Boundaries may consist of physical or abstract lines of demarcation that separate the system from the surrounding environment. The boundary filter may be very permeable or fairly impermeable, depending on the component it is screening in or out of the system.

For survival, all systems must receive varying types and amounts of matter, energy, and information from the environment. Through the process of selection, the system regulates the type and amount of *input* received.

The system uses the input through self-regulation to maintain the system's equilibrium or homeostasis. Some types of inputs are used immediately in their original state, while others require complex transformation *(throughput)* for use. Matter, energy, and information are continuously processed through the system and released as outputs.

After processing input, the system returns *output* (matter, energy, and information) to the environment in an altered state, affecting the environment.

The system continuously monitors itself and the environment for information to guide its operation. This *feedback* information of environmental responses to the system's output is utilized by the system in adjustment, correction, and accommodation to the interaction with the environment. Feedback may be positive, negative, or neutral.

Substances that occupy space and can be exchanged between the system and environment are considered *matter*.

The ability to perform, carry out tasks, and overcome resistance, in a physical and emotional sense, may be considered *energy*.

Through dynamic interaction with the environment, the system exchanges *information* in different forms, such as verbal and behavioral communication, visual media, taste, smell, and touch. Information is used by the system in the process of selection and decision making.

For survival, a system must achieve a balance internally and externally. *Equilibrium* depends on the ability of the system to regulate input and output with the environment to achieve a balanced relationship of the interacting parts. Since balance is continually changing, a self-regulating mechanism within the system monitors the interaction of inputs and outputs with the environment by using information from feedback. Through interactions with the environment, the system uses various *adaptation* mechanisms to maintain equilibrium. Adaptation may occur through accepting or rejecting the matter, energy, or information, and by accommodating the input and modifying the system's responses to maintain or regain equilibrium.

Systems theory is applicable in the nursing process of the individual, family, and community client. It is the most frequently used approach to assess and analyze a community. However, since it is so broad, supplemental approaches are often required to delineate input, throughput, and output.

Principles of learning and teaching

While working with clients, the nurse frequently teaches the client about health promotion activities. The nurse may instruct clients in understanding their dietary alterations, medications, and changes in activities of daily living. For effective teaching, there are certain principles of both learning and teaching that the nurse must consider in working with clients. Pohl[9] summarized these learning and teaching principles as follows.

Principles of learning

Perception is necessary for learning. Individuals use their five senses to grasp and interpret meaning in their environment. These senses must be intact and functional for learning to occur. Awareness of the client's perceptual abilities is extremely important in teaching, since reduced perception due to physical or emotional change alters the client's ability to fully and accurately perceive and process information. The nurse needs to continuously monitor the client's perception of information and make corrections in giving or altering the client's understanding of the situation.

Conditioning is a process of learning. In response to specific stimuli, individuals learn certain responses through conditioning (if repeated over time). Some responses may be elicited by different stimuli. On a more complex level, individual habits and patterns of behavior and thinking are learned through conditioning. In teaching clients, the nurse should consider which factors will facilitate and reinforce desirable learning responses.

The process of trial-and-error is a way of learning. In unfamiliar situations, learning may occur through trial-and-error. As the client achieves repeated success in achieving desired goals when using a specific approach, new learning patterns will develop.

Learning may occur through imitation. From infancy on, individuals observe the behavior of others and frequently imitate behaviors that appear appropriate for a given situation. Nurses may employ this principle in demonstrating techniques to clients or in role modeling.

The development of concepts is part of learning. Individuals use concepts to give meaning to their world. As Margaret Pohl states, "Conceptualization is a complex process involving six components: perception, emotions, verbal symbols or words, integration, generalization, and abstraction."[9] As a client learns new information, concept formation will occur, and the nurse should check for accuracy of the meaning of new concepts.

An individual must be motivated in order to learn. For learning to occur, the client must have a willingness or desire to learn or change. An individual may be motivated for numerous reasons, such as need, status, or achievement. Motivation may be constant, or temporary, strong or weak. Frequently the nurse needs to stimulate or incite motivation to learn in the client.

Physical and mental readiness is necessary for learning. An individual must have the physical and mental ability to learn the given task. Physical readiness is related to the individual's age and physical health status, while mental readiness refers to the level of the cognitive abilities to understand, assimilate, and apply. The level of the learner's physical and mental readiness must be evaluated in relation to the level of the learning task to be accomplished.

Effective learning requires active participation. Active involvement on the part of the learner through participation in the learning process facilitates more effective learning. Learning by doing is retained longer, since it involves using more than one sense organ and may incorporate cognitive, psychomotor, and affective learning processes.

New learning must be based on previous knowledge and experience. Learning is a sequential process that proceeds from basic or simple tasks to more complex skills. The nurse must first determine the client's current level of knowledge about a topic before providing new information. Assessing the client's previous knowledge reduces the chance of the client's misunderstanding new information when the client lacks specific information or is misinformed. Also, by determining the client's present knowledge, the nurse will be able to avoid repeating information the client is already familiar with, a repetition that might hinder the client's interest in learning.

The emotional climate affects learning. The emotions of the client toward learning environment have a strong influence on the client's ability to learn. The nurse should examine the client's feelings about the topic and the client's current emotional state before teaching. The nurse should also be aware of the learning environment, which may be stimulating, neutral, or distracting.

Repetition strengthens learning. Continued practice enhances the learner's retention of new information and formation of new behavior patterns. Different clients need different amounts of repetition for effective learning, depending on the complexity of the skill to be learned and the client's abilities to learn.

Satisfaction reinforces learning. When an individual receives satisfaction in learning new behaviors, these new behaviors will be retained longer. Personal pride in accomplishment is a strong incentive for learning and retaining new skills. The nurse should consider both internal (personal) and external factors that facilitate client satisfaction in learning, such as rewards or praise.

Principles of teaching

Good nurse-learner rapport is important in teaching. Client learning is facilitated when the nurse and client have a positive relationship that is cooperative, comfortable, and caring. A positive interpersonal relationship enhances learning.

Teaching requires effective communication. New information is learned through effective verbal and visual communication techniques. Effective communication is accomplished when the listener grasps the meaning conveyed by the speaker. The nurse must receive feedback from the client to validate that the client understands the information correctly.

Learning needs of clients and co-workers must be determined. Before the client is taught, the client's learning needs must be assessed. The client's learning needs vary based on previous knowledge and experience and the present situational needs.

Objectives serve as guides in planning and evaluating teaching. The client and nurse determine what learning needs are to be accomplished and establish an objective that states precisely and clearly the behaviors to be demonstrated. The objective serves as a criterion for evaluating achievement of learning.

Planning time for teaching and learning requires special attention. The nurse must set aside time to develop an effective teaching plan and collaborate with the client to find the most appropriate time for implementing the teaching plan.

Control of the environment is an aspect of teaching. The nurse must consider personal and environmental factors that influence client learning. The client's comfort and elimination of distracting interruptions are two important factors that promote an effective learning environment.

Learning principles must be applied appropriately. In developing a teaching plan, the nurse should review the principles of learning and apply these to the client's unique needs and specific situation.

Teaching skills can be acquired through practice and observation. The same principles that apply to learning may be used in learning to teach. The nurse must be motivated to learn the art and skills of teaching and have sufficient physical and mental readiness. Through observation, imitation, and the acquisition of new knowledge and practice, the nurse can learn to be an effective teacher.

Evaluation is an integral part of teaching. The fact that the nurse has taught the client does not mean the client has learned. The nurse should have the client demonstrate achievement of the learning objectives to validate that the client has achieved the newly learned behaviors.

•   •   •

Pohl's basic principles for learning and teaching describe methods of learning and factors that the nurse should consider when teaching clients. In the nursing process, these principles provide the scientific rationale that supports different teaching strategies in nursing implementation. These principles are not appropriate as a framework for assessing or analyzing data in the nursing process, but are an excellent scientific rationale to support the implementation strategies. Chapter 10 shows examples of their use.

REFERENCES

1 Duvall, E.M.: Marriage and family development, ed. 5, Philadelphia, 1977, J.B. Lippincott Co.
2 King, I.M.: Toward a theory for nursing, New York, 1971, John Wiley & Sons, Inc.
3 Levine, M.E.: Introduction to clinical nursing, ed. 2, Philadelphia, 1973, F.A. Davis Co.
4 Levine, M.E.: The four conservation principles of nursing, supplemental material for nursing theorists general sessions, The Second Annual Nurse Educator Conference, New York City, December 4-6, 1978.
5 Orem, D.E.: Nursing: concepts of practice, New York, 1971, McGraw-Hill Book Co.
6 Orem, D.E.: Nursing: concepts of practice, ed. 2, New York, 1980, McGraw-Hill Book Co.
7 Otto, H.A.: A framework for assessing family strengths. In Reinhardt, A.M., and Quinn, M.D., editors: Family-centered community nursing, vol. 1, St. Louis, 1973, The C.V. Mosby Co.
8 Peplau, H.E.: Interpersonal relations in nursing, New York, 1952, G.P. Putnam's Sons.
9 Pohl, M.L.: The teaching function of the nursing practitioner, ed. 3, Dubuque, Iowa, 1978, Wm C. Brown Co., Publishers.
10 Roy, Sr.C.: Introduction to nursing: an adaptation model, Englewood Cliffs, N.J., 1976, Prentice-Hall, Inc.
11 Roy, Sr.C.: The Roy adaptation model. In Reihl, J.P., and Roy, Sr.C., editors: Conceptual models for nursing practice, ed. 2, New York, 1980, Appleton-Century-Crofts.
12 Satir, V.: Peoplemaking, Palo Alto, Calif., 1972, Science and Behavior Books.
13 von Bertalanffy, L.: General systems theory: foundations, development, and applications, New York, 1968, George Braziller, Inc.

BIBLIOGRAPHY

Daubenmire, M.J., and King, I.M.: Nursing process model: a systems approach, Nurs. Outlook **21:**512, 1973.
King, I.M.: Conceptual frame of reference for nursing, Nurs. Res. **17:**27, 1968.
Nursing Theories Conference Group: Nursing theories: the base for professional nursing practice, Englewood Cliffs, N.J., 1980, Prentice-Hall, Inc.
Reihl, J.P., and Roy, Sr.C.: Conceptual models for nursing practice, ed. 2, New York, 1980, Appleton-Century-Crofts.
Satir, V.: Conjoint family therapy, Palo Alto, Calif., 1967, Science and Behavior Books.

II

Components of the NURSING PROCESS

NURSING ASSESSMENT
Overview of data collection

PAULA J. CHRISTENSEN

GENERAL CONSIDERATIONS

Data collection is the foundation of the nursing process. An accurate assessment leads to identification of the client's health status and concerns or nursing diagnoses. This provides direction for nursing implementation and alleviation of client concerns. The purpose of data collection is to identify and obtain pertinent data about the client.

Nursing's aim is to consider clients in a multifocal way. Individuals, families, and communities have multiple aspects that are interrelated and influence each other. The psychological, biophysical, spiritual, and sociocultural elements of the client must be considered to ensure a comprehensive and accurate assessment. To accomplish this, the nurse needs a strong knowledge base in a variety of disciplines. A knowledge base of the theories, norms, and standards of behavior provides a foundation to collect pertinent information from clients and make sound judgments about their health.

This chapter begins with a brief historical overview of data collection. Factors influencing data collection, the nurse-client relationship, and patterns of behavior are then discussed. Three major tools for data collection and specific examples of each are given. The most important points are then drawn together in a discussion of guidelines.

The assessment process is applicable to all groups of clients: individuals, families, and communities. Specific examples of data collection for each client group are provided in the next three chapters.

Historical perspectives

Nursing care has frequently included a limited assessment of clients' health-related concerns. Traditionally, the nurse depended on medical diagnoses to give direction to nursing care. Nurses also used intuitions made while in contact with their clients. These intuitions usually came out in forms such as: "I just have a feeling that Mr. Polaski is going downhill" or "Something tells me that I better check Ms. Armond's blood pressure more frequently." These intuitions were based on an important form of data collection that still exists today—subjective impressions—one that cannot be refuted yet also cannot be the sole source of data obtained. Behavioral and medical sciences have developed to the point of providing certain concrete indicators of health. These specific indicators of health give nurses a basis to collect data and make judgments.

The nursing profession has become increasingly accountable and responsible for basing implementation on a sound nursing assessment. Medical diagnoses and intuitions now serve as cues for further data collection. Since nursing practice focuses on maintenance, restoration, and promotion of health, the nurse must conduct a comprehensive and valid nursing assessment.

Nurse-client relationship

The nurse-client relationship is the means for applying the nursing process. This relationship is the vehicle by which the nurse works with the client. Carl Rogers[4] identifies three aspects that facilitate personal growth in a relationship: (1) genuineness, the ability to be aware of one's own feelings, or being real; (2) respecting the separateness of another, accepting the other unconditionally; and (3) a continuing desire to understand or empathize with the other. These aspects are applicable to all human relationships, especially the nurse-client relationship.

Trust, empathy, caring, autonomy, and mutuality are five concepts basic to the development of a nurse-client relationship.[5] These concepts need to be reciprocal during nurse-client interactions, but the nurse is responsible for setting the tone. Therefore, the nurse needs to identify specific actions that communicate trust (consistency, honesty), empathy (touch, sincerity), caring (genuineness, eye contact), autonomy (nonjudgmental, nonthreatening), and mutuality (inclusion of client in decision making).

Numerous communication techniques that foster the nurse-client relationship have evolved from psychological theory and practice disciplines. These techniques are useful during any nurse-client interaction to facilitate obtaining information and establishing rapport. The communication techniques are enabling devices that should be incorporated naturally into nurse-client interactions. The techniques chosen are based on the nurse's comfort with them. Examples of facilitative verbal and nonverbal communication techniques are found in Table 3-1. In many situations nonverbal communication reveals the true, often unacceptable message. Nonverbal messages can be unintentional as well as intentional. The nurse's goal in communication is to exhibit congruent verbal and nonverbal messages; in other words, the verbal and nonverbal messages should be saying the same thing. Definitions of the techniques shown in Table 3-1 are in the glossary. The use of these techniques does not guarantee a meaningful relationship. All aspects of the situation must be taken into account, such as the client's health state, environmental influences, and the nurse's knowledge and use of self.

Effective nurse-client relationships can be attained when nurses are willing to look at their own values, prejudices, strengths, and limitations. Nurses discover how this "self" affects interactions with others. This cannot be done through intellectual development alone; nurses must be open to the discovery of their own motivations and feelings through experience and relationships with others.

Table 3-1. Facilitative communication techniques

Verbal	Nonverbal
Open-ended statements and questions	Thoughtful silence
Related questions	Touch
Verbalization of the implied	Active listening
Clarification of statements	Watching and eye contact
Consensual validation	Open body language
Sharing of perceptions	
Restatement, repetition of main idea	
Reflection of feelings and content	
Focus	
Summary	

Patterns of behavior

All clients have common patterns of functioning. A pattern is viewed as a composite sample of traits or behaviors characterized by rate, rhythm, intensity, duration, and amount. The individual is a combination of biophysical, psychological, sociocultural, and spiritual aspects. The family has a certain definable structure and process. The community is made up of systems and subsystems that influence its functions.

The behavior patterns given in Table 3-2 are examples of similar characteristics each client group possesses.

Table 3-2. Patterns of behavior

Individual	Family	Community
Exercise	Communication	Socialization
Circulation	Roles	Power
Self-concept	Physical maintenance	System linkage
Valuing	Decision making	Boundary maintenance

Theories describe the healthy and unhealthy aspects of clients' patterns of behavior. These patterns can serve as guidelines for data collection. All clients possess certain basic patterns, yet each client may exhibit or combine patterns in a different way. Looking for differences and similarities among clients helps the nurse avoid using personal interpretation of data during the data collection process.

Factors influencing data collection

Several factors influence the process of data collection—how the data are presented by the client and how they are perceived by the nurse. Both the client and the nurse enter a situation with previous experiences and knowledge that influence their perceptions and interpretations. More specifically, the nurse and the client are influenced by their respective (1) physical, mental, and emotional states and needs; (2) cultural, social, and philosophical backgrounds; (3) number and functional ability of senses; (4) past experiences associated with the present situation; (5) meaning of the event; (6) interests, preoccupations, preconceptions, and motivational levels; (7) knowledge or familiarity with the situation; (8) environmental conditions and distractions; and (9) presence, attitudes, and reactions of others.[3]

These factors create a situation in which both clients and nurses automatically assign personal meanings or interpretations of the situation. Difficulty arises when the nurse's perception or interpretation is used as fact. The nurse's awareness and conscious willingness are needed to develop the skill of differentiating actual data from personal interpretation.

TOOLS FOR DATA COLLECTION

Data collection occurs through the use of three tools: interaction, observation, and measurement. Interaction data are considered any spoken word from the client, health care personnel, or significant others. Observations made through the senses, including written documents, are observation data. Measurement data are those obtained through the use of instruments that quantify information. Definitions and examples of these tools are given in the following discussion.

All these tools have strengths and limitations. They should not be used in isolation, since accurate assessments cannot be made through the use of one tool alone. In some situations the use of two tools will dominate, depending on the age and health status of the client and the given situation. Generally, the nurse should always use at least two of the three tools for data collection.

Interaction

Interaction is defined as a continuous exchange between the nurse and the client. The purpose is to obtain information or develop rapport or both. Nursing today is often based on a series of transient interactions with clients, rather than sustained relationships. The same characteristics discussed previously about growth-producing relationships also apply to isolated nurse-client interactions.

Interviews, or transitory relationships between two people for the purpose of gaining information or developing rapport, can be classified as directive-interrogative, rapport-building, or open-ended.[2] *Directive-interrogative* interviewing involves asking for specific information; the purpose is primarily to get data. The nurse maintains control of the direction of the interview, and the client becomes a passive participant. This type of interviewing is advantageous when a specific amount of data is needed in a short period of time, but disadvantageous in that the client is passive and may not be able to discuss concerns. History taking is an example of a directive-interrogative interview. *Rapport-building* interviews focus on building a relationship, not on getting information. Open, empathic responses are used by the interviewer to facilitate the client's control of the interview. Data emerge and a relationship develops, but rapport building takes time and specific data may not be obtained. The *open-ended* interview is a combination of the first two types; the goals are to get information from the client and to build rapport. The client's concerns emerge through the use of a variety of communication techniques.

The interviewer starts with the least amount of authority (open-ended statements and questions) to allow client directiveness and proceeds to increasing authority (more specific focus). All three types of interviews have a place in nurse-client interactions. In general, the nurse should use the least amount of authority necessary to obtain the information needed within the time allotted.

The outcome of interactions is data that reflect what the client said and what the nurse observed. Observations include the client's nonverbal behavior, appearance, and function, and the environment. Statements by the client should be noted as direct quotations. Paraphrasing what someone says tends to increase the probability of interpreting or placing one's own meaning to the data. Table 3-3 provides examples of objective statements of interaction data versus personal interpretations of them.

Table 3-3. Objective statements of interaction data versus personal interpretations

Objective interaction data	Personal interpretations
Individual client	
"I'd rather be left alone now."	Client is angry.
"I'm afraid of what they will find during surgery."	Client is afraid of surgery.
Family client	
"My mother is hardly ever at home."	Mother does not care about time spent with child.
"I'm expected to do all the housework around here with no help."	Family expects mother/wife to do all the work around the home.
Community client	
"The city council meets once a month."	Infrequent city council meetings.
"A lot of teenagers in this part of town are pregnant."	Epidemic of teenage pregnancies.

Observation

Observation is a process of noting pieces of information or cues through the use of the senses (sight, touch, hearing, smell, and taste). These senses are used in a variety of ways to observe the client's (1) general characteristics of appearance and physical function, (2) content and process of interactions and relationships, and (3) environment. Each sense is discussed in relation to these three categories.

The sense of sight is used to identify visual cues that clients and data sources project. Examples of data collected through the use of sight are as follows:

1. General characteristics of appearance and physical function: color, shape, amount, approximate size, gait, balance, and dress; data from written records about general characteristics (such as nurses' notes).
2. Content and process of interactions: nonverbal communication such as body movements, gestures, eye contact, personal space, use of touch.

3. Environment: neighborhood characteristics such as number of houses and cleanliness; characteristics of client's home such as rooms available, cleanliness, and furniture; data from written sources about client's environment.

The sense of touch is used to determine qualities of an object or person. Through simple touch or the use of palpation* and percussion* the following data can be obtained:

1. General characteristics: texture, moisture, temperature, density, and muscle and skin tone.
2. Content and process of interactions: not applicable.
3. Environment: temperature of air, moisture (humidity), and furniture.

Hearing is primarily used to actively listen to clients' verbal messages or to note interaction data. Other important uses of hearing are:

1. General characteristics: auscultation* of lung, heart, and bowel sounds, and percussion (along with touch) of tissue.
2. Content and process of interactions: amount of interacting with others, tone of voice(s), interruptions in conversations, and specific content of what is said.
3. Environment: house/neighborhood noise levels; usual sounds in home or community.

The senses of smell and taste are used less frequently. The odors of the client, home, and environment are detected through smell. The taste of local foods and, in some environments, chemicals in the air can be detected through taste.

Maintaining objectivity in observing clients is an important element of data collection. Examples of observation data that are objective versus notations of personal interpretations are given in Table 3-4. Recording specifi-

---

*The terms "palpation," "percussion," and "auscultation" are specific to the individual client. Refer to physical examination texts for an in-depth explanation of these concepts.

Table 3-4. Objective observation data versus personal interpretations

Objective observation data	Personal interpretations
Individual client	
Shoulder-length, dark brown hair with dull sheen.	Long, dirty brown hair.
Smiles frequently.	Appears to be happy.
Nail beds pink, rapid capillary refill of toes and fingers.	Good circulation of extremities.
Family client	
Mother does not look at son when he speaks.	Mother angry at son.
Parents laugh when speaking about sexual history.	Parents pleased with sex life.
Articles of clothing lying on floor and furniture.	Messy house.
Community client	
Sounds of two local factories present.	Noisy environment.
Garbage cans standing upright with lids on.	Neat neighborhood.
All board members present at meeting.	Active and interested people on board.

cally what one sees, feels, hears, smells, or tastes is more accurate than recording one's interpretation of it.

Measurement

Measurement is actually a form of observation. The tool is separated to indicate that certain data are conducive to more precise observation. Measurement is used to ascertain extent, dimensions, rate, rhythm, quantity, or size, frequently through the use of additional instruments along with the senses. Some forms of measurement data include laboratory values, vital signs, height, and weight for the individual client; number of family members, ages, and number of rooms in dwelling for the family client; and population, number of blocks in district, and epidemiological data for the community client. General observation data that can be quantified are also considered measurement data (for example, observation datum: smoked cigarettes during interview; measurement datum: smoked five cigarettes during 30-minute interview). Table 3-5 gives examples of objective, nonjudgmental measurement data in contrast with personal interpretations from measurement data.

Table 3-5. Objective measurement data versus personal interpretations

Objective measurement data	Personal interpretations
Individual client	
Blood pressure: 130/76.	Normal blood pressure.
Smoked 10 cigarettes in 1-hour interview.	Smokes a lot.
Height: 5'4"; weight: 120 lb.	Average height and weight.
Family client	
Four rooms in house with six family members.	Inadequate space for family.
Sister interrupted brother five times in 30 minutes.	Sister doesn't respect brother's right to talk.
Mother's age: 40 yr; father's age: 40 yr; child's age: 2 yr.	Late starting childbearing, didn't want child earlier or infertility problem.
Community client	
Fifteen homes located in one city block.	Crowded neighborhood.
Population of city: 3,000.	Small town.

Documenting interactions, observations, and measurements

The recording of interaction, observation, and measurement data is facilitated by the use of a columnar approach. This format allows the nurse to note the sequence and tools used to collect data. Depending on the client situation, two of the three tools are used more prominently. The size of the data collection columns can vary accordingly. For example, an infant client will provide minimum, if any, verbal data. Some interaction data may be obtained from the parent or staff, so the interaction column would be the smallest.

Example

Interaction	Observation	Measurement
Statements from parent/staff	Observations of client	Measurements of client

When recording data in the traditional form on a client's record, the nurse must note appropriate data from all three tools. Recording what the client said and what the nurse observed and measured are important in charting.

GUIDELINES FOR DATA COLLECTION

The American Nurses' Association standards for nursing practice[1] are the basis for most of the following guidelines for data collection.

1. *Data collected are comprehensive and multifocal.* The data need to reflect the life experiences of the client. Whatever the client group—individual, family, or community—the nurse should consider socioeconomic, political, biophysical, cultural, psychological, and spiritual influences. Given the amount of potential data that can be obtained from or about any client, a totally comprehensive data collection is unlikely to be obtained. Yet the data do need to represent a variety of factors that influence the client's patterns of living. The nurse must use judgment in focusing data collection on areas that are most pertinent to the client situation.

2. *A variety of sources are used for data collection.* The client is usually the prime source for data collection: but since perceptions of events and circumstances can vary, other sources should be used as well. Validation of data through a variety of sources strengthens the nurse's assessment. Specific examples of sources are given in the following chapters on data collection of individual, family, and community clients. Some general examples of data sources include client, family, and significant others, health care personnel, printed information concerning client, and written records.

3. *Appropriate tools are used for data collection.* At least two data collection tools should be used to ensure validity of data obtained. The appropriateness of the tools used depends on the client's age, status of health, and sources used.

4. *The data collected are objective and nonjudgmental.* The data gathered through the use of interaction, observation, or measurement should be nonjudgmental and objective. The nurse's personal interpretations or perceptions of a situation may lead to further data collection but should not be stated as data themselves.

5. *A systematic format is used for data collection.* Data collection should be systematic. Specific theoretical frameworks or conceptual models provide guides for data collection. Other, more eclectic approaches are useful as well. Specific examples of frameworks and models are given in subsequent chapters. Basically, the nurse begins data collection by assessing the client's major concern first, including multifocal influences on the concern. Then, a more general assessment of the client's health status is included if appropriate.

6. *The data collected reflect updating of information.* Data collection is continuous in nature. The data should reflect appropriate updating of information obtained from the variety of sources used. As new data are obtained, any changes in the health concerns or status of the client should also be noted.

7. *The data collected are recorded and communicated appropriately.* Data collection is virtually useless unless it is communicated appropriately in the client's record. To increase nurses' accountability and responsibility for data collection, information is written and kept in a retrievable record-keeping system.

SUMMARY

This chapter provided an overview of data collection. A variety of factors influencing this process were discussed, along with the importance of the nurse-client relationship. Interaction, observation, and measurement are the three tools used for data collection. The general guidelines identified for data collection are: (1) data are multifocal; (2) a variety of sources are used; (3) appropriate tools are used; (4) a systematic format is used; (5) data collection is continuous; and (6) data are recorded appropriately. The next three chapters provide specific examples of these guidelines as applied to data collection of the individual, family, and community.

REFERENCES

1 American Nurses' Association: Standards: nursing practice, Kansas City, 1973, The Association.
2 Enelow, A.J., and Swisher, S.N.: Interviewing and patient care, New York, 1972, Oxford University Press.
3 Murray, R.B., and Zentner, J.P.: Nursing assessment and health promotion through the life span, ed. 2, Englewood Cliffs, N.J., 1972, Prentice-Hall, Inc.
4 Rogers, C.: On becoming a person, Boston, 1961, Houghton Mifflin Co.
5 Sundeen, S.J., and others: Interaction: implementing the nursing process, St. Louis, 1976, The C.V. Mosby Co.

BIBLIOGRAPHY

Atkinson, L.D., and Murray, M.E.: Understanding the nursing process, New York, 1980, Macmillan, Inc.
Bates, B.: A guide to physical examination, ed. 2, Philadelphia, 1979, J.B. Lippincott Co.
Little, D.E., and Carnevali, D.L.: Nursing care planning, ed. 2, Philadelphia, 1976, J.B. Lippincott Co.
Malasanos, L., and others: Health assessment, St. Louis, 1977, The C.V. Mosby Co.
Marriner, A.: The nursing process: a scientific approach to nursing care, ed. 2, St. Louis, 1979, The C.V. Mosby Co.
Sierra-Franco, M.H.: Therapeutic communication in nursing, New York, 1978, McGraw-Hill Book Co.
Travelbee, J.: Interpersonal aspects of nursing, ed. 2, Philadelphia, 1971, F.A. Davis Co.

NURSING ASSESSMENT
Data collection of the
individual client

PAULA J. CHRISTENSEN

GENERAL CONSIDERATIONS

The individual client has historically been the focus of nursing care. Nurses now realize that caring for one individual involves working with more than the client alone. The client's family, significant others, beliefs, background, and psychological and physical states all influence the client and subsequent care. Data collected reflect information concerning the client's biographical status; and psychological, sociocultural, spiritual, and biophysical health. All three tools for data collection—interaction, observation, and measurement—are needed for a comprehensive and accurate set of data.

This chapter looks at types of biographical data needed and sources available. Examples of models for data collection of the individual client are provided along with sample questions.

Biographical data

Biographical information is obtained during the initial interview with the client. Most agencies have a specific form indicating what information is needed. The box on p. 39 gives an example of important biographical data. A directive-interrogative approach is frequently used to complete the data form. Ideally, much of the information could be obtained during an open-ended discussion.

Sources of data

The individual client is the primary source of data. Other sources used to collect data are:

Family and significant others
Survey of client's home and community
Medical records
Social records
Developmental records
Results of diagnostic tests

Nursing notes
Nursing rounds
Change of shift reports
Progress notes
Kardex

FRAMEWORKS FOR DATA COLLECTION

Theories, frameworks, models, and principles are used as approaches to data collection. These approaches give direction to obtaining systematic and purposeful data. The nurse decides which combination of approaches is appropriate to the client's age, health status, and situation. The nurse's knowledge of approaches and the client situation determine the choice.

Some agencies provide a guideline for getting information about the client's expressed concern. Those guidelines seldom identify how the concern affects the client's life-style. Additional information is needed to ensure multifocal and comprehensive data. The chosen format is a *general guide* for data collection, not a rigid tool.

Initial data collection focuses on the client's primary expressed concerns and how the concerns affect other patterns of living. For example, if the client's expressed concern is psychological related to coping with stress, the nurse begins by assessing psychological coping and health. To obtain multifocal data, the nurse uses other approaches to get information about how the client's stress affects other patterns of living.

Nursing model

A number of nursing models assist systematic data collection of individuals. The Nursing Theories Conference book[5] provides an overview of numerous nursing models and frameworks that are useful. Chapter 2 and Appendix C also provide examples of some nursing models.

Roy[7] provides a multifocal format in her discussion of areas of adaptive modes. Roy's adaptive modes are identified as basic physiological, self-concept, role mastery, and interdependence. The basic *physiological mode* includes exercise and rest, nutrition, elimination, fluid and electrolytes, oxygen, circulation, and regulation. The *self-concept mode* incorporates the physical self, personal self, and interpersonal self. *Role mastery* involves looking at others' expectations of the client as well as the client's self-expec-

---

BIOGRAPHICAL DATA

Name _____
Address _____
Age _____
Date of birth _____
Place of birth _____
Gender _____
Ethnic group _____
Religious preference _____
Primary language spoken _____
Marital status _____
Education _____
Occupation _____
Health insurance _____
Income _____

tations. The client's relationships and interactions with family and community are all parts of the *interdependence mode*. Examples of questions used for data collection based on this framework are shown in Table 4-1. The questions are arranged according to the data collection tools of interaction, observation, and measurement.

Table 4-1. Data collection of individual client based on Roy's assessment model

Area of data collection	Observations	Interactions	Measurements
A. Basic physiological mode			
1. Exercise	What is the tone of the client's muscles? Are height and weight proportional? Is any atrophy present?	What kinds of physical activity do you engage in? How long has it been since you've exercised? What type of work do you do for a living? Are you satisfied with the amount of exercise you get each week?	Frequency and regularity of exercise. Length of time of physical exercise. Length of time since client has exercised. Height and weight.
2. Rest	What is the client's nonverbal language? Posture Yawning Circles under eyes Concentration on discussion	How much sleep and rest do you get each 24 hours? Do you take naps? Do you feel rested with the amount of sleep you get? What helps you sleep (for example, backrubs or music)? How often do you wake up during the night?	Number of usual hours of sleep and rest. Number of hours sleep and rest needed to feel rested. Medications and dose used for sleep.
3. Nutrition	What are the tone, texture, and coloring of skin and mucous membranes? Do height and weight appear proportional? What is the texture of hair? Condition of scalp? What is the condition of nails?	How many meals do you eat per day? What is your knowledge of the four basic food groups? Whom do you eat with? Where do you eat your meals? How often do you eat at home? In restaurants? Do you take daily vitamins? With iron? With minerals? Any recent changes in diet or weight? Any increase or decrease in appetite? What kind of foods can and do you eat?	Three-day recall: record specific food and fluid take for 3 days. Height and weight. Lab results: CBC, electrolytes. Fat caliper reading.
4. Elimination	What are the color and odor of the urine? Describe the consistency and color of stools. (Physical exam: auscultation, inspection, palpation, and percussion of abdomen.)	How often do you urinate and have a bowel movement? What do your bowel movements look like (consistency, color)? What does your urine look like (clarity, color)? Do you have any burning or foul smell of your urine? Do you need laxatives to have a bowel movement? Enemas?	Frequency and amount of urination. Frequency of bowel movement. Amount and kind of laxative, bulk agent, or enemas.

Table 4-1. Data collection of individual client based on Roy's assessment model—cont'd

Area of data collection	Observations	Interactions	Measurements
5. Oxygen and circulation	What are the color and temperature of extremities? Note characteristics of respirations, use of accessory muscles, cough. (Physical exam: auscultation, inspection, palpation, and percussion of chest and back.)	Do you smoke cigarettes? Cigars? A pipe? Do you inhale the smoke? What do you understand about the effects of smoking? Are your arms or legs unusually cool to the touch? Do you have any bleeding problems?	Number of cigarettes, cigars, or pipes smoked per day. Lab results: CBC, protime. Number of seconds it takes for capillary refill.
	Is there rapid capillary refill when toe and fingernails are blanched? What is the color of mucous membranes? Are pedal pulses palpable?	Do you have high blood pressure? Do you experience chest pains, shortness of breath, or "fluttering" in your chest?	Blood pressure, pulses, respirations, temperature. ECG
6. Fluids and electrolytes	What is the client's skin turgor? What is the condition of the mucous membranes? Is dependent edema present?	How much fluid do you drink per day? Are you unusually thirsty? Do you have a history of high blood pressure? Are you receiving any medication to regulate your blood pressure or "water" in your body? Do you add salt to your food while cooking? At the table? Do you take any potassium supplements?	Amount of fluid drunk per day. Blood pressure, pulse, respiration, temperature. Medication and dose. Measurement of ankles. Lab results: CBC, electrolytes. Medication and dose.
7. Regulatory	(Physical exam: function of senses, reflexes.) Are height and weight proportional? What are the texture and appearance of hair on client's body? Are there any physical defects noted about the client's eyes, ears, nose, or tongue?	Do you have difficulty with your sight? Hearing? Touch? Taste? Smell? Do you have a history of diabetes? Thyroid problems? If so, what medications are you taking? Have you ever had any difficulty with your hormones? When was your onset of secondary sex characteristics? Are you taking birth control pills? How old were you when you started your first period? When was your last period? How often do you get your period? Do you know how to examine your own breasts? Do you have regular Pap smears?	Temperature. Names and doses of medications. Date of last menstrual period. Number of days in usual cycle. Frequency of self breast exam.

Continued.

Table 4-1. Data collection of individual client based on Roy's assessment model—cont'd

Area of data collection	Observations	Interactions	Measurements
B. Self-concept mode			
1. Physical self	What is the nature of the client's clothes? Tight or loose fitting?	What is your highest weight and lowest weight?	Height and weight.
	Does the client shield or avoid touching or looking at certain areas of the body?	Have you had any physical alterations of your body?	
	What is the nature of scars, deformed body parts, and alterations in function?	Was or is it difficult for you to accept those changes?	
	Whom does the client interact with?	How have those changes affected your relationship with others?	
	What is the client's affect?	How do you feel about your weight and appearance?	
2. Personal self	Note nonverbal communication: body language, eye contact, gestures, affect, voice tone.	What religion and values were you raised with?	Frequency of attendance at church-related functions.
		Do you practice them now?	
	How is the client groomed?	What kind of involvement do you have with your church?	
	Hair	Are you comfortable with that?	
	Clothes	How do you usually express your feelings and thoughts to others? Are there some times when you don't? When are they?	
	Nails		
	Makeup		
		Describe some characteristics of the type of person you'd most like to be. Do you see yourself as that person? Is your description realistic to you?	
		What do you do when you have a problem?	
3. Interpersonal self	Note nonverbal communication:	How do you see yourself in relation to other people? Better than? Equal to? Less than equal to?	
	Facial expressions		
	Gestures		
	Hand and foot movements	Describe a usual day for you. How much time do you spend alone?	Number of hours in a day spent alone.
	Posture		
	Congruence with spoken words	When you get angry, how do you deal with it? Hold it in? Yell? Hit someone or something? Talk to someone?	

Table 4-1. Data collection of individual client based on Roy's assessment model—cont'd

Area of data collection	Observations	Interactions	Measurements
C. Role mastery mode	Note activities of the client: Parenting Studying Reading Cooking Cleaning Leisure Being sick Occupation	What are your family's expectations of you? Significant others' expectations of you? Are these people clear in expressing their expectations? Are they expressed verbally, through actions, or hints? What do you think others expect of you? What are your expectations of yourself? How do they fit with what others expect of you? What do you do for a living? Are you meeting your own and others' expectations at work? Are they compatible? If not, do you talk with those concerned? Do you feel overextended? Underachieved?	How much time per day or week does the client spend in various activities listed?
D. Interdependence mode	Note nonverbals while interacting with others (such as family, friends, interviewer)	Who are the people in your family? Whom do you feel closest to in your family? For what reasons? Who are other people important to you? Who do you socialize with other than your family? How often? Are you satisfied with this contact? What activities in and outside the home are you involved with? How do you see yourself fitting into your family? Your group of friends? Do you feel in competition with family or friends (for example, material goods or status)?	How often does the client interact with family? How many people or activities does the client interact with outside work and family?

Eclectic data collection model

Specific assessment data to determine patterns of health are obtained using a variety of concepts in a multifocal model. Viewing the individual client as a biopsychosociospiritual being provides a basis for data collection. The box below shows a format based on this model.

Since the biophysical facets of the individual are numerous, assessing each individual facet is an overwhelming task. There are, however, some general patterns of biophysical health that serve as a starting point for data collection. Assessing the client's general appearance and daily activity patterns of nutrition, elimination, exercise, hygiene, sleep and rest, sexual activity, and substance use provides a general understanding of the client's bio-

---

**FORMAT FOR DATA COLLECTION
USING BIOPSYCHOSOCIOSPIRITUAL MODEL**

Informant _____
Major concern _____
History of major concern _____
Biophysical health
    General appearance _____
    Daily activity patterns
        Nutrition _____
        Elimination _____
        Exercise _____
        Sleep and rest _____
        Sexual activity _____
        Hygiene _____
        Substance use _____
    Review of systems _____
    Physical examination _____
    Past biophysical health
        Restorative interventions _____
        Allergies _____
        Immunizations _____
        Growth and development _____
        Foreign travel _____
        Family health history _____
Psychological health
    Interaction patterns _____
    Cognitive patterns _____
    Emotional patterns _____
    Sexuality _____
    Self-concept _____
    Coping patterns _____
    Family coping patterns _____
Sociological health
    Cultural patterns _____
    Significant relationships _____
    Recreation patterns _____
    Environment _____
Spiritual health
    Religious beliefs and practices _____
    Values and valuing practices _____

physical capabilities and limitations. Anatomy and physiology texts as well as sources on health maintenance and promotion give norms of physical appearance and function to guide data collection. Depending on the nature of the data collected, most are obtained through interaction and observation.

The review of systems and physical assessment are included as current biological data. Texts about physical examination provide a format and explanation for obtaining these data. Data from the review of systems are obtained through interviews and recorded as interactions. Data obtained through physical assessment are recorded as observations and measurements.

Past *biophysical* health data are important to gain a perspective on the client's current health status. Restorative interventions such as surgeries and major treatments, allergies, and immunizations should be known. Important past health data also include the presence or absence of alterations in growth and development; foreign travel; and family health history, including genetic and familial physical and emotional illnesses.

Psychological health is assessed through data collection related to the following patterns: interaction, cognition, emotions, coping, self-concept, sexuality, and family coping. References from mental health, psychology, family theory, sexuality, and communication provide norms of psychological health that guide data collection.

Sociological health patterns that are important to assess include cultural background, significant relationships, and recreation. Data concerning the client's environment are also included here. Social patterns are found in sources describing specific cultures, social influences, leisure theory, personal space, and interpersonal relationships. These sources provide a base for data collection.

Spiritual health includes religious beliefs and practices and values and valuing practices. The congruence between beliefs and belief practices is often important in maintaining spiritual health. Books that deal with "meaning to life" issues, specific religious practices, and valuing help the nurse collect data about spiritual health patterns.

Table 4-2 provides examples of questions that can be used for data collection based on an eclectic biopsychosociospiritual model.

Other models and frameworks	Several frameworks and models from other disciplines are useful in providing a systematic approach to data collection. More general or multifocal frameworks include Dunn's work on high-level wellness[2] and Maslow's work on hierarchy of needs.[4] Developmental frameworks are more specific and limited in scope. Erikson[3] discusses psychosocial development throughout the life span for individuals in a traditional family. Piaget[6] provides a framework for assessing cognitive development of children and adolescents. Selye's stress theory[8] is useful in looking at physiological and psychological coping. Aguilera and Messick[1] provide a framework to work with individuals in crisis. Some approaches are very limited in scope. The more limited in scope the approach, the greater is the need to combine it with others to provide a multifocal data collection of the client.

Text continued on p. 53.

Table 4-2. Data collection of individual client based on eclectic assessment model

Area of data collection	Observations	Interactions	Measurements
A. Biophysical health			
1. General appearance	What is the client wearing? Is it appropriate for the environment? Any visible alterations in physical function? Note the client's steadiness of gait. Note nonverbal communications: body language, eye contact, gestures, affect. Note characteristics of movement and speech.		
2. Daily activity patterns			
a. Nutrition	What are the tone, texture, and coloring of skin and mucous membranes? Do height and weight appear proportional? What is the texture of hair? Condition of scalp? What is the condition of nails? Gums? Teeth?	What kind of foods can and do you eat? How many meals do you eat per day? What is your knowledge of the four basic food groups? Whom do you eat with? Where do you eat your meals? How often do you eat at home? In restaurants? Do you take daily vitamins? With iron? With minerals? Any recent changes in diet or weight? Any increase or decrease in appetite?	Three-day recall: record of specific food and fluid intake for 3 days. Height and weight. Lab results: CBC, electrolytes.
b. Elimination	What are the color and odor of the urine? Describe the consistency and color of stools. (Physical exam: auscultation, palpation, percussion, and inspection of abdomen.)	How often do you urinate and have bowel movements? What do your bowel movements look like (consistency, color)? What does your urine look like (clarity, color)? Do you have any burning or foul smell of your urine? Do you need laxatives to have a bowel movement? Enemas?	Frequency and amount of urination. Frequency of bowel movements. Amount and kind of laxative, bulk agent, or enema used.
c. Exercise	What is the tone of the client's muscles? Are height and weight proportional? Is any atrophy present?	What kinds of physical activity do you engage in? How long has it been since you've done them? What type of work do you do for a living? Are you satisfied with the amount of exercise you get each week?	Length of time of physical activity. Length of time since client has exercised. Height and weight.
d. Hygiene	Are the person's clothes, hair, and nails groomed? What is the condition of scalp and hair?	Describe how you take care of your body.	Frequency of hygiene.

Table 4-2. Data collection of individual client based on eclectic assessment model—cont'd

Area of data collection	Observations	Interactions	Measurements
	Note odors (body and mouth), makeup, and appearance of teeth.	Do you prefer baths, showers, or sink baths? Morning or evening?	
		Do you use deodorant agents or cologne?	
		How often do you brush your teeth? Floss?	Frequency of oral care.
		When did you last visit your dentist?	Date of last dentist visit.
e. Substance use	What are the person's nonverbal messages while smoking? Jittery? Quick movements? Slow, relaxed movements? Attention span? Ability to understand spoken word? Response time?	Do you smoke cigarettes or cigars?	Number of cigarettes or cigars smoked during interview.
		What is your understanding of the effects of smoking?	Number of cigarettes or cigars per day.
		Do you inhale the smoke?	
		Do you drink alcoholic beverages?	Frequency of drinks per day or week.
	Note pupil dilation and constriction, hand tremors.	Whom do you drink with? Do you drink alone?	Number of drinks per day or week.
		Do you smoke marijuana or use any tranquilizers or stimulants (coffee, tea, cola)?	Frequency of use of marijuana and drugs.
		What is your understanding of the use of marijuana and drugs?	Number of cups of coffee, tea, or cola.
			Amount of marijuana or drugs used at one time.
		Do you use drugs and alcohol at the same time?	
f. Sleep and rest	What is the client's nonverbal language? Posture Yawning Circles under eyes Concentration on discussion	How much sleep and rest do you get each 24 hours?	Number of usual hours of sleep and rest.
		Do you take naps?	
		Do you feel rested with the amount of sleep you get?	Number of hours sleep and rest needed to feel rested.
		What helps you sleep (for example, backrubs, music, or warm milk)?	Medication and dose used for sleep.
		How often do you wake up during the night?	
g. Sexual activity	Note nonverbal communication during discussion: Eye contact Gestures Tone of voice	Do you feel that your sexual needs are being met?	Frequency of sexual contact.
		Do your needs coincide with those of your partner?	
		If not, how do you deal with the difference?	
		How are your sexual needs met? (for example, intercourse, touching, fondling, or masturbation)?	
		What are your menstrual cycles (periods) like (regularity and discomfort)?	Date of last menstrual period.
		How old were you when your first period started?	Usual duration of cycle.
		Do you know how to examine your own breasts?	Frequency of self breast exam.
		Do you have regular Pap smears?	

Continued.

Table 4-2. Data collection of individual client based on eclectic assessment model—cont'd

Area of data collection	Observations	Interactions	Measurements
3. Past bio-physical health			
a. Restorative interventions	Any apparent physical dysfunction or limitations?	What major illnesses and surgeries have you had? What treatment did you have for them? Was the recovery uneventful? Did these have an impact on your current life-style? Are you currently being treated for or affected by these incidents? How have these affected your physical functioning?	Dates of major illnesses, injuries, and surgeries. Length of each hospitalization.
b. Allergies	Note appearance of eyes and surrounding tissue, presence of sniffling, need to blow nose. Note condition of skin (redness, scaling) and scratching.	Are you allergic to any foods, medications, or other substances (dust or animals)? What is your usual reaction? Have you ever been treated for allergies?	
c. Immunizations	Observe documents of immunizations.	Are your immunizations up to date? Did you experience any unusual reactions to the immunizations?	Dates of immunizations.
d. Growth and development	Depending on client's age, is the person able to carry on a conversation, verbalize thoughts, and follow directions?	Were your growth and development as a child the same as for other children your age? Did you feel the same as friends and siblings in developing verbal and motor skills?	Child development measures (such as Denver Developmental Screening Test).
e. Foreign travel		Have you traveled out of this country? If so, were you exposed to or did you contract any diseases?	Dates and length of travel.
f. Family health history	Observe documents indicating familial diseases.	Do you have any chronic illness—physical or emotional—in your family (for example, tuberculosis, diabetes, cancer, hypertension, depression, anxiety, heart disease, kidney disease)?	
B. Psychological health			
1. Coping patterns	Note nonverbal communication (eye contact, gestures, body language, voice tone, affect).	Who are the people significant (who mean a lot) to you? Who can and do you talk to on a regular basis? How much time do you spend alone? How many people do you relate to each day? Do you go out with and see other people on a regular basis?	Number of hours each day spent alone. Number of times per day or week client sees family and friends.

Table 4-2. Data collection of individual client based on eclectic assessment model—cont'd

Area of data collection	Observations	Interactions	Measurements
		Do you keep to yourself most of the time?	
		Do you exercise regularly? What type?	
		Do you have anyone to go to in times of need (such as family, friends, clergy, social agency)?	Frequency of times client calls on these people.
		What do you do to handle stressful situations in your life (for example: *biophysical:* eat, smoke, become agitated, use nervous gestures, sleep, exercise, drink alcoholic beverages, desire sexual activity; *psychological:* become angry with self, become anxious, intellectualize, withdraw, deny, accept, solve the problem; *sociological:* talk with person involved with stress, talk with noninvolved person, blame others, become angry with others; *spiritual:* talk with clergy, pray, read religious books, read mind-soothing poetry or prose)?	
2. Interaction patterns	To whom does the client speak in family? Note nonverbal communication during interaction. Does client answer questions or make comments with direct "I" statements?	Who are the people in your family? How do you usually express your feelings and thoughts to others (for example, directly and verbally, or indirectly through hints and behavior)? What do you think about voicing your opinion or feelings to family? To friends? Do you find ways to blame others for some things you do? What do you do when others make plans that you aren't particularly interested in? Who initiates activities with family? With friends? How do you feel about the way you interact with others?	Ages of family members.
3. Cognitive patterns	Note verbal ability: Concrete thought Simple sentences Formal operational thought Complex sentences Vocabulary used Ability to conceptualize	How much formal education have you had? Can you read? Did or do you have difficulty with school or learning new things? How do you learn best (watching others or reading)? How are you doing in school or at work?	Level of education. IQ.

Continued.

Table 4-2. Data collection of individual client based on eclectic assessment model—cont'd

Area of data collection	Observations	Interactions	Measurements

4. Self-concept	Note nonverbal communication.
	What is the nature of the client's clothes? Loose, fitted? Clean? Visible soil?
	Does the client shield or avoid touching or looking at a certain area of the body?
	
	What is the nature of any scars, deformed body parts, or alterations in function?
	Whom does the client interact with?
	What is the client's affect?
	How is client groomed?
	  Hair
	  Clothes
	  Nails
	  Makeup
		What is your highest weight? Lowest weight?
		How do you feel about your weight and appearance?
		
		Have you had any physical alterations of your body?
		Was or is it difficult for you to accept those changes?
		How have those changes affected your relationships with family? friends? the way you look at yourself?
		How do you see yourself in relation to other people (such as family, coworkers, friends)? Better than? Equal to? Less than equal to?
		What religion were you raised with?
		What social values were you raised with?
		Are you comfortable with those beliefs and values now?
		How do you express your thoughts and feelings to others? Are there some situations when you don't? When?
		What are your goals in the next 5 years? How do you plan to achieve them?
		(or)
		Where do you see yourself 5 years from now? How do you plan to get there?
		Describe some characteristics of the type of person you'd most like to be. Do you see yourself as that person? Is your description realistic to you?
			Height and weight.

5. Emotional patterns	Note facial affect.	What type of mood are you usually in (such as calm, depressed, pleasant, happy, excited, or agitated)? How do you express yourself during mood changes? Do your relations with others change as your moods do? How? Are you satisfied with your usual mood? Are you satisfied with your behavior during mood changes?	

Table 4-2. Data collection of individual client based on eclectic assessment model—cont'd

Area of data collection	Observations	Interactions	Measurements
6. Family coping patterns	Note nonverbal communication.	How does your family handle stress? Be specific for each member of the family. (See B.1. Coping patterns, p. 48.) How does your family make decisions? Who has the last word? If someone in the family disagrees with another, what happens? If someone in the family gets sick, who is the caretaker? What is your role or place in the family?	
C. Sociological health			
1. Cultural patterns	What type of clothes does the client wear? How is the hair groomed? Stylish?	What social values were you brought up with? Which ones are important to you now? What are and were the traditions in your family? Family gatherings Celebrations Head of home Types of food eaten Religious activities Health care practices Which ones of these do you participate in?	Frequency of traditional family get-togethers.
2. Significant relationships	Whom does the client interact with? Note nonverbal communication during client's interactions with others.	Who are the significant people in your life? Family? Friends? (Name them.) Whom do you feel closest to? Why? How does your family get along as a whole? Is there any major conflict in your family? Whom do you go to when you have a concern or need help? How is your family reacting to your health-related concerns? Do they accept them? Are they supportive?	
3. Recreation patterns	Note leisure materials in environment: Books Craft material Woodworking Sport equipment Stereo Collections	What do you do for fun? How do you feel about leisure time? Do you have hobbies or interests outside of work (such as club memberships, sport activities, children's activities)?	Number of hours per day or week spent in leisure activities.

Continued.

Table 4-2. Data collection of individual client based on eclectic assessment model—cont'd

Area of data collection	Observations	Interactions	Measurements
3. Recreation patterns— cont'd		Do you have the resources to get involved with your interests? Materials Money Transportation Time What do you know about your community's recreation resources? How long has it been since you participated in any leisure activities? What do you feel or think about that?	Length of time since having leisure activity.
4. Environment	What is the appearance of dwelling in regard to: Safety Orderliness Cleanliness Note steps, placement of rooms, shower or tub, and availability; loose rugs. What are the usual sounds, noises, and odors of the environment?	What type of dwelling do you live in (multiple dwelling, single dwelling)? Are you comfortable in the place you live? Do you feel you have enough space to yourself? Is your place easy to move around in? Are there sounds, noises, or odors in the environment that are of concern to you? Do you have any pets? If so, what kind?	Number of people and rooms in dwelling.
	(The same observations can be made in regard to outpatient or inpatient settings.)	(The same interaction data are relevant to outpatient or inpatient settings.)	(The same measurement data can be made in outpatient or inpatient settings.)
D. Spiritual health			
1. Religious beliefs and practices	Are there any religious artifacts present in the environment? On the client?	What are your religious practices? What is your involvement with church groups and committees? Do you have a religious preference? Do you practice the same religion you grew up with? If not, do you feel any conflict about this? What does your family or significant others think about your differences?	Amount of time spent in religious activities per week.

Table 4-2. Data collection of individual client based on eclectic assessment model—cont'd

Area of data collection	Observations	Interactions	Measurements
2. Values and valuing	What are the indicators of values in the environment? Orderliness Cleanliness Safety Upkeep of furniture, belongings What are the indicators of values in interactions with others? Open dialogue Praise for others Active listening Touch Are there any books or pamphlets regarding things valued by client? Does the client incorporate values into life-style?	What things are important to you in life? Which ones would you say were most important? How do you incorporate these things into your life-style? If not, are you comfortable with this? How do you feel about the social morals you were brought up with? Does this present any conflict for you internally or with your family? How do you see yourself in relation to society? What do you think about helping people you don't know? People you do know?	

SUMMARY

Data collection of individual clients is systematic, comprehensive, and purposeful. The approach depends on the nurse's knowledge and skills, the client's age and health status, and the situation. A combination of approaches is needed to obtain multifocal data.

REFERENCES

1 Aguilera, D.C., and Messick, J.M.: Crisis intervention: theory and methodology, ed. 4, St. Louis, 1982, The C.V. Mosby Co.
2 Dunn, H.L.: High level wellness, Arlington, Va., 1961, R.W. Beatty Co.
3 Erikson, E.H.: Childhood and society, ed. 2, New York, 1961, W.W. Norton & Co., Inc.
4 Maslow, A.: Toward a psychology of being, New York, 1968, D. Van Nostrand Co.
5 Nursing Theories Conference: Nursing theories: the base for professional nursing practice, Englewood Cliffs, N.J., 1980, Prentice-Hall, Inc.
6 Piaget, J.: The psychology of intelligence, ed. 2, London, 1950, Routledge & Kegan Paul, Ltd.
7 Roy, Sr. C.: The Roy adaptation model. In Riehl, J.P., and Roy, Sr. C.: Conceptual models for nursing practice, ed. 2, New York, 1980, Appleton-Century-Crofts.
8 Selye, H.: The stress of life, New York, 1956, McGraw-Hill Book Co.

BIBLIOGRAPHY

King, I.M.: Toward a theory of nursing, New York, 1971, John Wiley & Sons, Inc.
Orem, D.: Nursing: concepts of practice, ed. 2, New York, 1980, McGraw-Hill Book Co.
Rogers, M.E.: The theoretical basis of nursing, Philadelphia, 1970, F.A. Davis Co.
Roy, Sr. C.: Introduction to nursing: an adaptation model, Englewood Cliffs, N.J., 1970, Prentice-Hall, Inc.
Selye, H.: Stress without distress, New York, 1974, Lippincott and Crowell, Publishers.

NURSING ASSESSMENT
Data collection of the
family client

LINDA L. DELANEY

GENERAL CONSIDERATIONS

An important aspect of nursing today is the emphasis on the family unit as the client. The family serves as a buffering zone or neutralizing agent between the individual and society. It provides psychosocial protection for its members and is the major vehicle for the transmission of culture. The health of the individual is interwoven with the relationships, beliefs, values, and duties in the family system. The family is a necessary and natural unit of service for the nurse.

Collecting data about a family system can be an overwhelming or a stimulating experience. The nurse is confronted with two or more individuals, each with his or her own unique qualities. Interacting together they form a whole that is greater than and different from the sum of the individual members. The environment influences both family and individual existence. The nurse collects data about the family structure, the family process, and the environment. To collect valid and accurate data, nurses must be aware of their own definitions and perceptions of family functioning. These unconscious values can skew nurses' observations and interactions.

Family definition

A family can be defined in many ways. Traditionally, the nuclear family was defined as a married couple and their children by birth or adoption. The family was an easily recognized unit or group in the community. This clean-cut definition no longer describes the majority of family systems. The nurse who provides service to the primary group in society must have a broader, less rigid definition of a family. In formulating this definition, the nurse considers legal, biological, sociological, and psychological factors.

Legally, an authorized consent or information release is confined to those related by blood ties, adoption, guardianship, or marriage. Biologically, any genetic or familial workup includes collecting data about the family of origin, biological kin networks, and the family of procreation. Sociologically, the group might include any group of people living together. A family might be a parent, two children, and a boarder; or it might be several people living in a common dwelling, such as a convent or monastery, a dormitory, or a boarding house. Psychologically, the family includes any group with strong emotional ties who consider themselves a family. The extended family is an important component of many cultures; grandparents, aunts, uncles, and cousins are considered integral parts of the family unit. The extended family also includes alternate family forms. Examples are the homosexual couple with or without children; two unmarried people who live together; and substitute family members such as foster children, foster parents or grandparents, roommates, close neighbors or friends, and in some instances, even pets.

The nurse's definition of family used for data collection depends on the employer's policies, personal values, and perceptual set. The definition may expand or contract according to the specific family situation. For example, a roommate may be allowed to visit a client in an intensive care unit where there is a "family only" visiting policy. However, this roommate would not be allowed to sign an authorized consent form or held accountable for the client's expenses.

In this book the family is defined as a dynamic system of two or more individuals who consider themselves a family. They share a history, common goals, obligations, instrumental and affectional bonds and ties, and a high degree of intimacy.

Perceptions

The nurse's perceptions of what constitutes a family influence data collection. The nurse must differentiate actual data from inferences. For example, a nurse with a close extended family might assume that a young woman accompanied by her mother on clinic visits is receiving positive support. In reality, the young woman may feel her mother sees her as incompetent and is checking up on her. A nurse can also skew data by faulty collection methods. If the nurse perceives the mother as the primary information giver on family health, she may direct all of her questions to the mother. Valuable data about the family may be missed.

FAMILY STRUCTURE AND PROCESS
Structure

Family structure refers to the family composition. Who makes up this family? What are the names, ages, health states, and occupations of the individual members? Are they residing in a common residence? Does anyone else live with them?

The extent and depth of data collection about the family health state are determined by the purpose of the family interview. Data can be collected about the immediate family members (the identified unit of service), the family of origin (the family into which the individual was born), the family of procreation (the family the individual helped create), and extended family members (grandparents, parents, aunts, uncles, and cousins).

The assessment guide for the individual can be used. The data can be collected and organized schematically for clarity and for the facilitation of data processing. This is called a genogram or family diagram. An example of this is shown in Fig. 2.

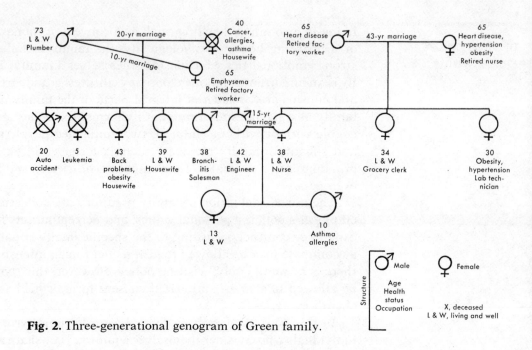

Fig. 2. Three-generational genogram of Green family.

Generation one of the Green family consists of one male plumber, age 73, married, living, and well. Mr. Green's first wife died of cancer at the age of 40. They were married 20 years. Mr. Green's present partner is a 65-year-old female with emphysema who is a retired factory worker. They have been married 10 years. Mr. Green and his first wife had six children, four of whom are living; a 43-year-old female with back problems who is a housewife; a 39-year-old female, living and well, who is a housewife and retired school teacher; a 38-year-old male with chronic bronchitis who is a salesman; and a 42-year-old male, living and well, who is an engineer. The engineer is married to a 38-year-old female, living and well, who is a nurse. They have two children; a 13-year-old female, living and well, and a 10-year-old male with asthma and allergies. As can be seen, Fig. 2 depicts three generations of a family with age, health status, and occupation of the members easily discernible.

Process

Family process refers to the functions and group interactions by which the family operates. It means those activities that differentiate a family from another collection of individuals. The number of persons examined for family process depends on the purpose of the family-nurse encounter. There are many frameworks in the literature that describe family processes. This chapter on data collection for the family describes the developmental, interactional, and systems approaches.

DEVELOPMENTAL FRAMEWORK

One way to assess family process is the developmental approach. Duvall[2] focuses on the family as a small group changing and evolving over time. Family life is divided into eight successive stages, beginning with the married couple and ending with the death of the surviving spouse. Critical family developmental tasks are defined for each stage. Duvall lists the following family developmental tasks as basic to all families*:

1. Physical maintenance: providing shelter, food, clothing, and health care for its members.
2. Resources: meeting family costs and allocating such resources as time, space, and facilities according to each member's needs.
3. Division of labor: determining who does what in the support, management, and care of the home and its members.
4. Socialization: assuring each member's socialization through the internalization of increasingly mature roles in the family and beyond.
5. Interaction: establishing ways of interacting and communicating (for example, expressing affection, aggression, and sexuality) within limits acceptable to society.
6. Expansion and reduction: bearing (or adopting) and rearing children; incorporating and releasing family members appropriately.
7. Societal links: relating to school, church, work, and community life; establishing policies for including in-laws, relatives, guests, and friends.
8. Morale and motivation: maintaining morale and motivation, rewarding achievement, meeting personal and family crises, setting attainable goals, and developing family loyalties and values.

According to Duvall all families have these basic tasks as long as they are in existence. Each family performs these functions in its own unique way. The nurse collects data to ascertain how the family is meeting each of these tasks.

The nurse using Duvall's framework qualifies the data collected with information gleaned from family structure. The number, ages, and needs of family members are taken into account. For example, a family taking home a grandmother who had a stroke would have different safety needs (such as bars around the toilet and bathtub, and oxygen storage) than a family with a toddler (medicines and chemicals locked up, electrical outlets covered). Also, Duvall focuses on the family life cycle in regard to the ages of the children. This theory is not applicable to nontraditional or variant family forms (such as cohabitating, homosexual, and communal families).

Table 5-1 illustrates how the nurse collects data using Duvall's framework with the tools of observation, interaction, and measurement. This table is developed as an example and is not intended to be inclusive.

---

*Adapted from Duvall, Evelyn Millis: Marriage and family development. Copyright © 1957, 1962, 1967, 1971, 1977 by J.B. Lippincott. Reprinted by permission of Harper & Row, Publishers, Inc.

Table 5-1. Data collection of the family client based on Duvall's framework

	Observations	Interactions	Measurements
Physical maintenance	Type of housing: apartment or house, odors, state of repair of abode, temperature of environment. Apparel of family members. (For example, if it is snowing, are clothes warm?) Physical appearance of family members. (Height and weight proportionate? Skin color? Teeth: decayed, clean, missing, white?)	Where do you live? How many rooms? Do you have a refrigerator and stove? What foods has your family eaten for the last 3 days? Do you have a family doctor? Do you have a dentist? What immunizations have your family members had? Do you get your eyes checked? By whom? How often?	 Three-day diet recall. Frequency of doctor visits. Frequency of dental visits. Height and weight of family members.
Resources	Are individual family members similarly clothed? Are individual rooms furnished similarly?	How do you make ends meet? Do you feel your home is adequate for your needs? How do you decide how the money will be spent?	Family income. Family expenses. Family savings. Ratio of rooms per person.
Division of labor	Who answers the telephone? Who tends the children? Pets?	Who does the chores? Who decides what will be done when? Who is the family breadwinner? Who takes care of the children? Who does the budgeting?	
Socialization	Social behavior of family members (such as 2-year-old climbing on furniture; 6-year-old sitting quietly during interview; 15-year-old belching loudly several times during interview). Mealtime behavior (such as 2-year-old eating with spoon; 10-year-old eating with fingers). Aggressive behavior (such as 2-year-old lying on the floor and kicking and screaming when a cigarette lighter is taken from him; 10-year-old cursing when told he cannot go for a bicycle ride). Vocabulary.	Are you satisfied with your children's behaviors? What would you like to change? What do you want to stay the same? How do family members express anger? What happens when someone doesn't get his way? Tell me about your mealtime. Do family members eat together? What are your bedtimes? What time do you get up? Do you think this is enough sleep? Are sleep patterns regular? Where do family members sleep?	
Interaction	When one person speaks do the others listen? Are there frequent verbal interruptions?	How do you get along? How do you settle arguments? Who's the boss? What happens when someone breaks a rule?	Number of times members interrupted each other. Number of times one member answered for another.

Table 5-1. Data collection of the family client based on Duvall's framework—cont'd

	Observations	Interactions	Measurements
	Who answers the questions? Are facial expressions happy? Sad? Blank? Are family members sitting close to one another?	Do individual members feel their needs are being met? How do you show to one another that you like or love each other? What do you think are your children's, parents', or grandparents' needs or concerns? Are other members sensitive in picking up cues regarding others' feelings and needs?	Number of affectionate gestures. Number of angry, hostile gestures.
Expansion and reduction	Nonverbal behaviors when answering questions (for example, husband and wife look at one another, clasp hands, and smile as they discuss future children; mother cries as she discusses oldest son's college departure; wife avoids eye contact with husband and in-laws as she talks about present living arrangements).	Do you plan to have children? Are you using birth control? Which kind? Is this method satisfactory? At what age do you feel your children will be on their own? How do you feel about your children leaving home? Where will they be going? Are you prepared to take in one or both of your parents if necessary? How will this affect your lifestyle?	Number of planned children. Number of children living outside the parental home.
Societal links	Displayed artifacts: trophies, medals, ribbons, and service pins.	Are you active in any clubs, organizations, or civic associations? What are they? In what school activities do children participate? After-school activities? How do your children choose their friends? How do you monitor their activities: Books? Television? Movies? Does the family attend church? How do church activities fit into your activity schedule?	Number of hours per week spent in outside activities.
Morale and motivation	Family affect. Intensity of tone and body posture when answering questions.	How do family members get positive strokes? How do you encourage members to do a better job? What's special about your family? What are your family goals? Are goals shared by all members? What happens in this family when the going gets tough?	

INTERACTIONAL THEORY

Another approach in family assessment is interactional frameworks. In interactional theory the focus is on the way family members relate to one another rather than on functions or tasks. Satir[4] presents a simple but effective framework describing family process. This framework permits observations of how family roles are enacted and how role performance is perceived in a particular family. Four aspects of family life are examined: communication patterns, rules about how people should feel and act, self-worth of the individuals in the family, and the family's links to society. Healthy families have open communication channels, flexible rules, high self-worth perceptions, and successful negotiations with those outside the family. This framework is broad enough to encompass all family forms. As stated earlier, structural aspects of the family and health needs must be added to this approach.

Table 5-2 illustrates how the nurse collects data using Satir's framework and the tools of interaction, observation, and measurement.

SYSTEMS THEORY

When families are assessed, the systems framework may also be used. It includes structure and function. Systems theory has been discussed extensively in the literature as an integral component of family theory. Stevenson,[5] Satir,[4] and Beavers[1] describe the family as an open system with definite boundaries, having structure and process. Hart and Herriott[3] devised a conceptual framework for family process assessment using three categories of process necessary for systems survival. The three essential processes are adaptation to the environment, integration of the parts, and decisions as to the modes of carrying out allocation of resources required by the first two processes.

The process of adaptation consists of the system's efforts to *obtain* "goods" (matter, information, and energy) from the environment, *contain* goods within the environment, *dispose* of goods to the environment, and *retain* goods within the system. Using this framework, the nurse gathers information about those things the family gets from the environment (*obtains* money, food, and entertainment), those things the family does not want to come into their family system (*contains* outside family: violence, drugs, new ideas, strangers), those things the family sends out to the environment (*disposes* of people who do not follow rules, music, energy for organizing community activities), and those things the family keeps in (*retains* family secrets, love and affection, energy).

Assessing the way the system integrates its parts is related to its patterns of *interaction and communication* (how do family members receive and send messages to one another? How does the family communicate with those outside the family system?), its *desired state* (what are the family goals? What does the family value?), and its use of *feedback mechanisms* (how does the family maintain its desired state? What kinds of things cause them to rethink or redefine its values and goals?).

Decisions as to how the system carries out the allocation of resources required by the first two processes (adaptation and integration) are related to the system's desired state and its use of output monitored back to the system as input through feedback mechanisms. (What is the family's decision-

Table 5-2. Data collection of the family client based on Satir's framework

	Observations	Interactions	Measurements
Communication patterns	Who answers questions? Involvement of individual family members in discussion: for example does one member sit with arms folded with no interaction? Do family members look at one another before answering? Is discussion spontaneous? Halting? Open? Closed? Are there frequent verbal interruptions? Do family members touch one another? Are there long silences? What happens when one member disagrees with another? Do family members sit close to one another? Do family members smile at one another? At the nurse? Is there laughter? Tears? Angry voices?	How does each family member feel about his or her relationship with each other person in the family? What kinds of things do you talk about in your family: money, moving, work, school, or sickness? Tell me about your fun times. Tell me what you fight about. How do you express anger, disgust, and love? Who starts the conversations? What kinds of things do you enjoy about one another as individuals?	Number of times one member answered for another. Number of interruptions.
Self-worth	Words used to describe others (such as "sweet," "so nice," or "mean"). Voice tone: for example, taut, flowery, authoritative, authoritarian, docile, harsh, or ingratiating. Feeling tone: for example, syrupy, harsh, or devoid of feeling. Body posture: rigid or relaxed.	What makes this family different from other families? What special things do you contribute to this family? What would you like to see changed in this family? What kind of feelings do other family members have about you? What kind of feelings do you have about other family members? What is your family's general emotional climate: happy, secretive, angry, or indifferent?	
Rules	Communication patterns while discussing rules: body posture, voice tone (for example, while mother emphasized that children had equal voice in television program choice, Mary folded her arms and looked at the ceiling; Tommy laughed, shook his head, and punched Mary; dad sat looking straight ahead).	What are the family rules about behavior? Communication? Chores? Money? Activities? Privacy? Sex? Territory? Deference? Who agrees with the rules? Who doesn't? Who makes the rules? What happens when one is broken? How are rules changed?	Number of family members agreeing with the rules.
Societal linkages		How do you contribute to the community? What kinds of support do you receive from the community? To what clubs, organizations, and churches do you belong? How do you decide the activities in which you will participate? Are outside activities family or individually focused?	Number of outside activities involved.

making mode? Do all members agree before action is taken? Are compromises reached? Does one person make the decisions?)

Nurses using this approach need to qualify the data collected by considering structural aspects and family health needs. Table 5-3 illustrates how the nurse would collect data using Hart and Herriott's framework and the tools of observation, interaction, and measurement.

Table 5-3. Data collection of the family client based on systems framework

	Observations	Interactions	Measurements
A. Adaptation			
1. Obtain	Dress of family members. Artifacts or ornaments worn. Health state of individual family members. Furniture and appliances in home.	What is the source of family income? What is the source of health care information? What social services are being provided? What are entertainment preferences? What schools are attended? What churches are attended? What services does the family want from the nurse?	Family income. Number of these health care services sought. Number of social services being provided.
2. Contain	Environmental measures to avoid contact with toxic environmental forces. Screens, windows, and fence. Air conditioner, furnace. Presence or absence of television, radio, and reading material.	What are the rules about information coming into the system? What (if any) television programs, movies, books, and magazines are censored? Are certain words prohibited? Are certain substances (food, beverages, or drugs) banned? What people are not welcome? What services does family *not* want from nurse?	
3. Dispose	Are old medicines saved and reused? Is garbage collected or lying around the house?	Where do unwanted family members go (for example, unwanted pregnant teen, grandparents, retarded son, or spouse)? What energy is available for suprasystem use: for example, family members' activities in community (coaching, Girl Scouts, and sports).	
4. Retain	Family collections. Pictures and scrapbooks. Topics avoided.	What goods are retained for future use or heritage: for example, money, silver, jewelry? Medicines? What are family secrets (for example, teenage daughter taking birth control pills or father an alcoholic)? Are family members allowed to leave the system? Who? When? How much energy must each family member devote to system maintenance?	

Table 5-3. Data collection of the family client based on systems framework—cont'd

	Observations	Interactions	Measurements
		What information does family not want to share with nurse? (such as sex or drugs)	
B. Integration			
1. Communication	See Interaction in Table 5-1 and Communication in Table 5-2.	See Interaction in Table 5-1 and Communication in Table 5-2.	See Interaction in Table 5-1 and Communication in Table 5-2.
2. Roles	Who answers the questions? Who tends the children? Pets? Who answers the telephone?	What roles does each of the family members fulfill? What tasks or expectations accompany these roles? Are these roles acceptable to family members? Are family members performing roles adequately? What happens when some member no longer can or wishes to fulfill previous task functions associated with a role? How do family members learn to enact their roles?	Number of roles of each family member. Number of tasks, expectations, and roles.
3. Desired state			
a. Values	Dress. Artifacts.	What are the family values? How do they compare with those of the suprasystem; for example, neighbors, extended family, friends, or ethnic group? What does the family believe about health? Illness? How do individual family members feel about "family values"? What happens when someone disagrees with the prevailing values?	
b. Goals		What are the family goals? Do all family members share family goals? How are individual family members' goals the same or different from family goals? Who decides family goals? How are goals achieved? Are goals explicit or implicit?	
c. Functions		What kinds of things need to be that aren't being accomplished? Is there someone in the family who is willing or able to do these? How can nurse ("I" or "we") facilitate need?	

Continued.

Table 5-3. Data collection of the family client based on systems framework—cont'd

	Observations	Interactions	Measurements
d. Feed-back		How does the family stay on the right course? What are the events that let you know it's time to re-evaluate family roles, goals, or functions (neighbors are doing it or developmental needs change through crisis, illness)? Do you plan ahead or live each day as it comes?	
C. Decision making	Nonverbal behavior of family members during discussion: Voice tone Body posture Eye contact	How does your family make decisions? Who is the chief decision maker? What happens when the family doesn't agree on which course to take? How are decisions changed? Who takes the blame for bad decisions? Who takes the credit for good decisions?	

SUMMARY

The data collection methods for family process using different frameworks result in similar data, although variations occur in the analysis. Nurses collecting family data must be aware of their definition of family and must look at both structure and process. The framework chosen to guide the data collection and the depth of the assessment depend on the setting and the purpose of the interaction. Comprehensive data collection includes data in the biological, psychological, social, and spiritual realms. More than one framework is usually needed in family assessment.

REFERENCES

1 Beavers, W.R.: Psychotherapy and growth: a family systems perspective, New York, 1977, Brunner/Mazel, Inc.
2 Duvall, E.M.: Marriage and family development, ed. 5, Philadelphia, 1977, J.B. Lippincott Co.
3 Hart, S.K., and Herriott, P.R.: Components of practice. In Hall, J., and Weaver, B., editors: Distributive nursing practice: a systems approach to community health, Philadelphia, 1977, J.B. Lippincott Co.
4 Satir, V.: Peoplemaking, Palo Alto, Calif., 1972, Science and Behavior Books.
5 Stevenson, J.S.: Issues and crises during middlescence, New York, 1977, Appleton-Century-Crofts.

BIBLIOGRAPHY

Ackerman, N.W.: The psychodynamics of family life, New York, 1958, Basic Books, Inc., Publishers.
Ackerman, N.W.: Treating the troubled family, New York, 1966, Basic Books, Inc., Publishers.
Aldous, J.: Strategies for developing family theory, J. Marr. Fam. **32:**250, 1970.
Anderson, R.E., and Carter, I.E.: Human behavior in the social environment, Chicago, 1974, Aldine Publishing Co.
Anthony, J., and Benedek, T., editors: Parenthood: its psychology and psychopathology, Boston, 1970, Little, Brown & Co.
Bell, N.W., and Vogel, E.F.: Toward a framework for functional analysis of family behavior. In Bell, N.W., and Vogel, E.F., editors: A modern introduction to the family, New York, 1968, The Free Press.

Bell, R.Q.: Parent, child and reciprocal influences, Am. Psychol. **34:**821, 1979.

Bishop, B.: A guide to assessing parenting capabilities, Am. J. Nurs. **76:**1784, 1976.

Blair, C.L., and Salerna, E.M.: The expanding family: childbearing, Boston, 1976, Little, Brown & Co.

Black, K.M.: Teaching family process and intervention, Nurs. Outlook **18:**54, 1970.

Friedman, M.M.: Family nursing: theories and assessment, New York, 1981, Appleton-Century-Crofts.

Glick, I.D., and Kessler, D.R.: Marital and family therapy, New York, 1974, Grune & Stratton.

Hall, J.E., and Weaver, B.R.: Distributive nursing practice: a systems approach to community health, New York, 1977, J.B. Lippincott Co.

Hymovich, D., and Barnard, M.U., editors: Family health care, vol. I, New York, 1979, McGraw-Hill Book Co.

Kantor, D., and Lehr, W.: Inside the family, New York, 1975, Harper & Row, Publishers, Inc.

LeMasters, E.E.: Parenthood as crises, Marr. Fam. Liv. **19:**352, 1957.

Lewis, J.A., and others: No single thread: psychological health in family systems, New York, 1976, Brunner/Mazel, Inc.

MacVicar, M.G., and Archbold, P.: A framework for family assessment in chronic illness, Nurs. Forum **15:**180, 1976.

Meister, S.B.: Charting a family's developmental status: for intervention for the record, Am. J. Mat. Child Nurs. **2:**43, 1977.

Miller, J.R., and Janosik, E.H.: Family—focused care, New York, 1980, McGraw-Hill Book Co.

Otto, H.A.: A framework for assessing family strengths. In Reinhardt, A.M., and Quinn, M.D., editors: Family-centered community nursing, vol. I, St. Louis, 1973, The C.V. Mosby Co.

Parad, H.J.: Crisis intervention: selected readings, New York, 1965, Family Service Association of America.

Parsons, T., and Bales, R.F.: Family socialization and interaction process, New York, 1960, The Free Press.

Robischon, R., and Scott, D.: Role theory and its application in family nursing, Nurs. Outlook **17:**52, 1969.

Satir, V.: Conjoint family therapy, Palo Alto, Calif., 1967, Science and Behavior Books.

Tapia, J.A.: The nursing process in family health, Nurs. Outlook **20:**267, 1972.

Troll, L.E., Miller, S.J., and Atchley, R.C.: Families in later life, Belmont, Calif., 1972. Wadsworth, Inc.

Turner, R.H.: Family interactions, New York, 1970, John Wiley & Sons, Inc.

Whall, A.L.: Congruence between existing theories of family functioning and nursing theories, Adv. Nurs. Sci. **3:**59, 1980.

NURSING ASSESSMENT
Data collection of the
community client

BONNIE L. SOMMERVILLE

**GENERAL
CONSIDERATIONS
Definition**

The word "community" is frequently used in a variety of contexts with varied frames of reference; its meaning has therefore become blurred and nebulous. In this text, community is defined as a specific population living in a geographical area, or a group that has common values, interests, or needs. The important concept in this definition is that community has both geographical and interactional aspects.

A major goal of nursing is the prevention of illness and impairment and the maintenance of health. There is an increasing emphasis on maintenance and prevention at the community level. To make the nurse knowledgeable about a specific community's health status and health care needs, a comprehensive, systematic assessment must be done. This gives direction for planning and implementation.

In community health nursing the community is the client. It is essential that the community nurse work collaboratively with professionals and lay persons to identify relevant health factors within the community. The approach to community data collection is unique because of the range of parameters, such as size, complexity, and other characteristics. There are many useful frameworks for collecting data and judging community health status.

Communities have many similarities: people, physical facilities, governmental system, businesses, and social systems. The assessment framework that nurses choose depends on their focus and preference. One systems assessment framework and two other useful assessment frameworks are described. A chart with guidelines for data collection follows each assessment framework; each shows the tools of observation, interaction, and measurement. These charts are designed to provide examples of data to collect.

**SYSTEMS
ASSESSMENT
FRAMEWORK**

A system is defined as "a set of components or units interacting with each other within a boundary which filters both the kind and the rate of the flow of input and output to and from the systems."[8] This definition implies that a system possesses both structure and process. The structure of a system is the "static arrangement of the system's parts at any moment in three-dimensional space."[7]

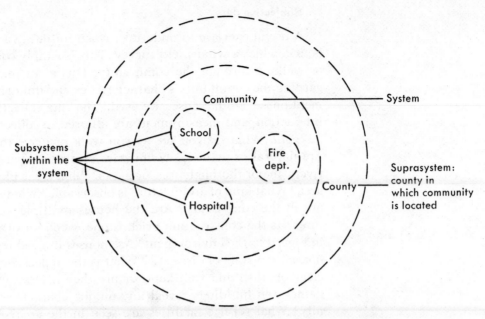

Fig. 3. Hierarchical arrangement of a community system.

Another characteristic of systems is their hierarchy. Every system has a subsystem (a component of a system that is in itself a system) and a suprasystem. For example, the assessed community is defined as the "system." The subsystems are the components of the system, such as the population, schools, hospitals, and fire department. The suprasystem is a larger system that includes the whole of which the focal system is a "part."[4] For example, this might be the county in which the system (community) is located, as in Fig. 3. When a community system (or any system) is assessed, both the structure and process must be addressed.

Structure

As stated earlier, structure refers to the arrangement of the system's (or subsystem's) parts at any given moment. These are the properties, both animate and inanimate, of the system. For example, the population, shopping resources, health resources, housing, protective services, ideas, values, and beliefs are structural parts.

When structural components of a system are assessed, both subjective and objective data collection methods are useful. Subjective data comprise information that may be biased by our life experiences since data are collected through observation and casual conversation with community residents. The reliability and validity of this method are questionable and may not hold up under scrutiny or scientific critique. However, subjective data are useful in that they lead to further inquiry under more scientific conditions. Objective data, on the other hand, are not biased. Data are collected using more valid and reliable methods. An example of objective data is the census of a community.

Subjective data

A useful exercise to undertake when initiating a community assessment is to conduct a windshield survey. This is simply collecting data by driving or walking through the community. This gives important information regarding the community's characteristics and uniqueness. During the assessment phase, all the senses are used.[1] The data collection tools of observation, interaction, and measurement are all used to collect subjective data.

Sight. What do you see as you walk or drive through the community? Are natural or artificial boundaries evident? What are these boundaries—rivers, major thoroughfares, or parks? What is the physical appearance of the area? What kind of architecture is observable? What style and size of housing are in the community? Are the houses multiple- or single-dwelling structures? Is the construction brick, stone, wood, or other? What is observable in regard to the environment? Are houses in good repair, or are there many houses in a state of disrepair? What is the appearance of the yards? Are they clear of trash and well kept, or are they littered with garbage? Do street names and buildings reveal any unique characteristics about the community? What service facilities are seen in the area? Are there social service agencies, grocery stores, pharmacies, health care providers, schools, and churches? What modes of transportation are available to the community residents? What are the conditions of the streets? Are there major highways in the area? Are service centers easily accessible? What recreation facilities are available in the community? Are there swimming pools, tennis courts, and ball fields, or are children playing in the streets or vacant lots? Whom do you see on the streets? Are there women with small children? Are there teens or older adults? How are they dressed? Are they black, white, or Asian? Are there ethnic neighborhoods? What animals do you see? Are there dogs? Are they on leashes or running loose? Can rats or other rodents be seen running about? What evidence of politics is visible? Are there campaign posters? Is there a party headquarters? Is there evidence of a predominant party affiliation? What protective services are seen in the community? Are there fire stations, police stations, and ambulances or other emergency vehicles?

Hearing. What can you hear when you drive or walk through the community? Is the area quiet? Can you hear birds singing and children playing, or are there loud industrial noises, traffic sounds, loud music, and airplanes?

Taste. Use the sense of taste to assess the flavor of the community. What kinds and numbers of food establishments are in the neighborhood? Are there multiple Italian, Greek, or Mexican restaurants? Are there many fast-food stores? Or are food services old, traditional, family-operated establishments?

Smell. How does the community smell (a paper mill smells much different from a bakery)? Are there noxious industrial emissions? Or are there pleasant odors of flowering trees and honeysuckle?

Touch. Use touch to understand how it feels to be there. Is the area surrounded by a barbed wire fence, or are there open fields of wild flowers? Do you feel uncomfortable? Do residents seem friendly? Are they willing to stop and chat, or do they ignore you and hurry on their way?

• • •

Another useful source of subjective data is informal conversations with the people in the community. How do they perceive the community? Do they feel it is a safe place to live? Is the crime rate high? Are resources accessible? Are taxes reasonable? How do they feel about living there? What needs do they feel they have?

The inferences and hunches that are generated by collecting subjective data give clues about the community and its health. When the nurse analyzes these data, hypotheses are generated that are further assessed using objective methods.

Objective data

Braden[1] suggests that objective data may be classified into three general categories: spatial, demographic, and resource identification. Much of this type of data is available through national, state, and local sources according to census tracts.

1. *Spatial data* comprise the geophysical characteristics of the community: rivers, mountains, altitude, temperature, humidity, pollution index, and highways. These data provide information about access to health facilities and about environmental factors conducive to specific diseases.

2. *Demographic data* comprise information describing an identified population. Included in these are age, sex, marital status, birth rate, mortality rate, socioeconomic status, occupation, educational levels, migration patterns, ethnic background, religion, and nationality. Knowledge of these demographic characteristics is essential in effective community planning. Comparison statistics about population characteristics are necessary to enable the nurse to recognize the significance of these data.

Tables 6-1 and 6-2 are examples of comparison data useful in making inferences regarding the community.

Table 6-1. Sex and race distribution

Race	Sex	City		County		State	
		No.	Percent	No.	Percent	No.	Percent
Nonwhite	Female	1,660	6.5	4,507	3.6	527,332	5.0
	Male	1,507	6.0	4,242	3.4	477,688	4.5
White	Female	11,389	44.9	47,786	46.2	4,961,312	46.5
	Male	10,817	42.6	58,522	46.8	4,685,685	44.0

Table 6-2. Income of families

Income	City		County		State	
	No.	Percent	No.	Percent	No.	Percent
Under $3,000	414	6.4	1,555	5.1	213,044	7.9
$3,000-$5,999	721	11.1	2,751	8.9	328,573	12.2
$6,000-$9,999	2,002	30.8	7,528	24.5	741,937	27.6
$10,000+	3,357	51.7	18,939	61.5	1,407,776	52.3
Median income	$10,197		$11,694		$10,313	

3. *Resource identification* refers to the existing facilities available to a community. The nurse should know what services are available and have knowledge about financial resources. Some resources to assess are the adequacy or inadequacy of the water and waste treatment, electricity, transportation, and protective services. Other resources are schools, churches, and shopping and health care facilities.

Most demographic and resource data are available from existing sources. The city planner's office, chamber of commerce, county extension office, and library are excellent resources in collecting these data. Publications of the Bureau of the Census, Public Health Service, and health systems agencies are also useful sources of demographic data.

Process

Process refers to the "dynamic change" in the components of the system—how the system functions. Hart and Herriott[2,3] developed a useful tool to assess community process. (This tool is also useful in assessing family process and has been discussed in that context in Chapter 5.) Three processes are identified as necessary for a system's survival:

1. Adaptation to the environment
   a. Obtain
   b. Contain
   c. Retain
   d. Dispose
2. Integration of the parts
3. Decision as to the methods of carrying out the allocation of resources required by the first two processes[2]

Assessment of these processes helps the nurse understand interaction within the system's components and between the system and its environment.

Adaptation

Adaptation is maintaining the boundaries of the system and filtering what comes in and goes out of the system. The process of adaptation consists of the system's effort to obtain, contain, retain, and dispose of goods.[2,3]

Obtain. What "goods" (matter, energy, or information) does the community obtain from the environment to help the system survive (obtain is parallel to input)? Examples of these goods are funding sources from the federal, state, and local government; health services; fire protection; manpower; and resources (Fig. 4). These data may be obtained through census information, resource directories, and government documents in a public library.

Contain. What goods is the community trying to contain within the environment (keep out of the community system)? Some examples of these might be a specific type of government, crime, drug abuse, annexation, industry, and expressways (Fig. 5).

Retain. What goods is the community trying to retain within its boundaries? Some examples of this might be strict housing codes (specified lot size, design, and price range), specific standards of education, adequate health facilities, and cultural and ethical aspects (Fig. 6).

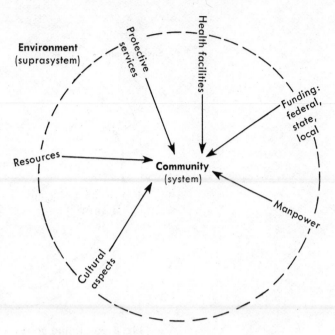

Fig. 4. Obtaining goods from the environment.

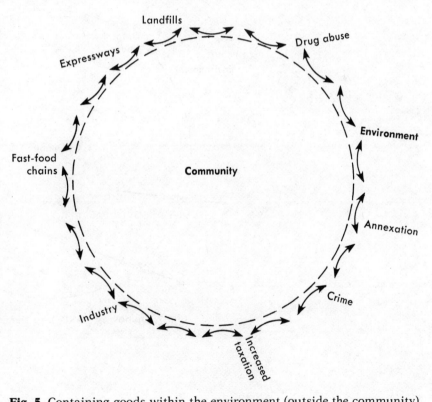

Fig. 5. Containing goods within the environment (outside the community).

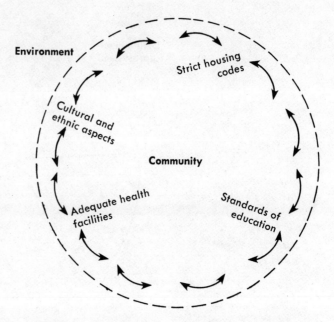

Fig. 6. Retaining goods within the community.

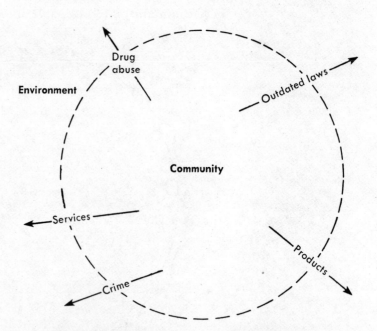

Fig. 7. Disposing goods into the environment.

Dispose. What is the community trying to dispose of into the environment? These aspects might be positive or negative. Does the community have a specific product it must sell that influences its survival? Other examples of what a community might want to "get rid of" are drug abuse, crime, a political personality, and outdated laws. Fig. 7 shows possible disposal goods of a community.

Integration

Integration refers to the way the community integrates its parts or components. What interactional and communication patterns has it found to accomplish what it wants? Within any community there are both formal and informal communication systems. Both must be understood to have a true picture of the community. Some avenues to explore are: How is information communicated to residents? Are there neighborhood newsletters, flyers, newspapers, radio announcements, television, and postal service? How is the notice of public meetings communicated? Are these meetings well attended? Who attends? What is done with citizens' feedback? According to the organizational chart, who is the person of power? Is this the case, or does the real power lie with someone else? What are the relationships between community resources, such as the fire and police departments? Do they share resources or is there duplication in service?

Assessing and understanding the interactional and communication patterns of a community give valuable information about its value system, priorities, and goals. These data give information to health care workers as to what changes the community would value and support and also what strategies would be most effective in implementing change.

Decision making

Decision making refers to the way the system goes about making decisions regarding getting and using resources to carry on the first two processes (adaptation and integration).

The process through which decisions are made may be called "transactional modes" or strategies. The system uses these modes to obtain its wants or needs. It is important to assess the community's transactional modes to see if they are working effectively to meet their needs. Five transactional modes have been identified[7]:

1. *Coercion:* This method uses force, fraud, and deception to convince others to comply. For example, a restaurant owner in a community may be forced to vote for a particular official to pass inspection.
2. *Bargaining:* This method is used to obtain compliance by offering "something for something," a "quid pro quo." For example, one community may have a large, well-equipped fire department, but a weak police force. It may negotiate with another community for police protection in return for fire protection.
3. *Legal-bureaucratic:* Compliance is obtained by an outside power; for example, the state may *mandate* that certain health standards be maintained by the community. An example would be that all school-age children must have specific inoculations before entering public school.

4. *Team-cooperative:* Compliance is obtained and goals are met by convincing others that they share common interests and goals. For example, community residents may oppose the building of a landfill within the community because they feel it may be detrimental to resale value of nearby homes.

5. *Gemeinschaft:* This mode of transaction involves the sentiments of others, convincing them to go along because of loyalty to the system. For example, community residents may spend much time, energy, and money fighting annexation, because they feel loyalty to the system.

Identification of various modes or strategies used by a community system provides clues about matches and mismatches between the status quo and the community's goals.

Assessment data regarding process information are obtained primarily by observation and interaction. Nurses can attend community meetings, political rallies, special interest group meetings, and if possible, bazaars and festivals. Insight into community process can be gained by reading newspapers, flyers, and bulletin boards. It is also useful to talk with residents of all ages and occupations. Information about community functions can be obtained through informal conversation with its citizens. Table 6-3 illustrates how the nurse can collect data using observation, interaction, and measurement. *Text continued on p. 79.*

Table 6-3. Data collection of the community client based on systems assessment framework

	Observations	Interactions	Measurements
A. Structure			
1. Subjective data			
a. Sight	What do you see as you walk or drive through the community? Are natural or artificial boundaries evident? What are these boundaries—rivers, major thoroughfares, or parks? What is the physical appearance of the area? What kind of architecture is observable? What style and size of housing are in the community? Are the houses multiple- or single-dwelling structures? Is the construction brick, stone, wood, or other? What is observable in regard to the environment? Are houses in good repair, or are there many houses in a state of disrepair? What is the appearance of the yards? Are they clear of trash and well kept, or are they littered with garbage? Do street		

Table 6-3. Data collection of the community client based on systems
assessment framework—cont'd

	Observations	Interactions	Measurements
	names and buildings reveal any unique characteristics about the community? What service facilities are seen in the area? Are there social service agencies, grocery stores, pharmacies, health care providers, schools, and churches? What modes of transportation are available to the community residents? What are the conditions of the streets? Are there major highways in the area? Are service centers easily accessible? What recreation facilities are available in the community? Are there swimming pools, tennis courts, and ball fields, or are children playing in the streets or in vacant lots? Whom do you see on the streets? Are there women with small children? Are there teens or older adults? How are they dressed? Are they black, white, or Asian? Are there ethnic neighborhoods? What animals do you see? Are there dogs? Are they on leashes or running loose? Can rats or other rodents be seen running about? What evidence of politics is visible? Are there campaign posters? Is there a party headquarters? Is there evidence of a predominant party affiliation? What protective services are seen in the community? Are there fire stations, police stations, and ambulances or other emergency vehicles?		
b. Hearing	What can you hear when you drive or walk through the community? Is the area quiet? Can you hear birds singing and children playing, or are there loud industrial noises, traffic sounds, loud music, and airplanes?		

Continued.

Table 6-3. Data collection of the community client based on systems assessment framework—cont'd

		Observations	Interactions	Measurements
	c. Taste	Use the sense of taste to assess the flavor of the community. What kinds and numbers of food establishments are in the neighborhood? Are there mulple Italian, Greek, or Mexican restaurants? Are there many fast-food stores? Or are food services old, traditional, family-operated establishments?		
	d. Smell	How does the community smell (a paper mill smells much different from a bakery)? Are there noxious industrial emissions? Or are there pleasant odors of flowering trees and honeysuckle?		
	e. Touch	Use touch to understand how it feels to be there. Is the area surrounded by a barbed wire fence or are there open fields of wild flowers? Do you feel uncomfortable? Do residents seem friendly? Are they willing to stop and chat, or do they ignore you and hurry on their way?		
2. Objective data				
	a. Spatial data	What is the topography—what rivers, mountains, and highways are in the community?		What are the altitude, temperature range, humidity range, and pollution index?
	b. Demographic data			What are the statistics relating to age distribution, sex ratio, marital status, birth rate, mortality rate, income level, occupation, educational levels, migration patterns, ethnic background, religion, and nationality?
	c. Resource identification data		What services are available to residents? What financial resources are available? How adequate are waste treatment, electricity, transportation, and protective services?	

Table 6-3. Data collection of the community client based on systems assessment framework—cont'd

	Observations	Interactions	Measurements
B. Process			
1. Adaptation			
a. Obtain	What health facilities are seen in the community?	What other services do these facilities make available to the residents? How are they funded?	What is the amount of funding?
	What protective services are visible?	How are they funded?	What is the amount of funding?
	What educational facilities are available?	Are they public or private? How are they supported?	How many educational facilities are available? How many students attend these facilities?
	What religious facilities are available? What denomination are they?		How many religious facilities are available?
	What cultural facilities are available?	How are they supported?	
		What is the tax structure of the community?	What is the average amount of tax paid per family?
		What is the major source of income to the community?	
	What shopping facilities are available? Where are they located? Are they easily accessible?		
b. Contain		Is there a drug problem? What efforts are being made to keep this problem under control?	
		Is annexation being opposed?	
		Is crime a problem? What is the major source of crime? What is being done to eliminate this?	
		Is there a type of housing that is being opposed (such as apartments or low-income housing)?	
		Is a shopping mall, industry, or health facility being opposed? Why? What are the perceived consequences of these?	
		Is there a political system that is being opposed? Why?	
c. Retain		Does the community strive to maintain specific housing codes to maintain as a standard of living (including specifications as to size of lot, type of structure, and price range)?	

Continued.

Table 6-3. Data collection of the community client based on systems assessment framework—cont'd

	Observations	Interactions	Measurements
c. Retain—cont'd		Is the community working to maintain a standard of health care and education? Are there specific cultural aspects that are valued and being maintained? Is there a governmental structure being supported and maintained? Are there cultural and ethnic groups that are valued and maintained?	
d. Dispose		Is there industry that produces a product that the community depends on for its survival? Is there a school that graduates large numbers of students? Are there outdated laws that the system is trying to dispose of? Are there crime and drug problems? What is being done about these? Does the system have a specific service it is trying to market?	
2. Integration			
a. Role relationships		What are the norms of the community? What is expected and tolerated within the system? What does it value? What are its priorities? What are its goals? What is the organizational structure? Where is the locus of power? What is the relationship between community organizations: cooperative or hostile? What is the relationship between protective services such as fire and police?	
b. Communication	What are the newspaper, flyers, newsletters, and bulletins that provide information about community concerns and schedules of activities and meetings?	How is information transmitted in the community (newspaper, newsletters, flyers)? Are there radio and television stations that provide public information announcements? Are there public meetings to discuss community concerns? Who attends these? What is done with feedback? Are community officials easily accessible? Do they respond to residents' concerns?	

Table 6-3. Data collection of the community client based on systems assessment framework—cont'd

	Observations	Interactions	Measurements
3. Decision making		What are the community's decision-making patterns? Are decisions made by a group of leaders or by a few individuals?	
a. Coercion		Is there evidence or perception of residents being forced to comply for fear of reprisal? Do people feel they have been deceived about political issues?	
b. Bargaining		Are there negotiations between community services to meet needs and accomplish goals?	
c. Team-cooperative		Is there a feeling of teamwork among community residents? Do they feel they are working together to accomplish a common goal?	
d. Gemeinschaft		Is there a feeling among residents and business people that they will "go along" with community functions for the good of the community? An example would be that citizens support fund-raising activities of schools to buy new band uniforms or to make improvements.	

INTERACTIONAL ASSESSMENT FRAMEWORK

Irwin Sanders developed a model of community assessment that focuses on social relationships: interactional networks through which daily activities of the community are performed.[6] The demographic, cultural, ecological, and personality aspects are viewed as part of the total environment in which the community as a social system functions.

Sanders' framework views the community in three dimensions:
1. As a social system
2. As a place
3. As a collection of people

Community as a social system

The data collected for this dimension have to do with the patterns of behavior, or interactions, within the system that keep it functioning as a system. The major functions Sanders identifies include:

1. Recruitment of new members for participation in the system
2. Socialization of new members for participation in the system
3. Communication: the flow of ideas by which decisions are made and opinions formed
4. Differentiation of community needs and assignment of personnel to meet these needs
5. Allocation of goods and services within the community
6. Social control mechanisms for maintaining order and controlling deviant behavior
7. Allocation of prestige: ranking of community members' prestige
8. Allocation of power: filling of leadership positions crucial to the functioning of the community system
9. Social mobility
10. Integration of components resulting in social cohesion and solidarity

This type of data collection is a complex process. It involves interviewing community leaders, talking with business people and other residents, reading the paper, and attending meetings and community activities.

Community as a place

When the nurse is collecting data for this dimension, both physical and cultural environments must be considered. Data to collect in the physical aspect include community location, shape, topography, size, presence of waterways and highways, and land use. The cultural environment includes resources available to community residents, such as hospitals, clinics, pharmacies, health departments, fire and police protection, emergency services, and shopping facilities.

These data are available through the United States Census materials, city planner, transit boards, department of health, and telephone directory.

Community as a collection of people

When the nurse views the community as a collection of people, the people are viewed collectively as a population rather than individually as personalities. The study of population is *demography*. Demographic data include population, size, age, age distribution, sex ratio, racial composition, marital status, nationality, language, religious groupings, educational composition, rural-urban distribution, and occupational distribution.

The study of demographic data provides a basis for analysis. It is used to determine the health status of the community and to plan ways to meet its health needs.

This framework focuses on the interactional networks in which the community's daily activities are carried out. The people and the physical and cultural aspects of the community serve as the setting in which the community as a social system operates. Table 6-4 shows examples of data the nurse collects using Sanders' framework.

Table 6-4. Data collection of the community client based on Sanders'
interactional framework

	Observations	Interactions	Measurements
A. Community as a social system			
1. Recruitment of new members			What is the birth rate in the community? What is the death rate? What is the pattern of migration? What is the rate of immigration? What is the age distribution of these people? Is there a replacement of people at all age levels?
2. Socialization		How are newcomers and young people made ready to assume adult responsibilities? Are mechanisms to teach technical efficiency provided? How does instillation of values occur? How are roles learned? How are community goals made known?	
3. Communication	What newspapers, newsletters, flyers, and bulletins are available to community residents?	What are formal communication channels? What are the informal communication channels? Is information communicated to residents? How? Through newspapers, newsletters, radio, and television? Are community leaders available for citizens' input? Do they respond to citizens' demands? Do residents attend community meetings? Do they give input? What is done with this?	
4. Differentiation of community needs		What are the needs and goals of the system? Who decides what these needs are? Are they decided by a few individuals, or is there input from a large group of residents? How does the system go about getting these needs met? How does it fill positions in the system to meet the needs?	
5. Allocation of goods and services		What is the economic structure of the community? Are community members able to provide for the minimum essentials of food, shelter, clothing, and education? Is the allocation of material goods fairly evenly distributed or is it very one-sided?	What is the median income of community residents? What is the income distribution? What is the educational distribution?

Continued.

Table 6-4. Data collection of the community client based on Sanders' interactional framework—cont'd

	Observations	Interactions	Measurements
6. Social controls		What is the major area of concern? How is deviant behavior controlled? Who decides on this method? Is this method successful?	What is the crime rate? Is it increasing or decreasing?
7. Allocation of prestige		How is prestige allocated? Is it affiliated with possession of wealth, or is it political or social? What responsibilities are associated with this: service and guidance?	
8. Allocation of power		What is the power structure? Is this socioeconomically based? Are people in harmony with distribution of power? Do community residents perceive the leadership selection process to be a democratic one?	
9. Social mobility		What is the process of movement of people from one stratum to another? Is it a demonstration of interest and ability or is it the result of other, less positive forces?	
10. Integration		What holds the community as a system? What are the common traits, cultures, values, and norms that are shared?	
B. Community as a place			
1. Physical environment	What is the location of the community? Is it near some waterway or harbor? Is it in the mountains? Is there rich farmland or mineral resources?		
	What is the shape? Are there limitations set by its topography?		
	What is the size?		How big is it in square miles?
	Are there highways that allow easy access to the community?		
2. Cultural environment	What resources are available to the residents? Are there shopping facilities nearby? What religious denominations are represented? Are there protective services such as police and fire departments? Are there emergency services? Are there medical centers, clinics, and pharmacies? What kinds and		

Table 6-4. Data collection of the community client based on Sanders'
interactional framework—cont'd

	Observations	Interactions	Measurements
	number of schools are in the community? What recreational facilities are in the area (swimming pools, tennis courts, parks, playgrounds, and ball fields)?		
C. Community as a collection of people		What languages are primarily spoken? What religious groups are in the community? What is the educational composition?	What is the population? What is the age distribution? What is the sex ratio, racial composition, marital status, and nationality composition? What is the rural-urban distribution? What is the occupational distribution? What are the birth, morbidity, and mortality rates?

<table>
<tr><td style="width:25%">KLEIN'S
INTERACTIONAL
FRAMEWORK</td><td>Another interactional framework for collecting data about a community is Donald Klein's model.[5] This model is strongly influenced by interpersonal theories in psychology.

    Klein's theoretical perspective of a community includes:</td></tr>
</table>

KLEIN'S
INTERACTIONAL
FRAMEWORK

Another interactional framework for collecting data about a community is Donald Klein's model.[5] This model is strongly influenced by interpersonal theories in psychology.

Klein's theoretical perspective of a community includes:
1. The community as a social system
2. Population and environment

Community as a social system

In this perspective, four processes are identified as necessary for community functioning:
1. Communication
2. Decision making
3. System linkage
4. Boundary maintenance

Communication

In every social system, both formal and informal communication channels exist. Both types must be assessed to understand the system; some areas to assess include what is recognized publically and what happens informally. It is also useful to determine who has the greatest access to communication, who talks to whom about what, and what mass media are available. In most communities there are places where people congregate to share information and ideas; where are these places, who attends, and what is done with the information?

Decision making

Numerous decisions are made in the typical community each year. There is usually a unique style of identifying important issues and making decisions. When these data are collected, it is helpful to assess *who* makes *what* decisions, and the degree of consensus on the "how" of these decisions. This type of information is collected by talking to residents and by reading: learning their value systems, political preferences, and power structure.

System linkage

System linkage refers to the various relations of interdependence that exist between groups and organizations within the community. What subsystems exchange their functions or products? What benefit is derived from this relationship? An example of this is the school system and health department collaborating to provide health screening for the community student population.

Boundary maintenance

Every system has boundaries that separate it from other systems. These may be topographical, politicosociological, and sociopsychological in nature. Whatever the nature, the function is to regulate passage of ideas, information, and people from one area to another.

To understand the system, one must assess the way the community protects its boundaries and maintains its separate existence. Data in this area include physical accessibility to the area, such as highways, waterways, airways, and railways. The assessor must be knowledgeable about the community's laws, rules, regulations, zoning ordinances, and political and social norms.

Population and environment

Population characteristics and environmental factors influence the types of problems communities face, the resources they possess, and the problem-solving approaches used.

Population characteristics

Certain characteristics have specific relevance to the health of the community. Some characteristics to be assessed are age distribution, sex ratio, marital status, migration patterns, literacy rate, level of education, and morbidity patterns. Other sociological characteristics are the income, occupation, ethnic background, religion, and nationality.

Environmental factors

Klein's mental health focus is emphasized in his discussion of the ecological aspects of community. He addresses the need to look at both the physiological and psychological components of the environment.

1. *Physical environment.* When the physical environmental aspects in this framework are assessed, spatial distribution and configuration are stressed. Klein contends that location of buildings, definition of boundaries, layout of roads, and space allocation for playgrounds

and parks reflect community dynamics and the valuing or devaluing of people within the area. For example, the location of a superhighway through an established neighborhood may be perceived by the assessor as the inhabitants' inability to influence their environment. This may reflect the residents' lack of significance to the community.

2. *Psychological environment.* When an assessment of a community is undertaken, it is imperative to understand the values and beliefs it embodies. The differences in values and beliefs that exist from one community to another are based largely on socioeconomic, cultural, geographical and ethnic factors. These unique factors influence priorities of a community and the way it deals with issues.

When collecting community data, the nurse determines how the members of the community perceive themselves in conjunction to nature. Do they perceive themselves as able to alter some of their environmental surroundings or do they feel powerless in the situation? In reference to time, is the community primarily oriented to past history? Is there planning, building, and talking about future occurrences?

This framework for data collection is strongly based on mental health concepts. It focuses on the interaction between individuals and social organizations. Table 6-5 illustrates the way the nurse collects data using observation, interaction, and measurement.

Table 6-5. Data collection of the community client based on Klein's interactional framework

	Observations	Interactions	Measurements
A. Community as a social system			
1. Communication	What newspapers, bulletins, flyers, and newsletters are available to community residents?	What are the formal communication channels? What are the informal communication channels?	
	Where are the meeting areas: bars, meeting halls, laundromat, or parks?	Do communications flow freely in the community? What are the methods by which ideas, thoughts, plans, and meetings are transmitted to residents? Are there newspapers, newsletters, and flyers available?	
		Are there specific gathering places where communications are shared? What are they? Who goes there? What is done with the information?	
2. Decision making		What are the community's decision-making patterns? Are decisions made by a group of leaders, or is there traditionally open and bitter fighting regarding even the smallest issues?	

Continued.

Table 6-5. Data collection of the community client based on Klein's interactional framework—cont'd

	Observations	Interactions	Measurements
2. Decision making— cont'd		Who are the decision makers in the community? Do they elicit input from citizens before making decisions?	
3. System linkage		What subsystem interaction is evident in the community? Do police and fire departments have a complementary relationship? Do business people support money-making projects of school children? Do they sponsor sporting activities? Do the board of education and board of health work cooperatively to provide health services for school children? Do churches allow the health department to operate clinics on their premises? Does the transit board cooperate with senior citizen groups in providing service to the elderly for recreation and health care? Do radio and television provide time for announcing community interest activities?	
4. Boundary maintenance	What are the physical boundaries of the community? Are they natural, such as a river, lake, mountain range, or are they manmade, such as a freeway, monument, or sign? What socioeconomic boundaries are seen? Is there an area in the community with large estates that only the economically advantaged families can maintain?	What political, religious, and social groups exist in the community that have specific admission criteria? What psychological boundaries exist in the community? Is it receptive to newcomers and new ideas? What socioeconomic groups are acceptable? What ethnic groups are welcome? What political and religious beliefs are acceptable?	

Table 6-5. Data collection of the community client based on Klein's interactional framework—cont'd

	Observations	Interactions	Measurements
B. Population and environment			
1. Population characteristics			Population. Age distribution, sex ratio, marital status, migration patterns, literacy rate, educational composition, birth rate, morbidity and mortality rates, income level, occupation composite, ethnic background, and nationality.
2. Environmental factors			
a. Physical	Is there a design to the location of buildings? Is preservation of natural parks included in the design? Are community beautification projects evident?	What zoning ordinances exist for new buildings? Are residential areas protected from industrial buildings? Are emission controls enforced? Are noise ordinances enforced?	Size of community in square miles. Population per square mile. Migration pattern into community. What is the pollution index?
b. Psychological		What is the history of the community? How did it come into existence? What are some of its traditions? What is its ethnic background? What is valued by this population? How does it perceive itself in regard to nature? Do the people make plans to alter the environment in order to meet their needs? Are they oriented to the past or future? Is there no building in the community, or is there much building, with long-range plans for the future?	

SUMMARY   Three models have been presented for collecting assessment data in a community system. Although different frameworks are used, many of the data are similar. Each framework addresses both structural and process aspects of the community. The framework the nurse chooses for the assessment depends on the community setting, the focus, and preference.

REFERENCES

1 Braden, C.J., and Herban, N.: Community health, A systems approach, New York, 1976, Appleton-Century-Crofts.
2 Hall, J.E., and Weaver, B.R., editors: Distributive nursing practice: a systems approach to community health, Philadelphia, 1977, J.B. Lippincott Co.
3 Hart, S.K., and Herriott, P.R.: Components of practice. In Hall, J.E., and Weaver, B.R., editors: Distributive nursing pratice: a systems approach to community health, Philadelphia, 1977, J.B. Lippincott Co.
4 Hazzard, M.E.: An overview of systems theory, Nurs. Clin. North Am. **6:**385, 1971.
5 Klein, D.: Community dynamics and mental health, New York, 1968, John Wiley & Sons, Inc.
6 Sanders, I.T.: The community: an introduction to a social system, New York, 1966, The Ronald Press Co.
7 Smoyak, S.: Toward understanding nursing situations: a transactional paradigm, Nurs. Res. **18:**407, 1969. (Brademeur cited by Smoyak.)
8 von Bertalanffy, L.: General systems theory, New York, 1968, George Braziller, Inc.

BIBLIOGRAPHY

Anderson, R., and Carter, I.: Human behavior in the social environment: a social systems approach, Chicago, 1974, Aldine Publishing Co.
Bennis, W.G., and others: The planning of change, New York, 1976, Holt, Rinehart & Winston.
Bertrand, A.: Social organization: a general systems and role therapy perspective, Philadelphia, 1972, F.A. Davis Co.
Reinhardt, A.M., and Quinn, M.D.: Current practice in family-centered community nursing, vol. I, St. Louis, 1977, The C.V. Mosby Co.
Tinkham, C.W., and Voorhies, E.R.: Community health nursing, evaluation and process, New York, 1977, Appleton-Century-Crofts.
von Bertalanffy, L.: General systems theory and psychiatry. In Arieti, S., editor: American handbook of psychiatry, vol. 3, New York, 1966, Basic Books Inc., Publishers.

Analysis and synthesis

PHYLLIS BAKER ANDREWS

GENERAL CONSIDERATIONS
Definition

Analysis is the categorization of data, identification of data gaps, and determination of patterns from pieces of data. Synthesis is the putting together of parts or elements to form a whole. The nurse puts together and compares knowledge of the client with standards, norms, theories, frameworks, and models to identify a particular relationship unique to that client. The relationships are not explicit from the start; they must be discovered or deduced.

Analysis/synthesis is used to interpret and give meaning to collected data. Both subjective and objective data are "gathered together, shuffled, sorted, scrambled and spit out in composite form."[3] La Monica[10] refers to this component as data processing; Little and Carnevali[11] define it as the ruling out and ruling in process. Analysis/synthesis is a decision-making process that ensures individualized nursing care. Client data are evaluated by categorizing, identifying data gaps, determining patterns, applying standards (comparing), establishing relationships, and identifying strengths and health concerns. The analysis/synthesis phase of assessment culminates in a summary statement or nursing diagnosis.

Historical perspectives

Analyzing/synthesizing is the professional nurse's responsibility. Nurses have used this method of decision making for years. In the 1960s analysis/synthesis was identified as a separate step in the assessment phase of the nursing process.

Analysis/synthesis is influenced by the nurse's background of scientific knowledge, past nursing experiences, and definition of nursing.[4] This scientific knowledge base includes anatomy, physiology, pathology, psychology, sociology, anthropology, epidemiology, bacteriology, and nursing theories. Knowledge of theoretical approaches, along with skills in critical thinking and decision making, is also necessary.

Overview	This chapter begins with a discussion of the intellectual process of analysis/synthesis. Application of theoretical frameworks and conceptual models is described. Guidelines and examples are then given for application to the individual, family, and community clients.

INTELLECTUAL PROCESS	This section discusses the cognitive skills involved in developing the analysis/synthesis. It includes discussions of objectivity, critical thinking, decision making, and inductive and deductive reasoning. In this text, the thought process and structural steps (guidelines) are discussed separately for clarification. In practice, they occur simultaneously.

Objectivity	The nurse maintains objectivity in interpreting client data to ensure accuracy. Nurses need an awareness of the effect of their values and beliefs on their perception of the data as they analyze the implied or inferred values and beliefs of the client.

Critical thinking	Critical thinking is sifting through the data and generating ideas about what it means. Processes such as imagining, conceiving, or inferring are used to join ideas. From these processes, an opinion or judgment is formed to interpret the data.

Decision-making process	Decision making is discriminative thinking and is used to choose a particular course of action. It is the process of identifying and selecting the best alternative and includes phases of deliberation, judgment, and choice. Nurses use decision making throughout the nursing process. It is especially relevant in analysis/synthesis.

Deliberation

Deliberation is a careful consideration of the data. The purposes of deliberation are to categorize the data; identify data gaps and incongruencies; determine patterns; and apply theories, models, frameworks, principles, norms, and standards.

Inductive or deductive reasoning is used to accomplish the purposes of deliberation. The inductive method involves putting assessment data into patterns that are then interpreted as within norms or not. It is reasoning from specific facts to a general conclusion. An example of induction is taking the cues, including signs and symptoms, and forming a pattern. Deduction is reasoning from an accepted principle to a particular instance, from the general to the specific. An example of deduction is starting with a conceptual model and categorizing client cues into that particular model.

The result of the deliberation phase is a series of statements concerning the way data patterns relate to the approaches used. The process of deciding health concerns and strengths is initiated.

Judgment

Judgment is an opinion regarding the health concerns and strengths of the client. The purposes of making judgments are to identify health concerns and strengths and establish relationships with these concerns and strengths. During the judgment phase the nurse analyzes the statements made in the deliberation phase and makes inferences or hypotheses.

Discrimination

The next phase is discriminating, or choosing among the options of strengths, health concerns, and relationships. In this phase the nurse decides what the health status is. This is accomplished by selecting the summary statement identifying the nursing diagnoses. The nursing diagnosis contains an identification of the client response to a condition, situation, or event, and the related contributing factors, if known. The nursing diagnoses are then validated and arranged in order of priority with the client. Validation provides feedback about the nurse's analysis/synthesis and decisions.

GUIDELINES FOR ANALYSIS/ SYNTHESIS

This section describes steps in analyzing/synthesizing data. These guidelines are suggestions for approaching this phase of the nursing process. Although most of the steps follow sequentially, one exception is the identification of data gaps and incongruencies (step 2), which may occur after the categorization of data (step 1) as indicated or after the establishment of relationships (step 6).

1. *Categorize all data.* The first step in analyzing data is to organize, group, or sort them in a logical, systematic way. Bower and Bevis[2] state that "the method of categorization is not nearly as important as having some systematic way of handling data that everyone knows and understands."

Theoretical frameworks and conceptual models appropriate for categorizing data of individuals, families, and communities are described later in this chapter. The nurse must decide which conceptual model is appropriate and how to group data in logical clusters.

2. *Identify data gaps and incongruencies.* Data gaps and incongruencies indicate areas in need of further assessment. Data gaps are missing data necessary to determine patterns and specific approaches. A data gap also exists when there are insufficient data to determine a pattern based on the approach. Examples of data gaps are nutrition (3-day recall), spiritual needs, family history, health history, past coping patterns, and resources. To determine data gaps, the data should be observed for obvious omissions. The list of data gaps may appear under a nursing diagnostic category as either "incomplete data base" or "incomplete information." An incongruency occurs when there are conflicting data. An example of an incongruency would be a client's denying a history of smoking while having an open pack of cigarettes and matches in a pocket, plus brownish stains on two fingers. This is an incongruency that needs to be clarified or validated before defining specific client concerns.

3. *Determine patterns.* The subjective and objective data are examined for cues, signs, and symptoms to determine whether the client's behavior is an isolated incident or indicates a pattern. The data are categorized to see what pieces or cues fit together and which is the best or most appropriate fit. Although this is still the deliberation phase of decision making, judgments and choices are constantly being made in the selection of cues that form a pattern. This is also the beginning of synthesis. Examples of identified patterns are those related to eating, smoking, sleeping, exercising, adapting, coping, communicating, health care practices, medical supervision, parenting, and resources.

4. *Apply theories, models, frameworks, norms, and standards.* In this step the categorized data and patterns are compared with theories, models, frameworks, norms, and standards to identify congruence with the approach. This is the major part of the synthesis process; it is incorporating the data into a model or framework to form a whole. The nurse uses knowledge of developmental and physiological norms and psychological parameters. Knowledge of theories and concepts of nursing, communication, adaptation, stress, crisis, role, group, family, leadership, and change are also important.

Standards used for individuals are the Metropolitan Life Insurance Company height and weight chart, the basic four food groups, normal ranges of vital signs and laboratory values, and developmental stages (such as the Denver Developmental Screening Test). The data are compared with normal ranges, values, expectations, and the client's previous condition. An important aspect of this step is the client's perception of "normal," as this may differ from the nurse's assumptions and perceptions. The nurse must learn the client's health standards as well as the cultural standards and take them into account. When the client and nurse agree, it is more likely that mutuality and cooperation will occur. If they do not agree, there may be a need for further assessment or negotiation.

5. *Identify health concerns and strengths.* After applying approaches, norms, and standards the nurse differentiates concerns and strengths and weighs the results. This is the primary judgmental phase, in which the nurse analyzes and interprets the data according to client strengths and concerns, based on scientific knowledge. The term "concern" is preferable to "problem," "disability," "deficit," or "limitation," all of which have negative connotations. Inferences are made about the client's health state, condition, or situation. The nurse judges the client's health status, which includes any actual, potential, or possible concerns reflected by the client's responses to the situation, condition, or state. After summarizing the data, the nurse makes one or more of the following judgments, and plans accordingly:

1. No concern exists and the client's health state is confirmed.
2. No concern exists but there is a potential concern.
3. A concern exists but the client is coping successfully.
4. A concern exists that the client needs assistance in handling.
5. A concern exists that the client cannot deal with at this time.
6. A concern exists that requires further diagnosis and study.
7. A concern exists that is not incapacitating but will be at a later date if it is not treated.
8. A concern exists that places heavy stress on the client's ability to cope.

9. A concern is critical to the client.

10. The concerns are long term and permanent.[22]

The client's abilities are identified as assets, strengths, or resources. These strengths are integrated in the plans for nursing care. Examples of strengths and concerns for the individual, family, and community are shown in Table 7-1.

Table 7-1. Examples of strengths and concerns applied to the individual, family, and community

Client	Strengths	Concerns
Individual	Ability for self-care	Decreased self-care
	Feelings of independence	Dependence
	High morale	Lack of self-esteem
	Family support	No family
	Many friends	Social isolation
	Adequate housing	Inadequate housing
	Education	Lack of job skills
Family	Past coping experience	Crisis
	Open communication	Dysfunctional communication
	Adequate financial resources	Inadequate resources
	Extended family presence	No support system
	Flexible rules	Rigid rules
	Defined roles	Confused roles
Community	Adequate funding to meet health needs	Inadequate funding
	Enthusiastic leadership and interest in health concerns	Disinterest
	Health services available	Unavailable
	Health services accessible	Inaccessible
	Health services acceptable	Unacceptable

6. *Establish causal relationships.* In this step the nurse explores and identifies factors influencing or contributing to the list of concerns. The nurse makes inferences and hypotheses about the causal relationships of client concerns. The establishment of these etiological factors gives direction to nursing interventions. Examples are "anxiety related to impending surgery" and "noncompliance with medication regimen related to lack of knowledge."

After relationships are identified, the concerns are organized in diagnostic statements. These are discussed in the next chapter.

APPLICATION OF THEORETICAL FRAMEWORKS AND CONCEPTUAL MODELS

The choice of a model or framework for the nursing process is made before or after data collection. The model or framework provides a structure for categorizing and interpreting the data. It influences the wording of the diagnostic statement. Examples of frameworks and models are given for the individual, family, and community.

Individual

When Roy's adaptation model is used, data are categorized according to basic physiological needs, self-concept, role mastery or function, and interdependence.[17] The patterns are interpreted as adaptive or maladaptive. An example of analysis/synthesis using Roy's model is shown later.

Another way of grouping data is Maslow's hierarchy of needs.[13] These needs include physiological, safety and security, love and belonging, esteem, and self-actualization. If the client's needs are not being met, there is a needs deficit. An example of Maslow's framework is shown later in this chapter.

Erikson's eight developmental stages[6] are another approach for analyzing client data. They include sense of trust, autonomy, initiative, industry, identity, intimacy, generativity, and integrity. These stages are one way of identifying a client's developmental level. At least one of these stages should be used in analyzing each client, since the causes of a client's health concerns frequently relate to the developmental or maturity level. For example, a 63-year-old may be at the trust versus mistrust level; this would certainly have an effect on the nurse's approach and interventions. A developmental analysis identifies the stage in which the client is operating and the developmental lags or needs.

The biopsychosociospiritual model is also applicable to categorizing data. The data are grouped according to these categories and then compared with standards and norms. Patterns are identified and relationships determined; judgments are made as to strengths and assets or health concerns.

Family

Families are analyzed using different conceptual frameworks. Four well-established frameworks are systems, structural-functional, interactional, and developmental. Regardless of the framework selected, the family is being evaluated as functional or dysfunctional. Patterns that make the family functional are family strengths. Patterns that are dysfunctional need to be clarified and identified as concerns.

If a systems approach is used, the family is evaluated as an open or closed system with rigid, diffuse, or permeable boundaries; functional or dysfunctional self-regulatory mechanisms (throughput); and system overload or deprivation (input or output).

The structural-functional approach is a variation of systems. In analysis, the functional and structural components are categorized separately. Structure may be grouped and evaluated according to:

1. Role structure (position, behavior, conflict, strain, sharing and modification)
2. Value systems (overt or covert rules, priorities, conflicts, and restrictive or flexible)
3. Communication patterns (functional or dysfunctional)
4. Power structure (coalitions and decision making, classified as dominated, autonomic, or leaderless)

The functional categories are either adequate or inadequate, functional or dysfunctional. These distinctions apply to Friedman's categories of family function[7]: affection (personality maintenance); socialization and social placement; reproduction; family coping; economy; and provision of physical necessities. An example of this approach is shown later.

The interactional approach focuses on ways family members interrelate. Internal family dynamics are analyzed in this approach as functional, potentially alterable, or altered. Processes or dynamics interpreted are role, status, communication patterns, decision making, coping patterns, and socialization. This approach is limited and needs to be used in conjunction with another approach. Satir[18] uses the interactional process to identify four categories: rules, self-worth, communication, and links to society.

Duvall[5] and Stevenson[20] use the developmental approach with family tasks and stages of progression through the life cycle. The collected data are analyzed for cues that identify the stage. Then a descriptive statement is made, noting the developmental needs.

Community

Approaches that are used for analysis/synthesis of community data are epidemiological, interactional, structural, functional, and systems. Regardless of the framework used, analysis indicates patterns, resources, and influencing factors that identify strengths, concerns, and high-risk populations. An example of Klein's interactional framework[9] appears later.

Community data are interpreted from histograms, frequency graphs, pie charts, statistical maps, tables, or narrative statements. The use of energy flow charts can graphically show interrelationships among systems. One of the problems in assimilating and analyzing community data is that the vital statistics or census data may not be current; this should be noted. The National Commission on Community Services[15] recommends the following criteria to evaluate overall health services of a community:

1. Health services should be comprehensive.
2. Health care should be continuous and coordinated.
3. Health care must be available, accessible, and acceptable.
4. Health care requires adequate facilities, personnel, and finances.

EXAMPLES OF APPLICATION

This section gives examples of ways to use the guidelines of the analysis/synthesis process. Tables 7-2 through 7-5 incorporate the decision-making process with the steps of the analysis/synthesis process. Column I categorizes the data into patterns according to the specific approach stated in column II; column III lists strengths and concerns; column IV lists the relationships; column V lists data gaps; and column VI lists the nursing diagnoses.

The data given for the individual, family, and community reflect one visit with the client. Written summaries of analysis/synthesis are given for each type of client, and the written summation identifies the approach and its components. Patterns of supporting data are cited with data gaps noted, and conclusions are drawn of strengths or concerns in relation to the concept of the approach. Thereafter, each concept of the approach is analyzed. At the end of this process, a list of overall client strengths is given, followed by the nursing diagnoses list.

vidual

Two brief case studies are presented and analyzed/synthesized. In the first (Table 7-2) a 75-year-old woman with medical diagnoses of hypertension and cataracts is interpreted according to Roy's adaptation model. The second (Table 7-3) is the application of Maslow's hierarchy of needs to a 50-year-old man with a history of alcoholism. Each model presentation includes an example of the analysis/synthesis process and a written summation.

Table 7-2. Analysis/synthesis of the individual client: Roy's adaptation model applied to 75-year-old woman with hypertension and cataracts

Deliberation		Judgment			Choice
I Data	II Model application (adaptive modes)	III Strengths and concerns	IV Relationships (influencing factors)	V Data gaps	VI Nursing diagnoses
"My feet are so swollen I can't wear shoes."	**A.** Physiological 1. Exercise and rest Maladaptive	Mobility impaired Safety	Edema of feet	Safety measures	Decreased mobility related to edema of feet Potential safety concern related to decreased mobility
Ht, 5'3". Wt, 160 lb.	2. Nutrition Maladaptive, according to Metropolitan chart	Increased wt	Unknown	24-hr recall of eating habits	Alterations in nutrition, cause unknown
Edentulous.	Potential maladaptation	Possible chewing concern	Edentulous	Assess if problem	Potential alterations in oral integrity related to edentulous condition
	3. Elimination 4. Fluid and electrolytes			Assess	
4+ pitting edema, both ankles, feet.	Maladaptive			Fluid intake, salt in diet	
Circumference of ankles: R, 10"; L, 10½".	Maladaptive				
"I haven't taken my medicine in 2 weeks."	Maladaptive		Lack of medication		Increased fluid volume related to lack of medicine

Table 7-2. Analysis/synthesis of the individual client: Roy's adaptation model applied to 75-year-old woman with hypertension and cataracts—cont'd

Deliberation		Judgment			Choice
I	**II**	**III**	**IV**	**V**	**VI**
	Model application (adaptive modes)	Strengths and concerns	Relationships (influencing factors)		
Data				Data gaps	Nursing diagnoses
P, 72; R, 20. Lungs clear. BP 200/100. Extremities cool to touch. 4+ edema of lower extremities.	5. Oxygen Adaptive Adaptive 6. Circulation According to Bates.[1] Elevated BP Maladaptive 7. Regulation		Hypertension	Past medical history: knowledge of disease	Alterations in circulatory system related to hypertension
T, 98.6°. Wears glasses. Has history of cataracts.	Adaptive now	Potential concern	Cataracts	Date of last eye exam	Potential for decreased vision related to cataracts
"I haven't taken my medicine in 2 weeks. I forget to take it."	Maladaptive	Noncompliance	Forgetfulness	Knowledge of medications, daily schedule	Noncompliance with medication related to forgetfulness
"My name is Sarah. I'm in the hospital for high blood pressure."	**B.** Self-concept Adaptive	Strength: coping with hospitalization			
Retired clerk. Knits for grandchildren.	**C.** Role function Erikson's ego integrity Adaptive	Strength: meeting developmental needs			
Husband died 3 months ago.	Adaptation unknown	Potential concern	Widowhood	Past coping	Potential dysfunctional grieving related to loss of husband
Lives alone with dog. Receives Social Security, pension, and Medicare.	**D.** Interpendence Adaptive now Adaptive	Potential concern	Living alone Decreased mobility Care of pet	Friends Family Leisure Socialization Pet care giver	Potential for social isolation related to living alone and decreased mobility
Belongs to Methodist church.	Adaptation unknown			Spiritual needs	

Analysis/synthesis: Roy's adaptation model

According to Roy's adaptation model[17] there are four adaptive modes or ways to cope with environmental changes. This client's data are analyzed according to these four categories: physiological needs, self-concept, role function, and interdependence.

Physiological needs include exercise and rest, nutrition, elimination, balance of fluid and electrolytes, oxygen, circulation, and regulation. In the category of *exercise and rest*, this client complains of her "feet being so swollen" that she cannot wear shoes. This is maladaptive in that it impairs her mobility.* There is also a potential safety concern related to her decreased mobility.* The data gap includes safety hazards. In the category of *nutrition*, the client's height (5'3") and weight (160 lb.) indicate that she is approximately 40 lb. overweight according to the Metropolitan chart.[21] This is maladaptive, leading to alterations in nutrition with cause unknown.* There is a data gap concerning *elimination* that needs to be assessed.* *Fluid and electrolytes* are maladaptive,* as exhibited by her 4+ pitting edema of both feet and ankles: right ankle circumference is 10", left ankle 10½". The influencing factor may be her not taking hypertension medication in two weeks. Data gaps include fluid intake and salt in diet. Her *oxygen* needs are adaptive according to the limited data of pulse 72, respirations 20, and clear lungs. According to Bates,[1] her blood pressure of 200/100 is elevated (maladaptive).* The fact that her extremities are cool to the touch and edematous indicates alterations in *circulation*.* The influencing factors and focal stimuli are her history of hypertension and noncompliance with medication. Data gaps include medical history and knowledge of disease. In the *regulation* category, the client's temperature of 98.6° is adaptive. The fact that she has cataracts and wears glasses is adaptive now, but there is a potential for decreased vision related to the cataracts.* Data gaps include dates of last eye examination and glaucoma test. Since she has forgotten to take her hypertension medication in 2 weeks, she may have a sensory overload, which is maladaptive.* Data gaps include daily schedule and knowledge of medications.

Data relating to the client's *self-concept* appear adaptive in that she is oriented to person, time, and place, and responds to questions appropriately. She seems to be coping with hospitalization.

Her *role function* is exhibited by the data that she is a retired clerk and knitting for her grandchildren. According to Erikson,[6] she is coping (adapting) with the ego integrity stage of development. There is a potential role adjustment related to the death of her husband 3 months ago, since her adaptation is unknown.* Data gaps include past coping and grieving.

Interdependence data (Social Security, pension, and Medicare) indicate that she has adequate income, which is adaptive. She lives alone with her dog. Her living arrangement has been adaptive; however, there may be a potential concern of social isolation due to her decreased mobility, living alone, and managing the care of her pet.* Data gaps include friends, family, and pet care giver. She belongs to the Methodist church but her spiritual needs are unknown.*

---

*Asterisk indicates concerns for nursing diagnoses.

This client's strengths are adequate oxygen, temperature regulation, orientation, coping with hospitalization, meeting most developmental needs, and adequate income.

The nursing diagnoses are:
1. Decreased mobility related to feet and ankle edema.
2. Potential safety concern related to decreased mobility.
3. Alterations in nutrition, cause unknown.
4. Potential alterations in oral integrity related to edentulous condition.
5. Increased fluid volume related to lack of medication.
6. Alterations in circulatory system related to hypertension.
7. Potential for decreased vision related to cataracts.
8. Noncompliance with medications related to forgetfulness.
9. Potential dysfunctional grieving related to loss of husband.
10. Potential for social isolation related to living alone and decreased mobility.
11. Incomplete data base†: elimination, spiritual needs, knowledge of hypertension and medication, and frequency of medical supervision.

†See Chapter 8, p. 120, for explanation of this category.

Table 7-3. Analysis/synthesis of the individual client: Maslow's model applied to 50-year-old man with history of alcoholism

Deliberation		Judgment			Choice
I Data	**II** Model application (needs categories)	**III** Strength and concerns	**IV** Rela- tionships	**V** Data gaps	**VI** Nursing diagnoses
Ht, 6′. Wt, 130 lb. Eats one meal daily.	**A.** Physiological According to Williams,[21] area of need	Decreased wt	Inadequate intake	Three-day recall of eating habits	Alterations in nutrition related to inadequate intake
Sleeps 2-3 hours.	Needs 5-6 hours	Inadequate sleep		Possible causes	Sleep pattern disturbances, cause unknown
"I haven't had sex in 10 months."	According to Masters and Johnson,[14] may be need	Potential concern		Sexual history, feelings	Potential sexual dysfunction
T, 98.6°. P, 64; R, 18.		Strength			
	B. Safety and security				
Smokes 2-3 packs of cigarettes daily.	American Cancer Society says unhealthy	Potential respiratory concern	Smoking	Duration, knowledge of adverse effects	Potential for respiratory impairment related to smoking
Has drunk 10-12 beers daily for 3 years.	Alcoholic's Anonymous states possible concern	Concern	Unknown	Drinking history, concerns caused	Excessive alcohol consumption

Continued.

Table 7-3. Analysis/synthesis of the individual client: Maslow's model applied to 50-year-old man with history of alcoholism—cont'd

Deliberation		Judgment			Choice
I Data	II Model application (needs categories)	III Strength and concerns	IV Rela- tionships	V Data gaps	VI Nursing diagnoses
States very de-pressed for 2 weeks. "I can't go on like this." Sits with head bowed.	According to Haber,[8] pos-sible suicidal pattern	Potential safety con-cern	Unknown	History of de-pressed state Meaning Assess suicidal plans	Potential suicidal pattern
	C. Love and belong-ing				
"No one cares for me." Has not seen children in 1 year. Sits with head bowed. Unemployed for 6 mo.	Need	Concern	Life-style	Situational sup-ports Significant others	Loneliness related to life-style
Divorced.	Need	Poor self-concept	Lack of self-esteem	Feelings of self-worth	Disturbance in self-concept related to lack of self-esteem
Dressed in torn shirt and soiled jeans with holes in knees. Heavy odor of perspira-tion.	Need	Personal hygiene concern		Feelings Daily schedule	Self-care deficit re-lated to personal hygiene
	D. Self-actualization				
Unemployed. Eighth-grade education.	According to Erikson, area of concern	Developmental concern	Unknown	Personal goals Employment history	Disturbance in self-concept
Came to hos-pital volun-tarily.		Strength			
Knows reason for hospital-ization.		Strength			

Analysis/synthesis: Maslow's hierarchy

According to Maslow's hierarchy,[13] individuals have physiological, safety, love and belonging, esteem and recognition, and self-actualization needs. (For a more detailed discussion of Maslow's hierarchy see Appendix C.) This client's data in the *physiological* category include: height 6', weight 130 lb.; eats one meal daily; sleeps 2 to 3 hours per night; has not had sex in 10 months; T, 98.6°; P, 64; R, 18. According to the Metropolitan chart,[21] the client is approximately 30 to 40 lb underweight. According to Williams,[21] one meal per day is inadequate.* Therefore this client has a need related to inadequate food intake. Data gaps include 3-day recall, and eating habits. According to Shortridge,[19] 2 to 3 hours' sleep per night is inadequate for most people. This client has a need related to decreased sleep.* The data gap includes possible causes. According to Masters and Johnson,[14] his sexual inactivity may indicate a need,* possibly related to his lack of self-esteem or alcohol consumption. Data gaps include sexual history and feelings. According to Malasanos,[12] his temperature, pulse, and respirations are within normal limits.

Data relating to *safety and security* include: client smokes 2 to 3 packs of cigarettes daily, has drunk 10-12 beers daily for the past 3 years, and has been very depressed for 2 weeks, stating "I can't go on like this." According to Haber,[8] the fact that the client has been very depressed, with an expression of potential suicide, indicates a possible safety need.* Data gaps include history of depressed state, assessment of its meaning, and assessment of suicidal plans. According to the American Cancer Society, smoking 2 to 3 packs of cigarettes daily is injurious to one's health. This is a safety and physiological need.* Data gaps include duration of habit and knowledge of adverse effects. Alcoholics Anonymous states that if drinking over a long period of time causes problems in daily living, a concern exists.* The duration of the habit for 3 years indicates a pattern of long standing. This is a safety as well as physiological need; since he smokes and drinks there may be a fire hazard. Data gaps include drinking history, the concerns it causes, developmental level, and values.

The client's need for *love and belonging* is evident by his statement that no one cares for him and that he is estranged from his children.* Data gaps include situational supports and significant others.

Data indicating *esteem needs* are: client sits with head bowed, has been unemployed for 6 months, is divorced, is dressed in torn shirt and soiled jeans with holes in both knees, and has heavy odor of perspiration.* Maslow[13] says that when love and belonging needs remain unsatisfied, the individual may feel alone, alienated, and distant from friends and relatives. Data gaps include feelings of self-worth and daily schedule.

Self-actualization data include: client's eighth-grade education, his statement that he came to the hospital voluntarily, and his knowledge of the reason for his hospitalization. According to Erikson,[6] the client has developmental needs related to identity, which is typical of the adolescent rather than adult stage.* The client's lack of education probably is affecting his employment chances. Data gaps include personal goals. His main strengths are that he is oriented and that he sought medical care.

The nursing diagnoses are:
1. Alterations in nutrition related to inadequate intake.
2. Sleep pattern disturbances, cause unknown.
3. Potential sexual dysfunction.
4. Potential for respiratory impairment related to smoking.
5. Excessive alcohol consumption.
6. Potential suicidal pattern.
7. Loneliness related to life-style.
8. Disturbance in self-concept related to lack of self-esteem.
9. Self-care deficit related to personal hygiene.
10. Incomplete data base: medical history and physical assessment.

---

*Asterisk indicates concerns for nursing diagnoses.

Table 7-4. Analysis/synthesis of the family client: structural-functional model applied to young family with one son, expecting second child

		Judgment			Choice
Deliberation					
I Data	II Model application	III Strengths and concerns	IV Rela- tionships	V Data gaps	VI Nursing diagnoses
	A. Structure 1. Role				
34-yr-old preg- nant wife; co- support, works in architec- tural firm.	Mother Cohead Wife	Potential concern		Anticipatory plans, feelings	Potential stress related to role change
35-yr-old hus- band; cosup- port, owns small busi- ness.	Husband Cohead Father				
"We alternate and share chores."	Complementarity	Strength			
3-yr-old child.	Son Grandchild				
	Potential brother	Concern	New baby	Anticipatory plans, feeling	Potential for sib- ling rivalry re- lated to baby
	2. Values				
Husband's busi- ness, wife's job.	Work	No conflict			
Shares chores and decision making; alone time in PM.	Democracy	No conflict			
Husband and wife college graduates.	Education	No conflict			
Wife weekly prenatal care.	Health	No conflict			
Family attends church regu- larly.	Religion	No conflict			
Child care by grandpar- ents.	Responsibility	No conflict			
	3. Communication patterns				
Couple take turns speak- ing, listen, include child.	According to Satir,[18] func- tional	Strength			
	4. Power structure				
Couple make de- cisions jointly.	Shared	Strength		Past decision out- come, process, relationship with extended family	

Table 7-4. Analysis/synthesis of the family client: structural-functional model applied to young family with one son, expecting second child—cont'd

Deliberation		Judgment			Choice
I **Data**	**II** **Model application**	**III** **Strengths** **and concerns**	**IV** **Rela-** **tionships**	**V** **Data gaps**	**VI** **Nursing diagnoses**
	B. Function 1. Affective				
Child sitting on mother's lap. Couple sitting close, occasionally touch.	Mutual nurturance	Strength		Need-response, family connectedness (recreation)	
	2. Socialization				
Child talks, walks; ht and wt proportionate.				Child-rearing practices, Denver Developmental Screening Test	
College graduates; husband in Big Brothers; wife neighborhood representative. Church attendance.	Community participation	Strength		Family history, culture	
	3. Reproduction				
3-yr-old; pregnancy.				Sexual history, family planning, maternal reproduction history	
	4. Family coping				
Pregnancy.	Life crisis	Potential		Past crises and coping mechanisms, resources Plans, feelings	Potential stressor related to addition of new family member
	5. Economic				
Husband's small business; wife's working.		Potential	Loss of income	Plans	Potential economic concern related to loss of income
	6. Provision of physical necessities				
Own 3-bedroom brick home. Weekly prenatal care.	Adequate	Strength Strength		Eating habits, 3-day recall; immunizations; dates of last dental, vision, breast exam, and Pap smear; use of alcohol, other substances; exercise; family and individual health history and knowledge of labor and delivery.	Maintenance of family health

Family   **Analysis/synthesis: structural-functional model**

This nuclear family is analyzed using the structural-functional approach. According to Friedman,[7] family structural dimensions include role, values, communication patterns, and power structure. Family functions are affective patterns, socialization, reproduction, family coping, economy, and provision of physical necessities (food, clothing, shelter, and health care).

In the *structural* component, *role* implies ascribed or achieved position in a family. Data from this family indicate that the 34-year-old woman has the roles of wife, pregnant mother, and cosupporter. The 35-year-old man is husband, father, and cosupporter. The 3-year-old boy is son, grandchild, and potential brother. The couple's statement that they alternate and share chores indicates complementarity, according to Parsons.[16] With the arrival of the new baby, there are two potential concerns. First, the changes in the woman's role from employment to unemployment may cause increased stress.* Data gaps include anticipatory plans and feelings. Second, there is a potential for sibling rivalry in the 3-year-old.* Data gaps include anticipatory plans and feelings.

Values are ideas, attitudes, or beliefs about worth that bind the family together, according to Friedman. Values influence rules and priorities. Values reflected by the data in this family are:

1. Work (both husband and wife are employed).
2. Democracy, equality, and freedom (husband and wife share chores and decision making; have time alone in evening; each has separate community interests).
3. Education (both husband and wife are college graduates).
4. Voluntarism (husband belongs to Big Brothers; wife is a neighborhood representative on a priority board).
5. Health (wife has weekly prenatal care).
6. Religion (family attends church regularly).
7. Responsibility (child is placed with grandparents while parents are at work).

At present there do not appear to be any conflicts in values in this family, which is a strength.

Communication patterns are reflected in the following family data: couple take turns speaking; they listen to each other and include their child in their conversation. According to Satir,[18] these are functional communication patterns, which is a family strength.

Power structure includes coalitions and decision making. There is only one datum indicating this component: husband and wife make decisions jointly. Data gaps include past decision-making process and outcomes, and relationship with extended family members.

The first dimension in *family functions* is *affective patterns*. According to Friedman, this one involves the family's perceptions, respect, and care of the psychological needs of its members. Family data reflective of this compo-

---

*Asterisk indicates concerns for nursing diagnoses.

nent include the child sitting on the mother's lap and husband and wife sitting near one another with occasional touching between them. Data gaps are a need-response and family connectedness (such as recreation). Mutual nurturance and closeness are identified as a strength.

Socialization includes child-rearing practices, education, and community contacts. There are data gaps in child-rearing practices and the developmental level of the child (Denver Developmental Screening Test). However, the child walks and talks, and height and weight appear proportionate.

Both husband and wife are college graduates, which probably influences their vocabulary and motivation for achievement. Data gaps include family history and culture. Both husband and wife participate in community activities (husband in Big Brothers and wife as neighborhood representative). The family also attends church regularly, which will influence the child's socialization. According to Satir,[18] family links to society are a strength.

Reproduction is another family function in which this family is participating (3-year-old and pregnancy). Data gaps include sexual history, maternal reproduction history, and family planning.

Family coping refers to the family's abilities to adapt to stress and stressors. Data gaps include past crises, coping mechanisms, and family resources. There is a potential stressor related to the addition of a new member to the family.* Data gaps include anticipatory plans and feelings.

The *economic* function involves the provision and allocation of finances, space, and materials. Data reflecting the economic function include husband's owning small business and wife's working in architectural firm. There is a potential concern related to the expected loss of the wife's income during confinement.* The data gap includes anticipatory plans.

The last function is the *provision of physical necessities,* including health care. Data indicating this function are: they own their three-bedroom home, and wife gets weekly prenatal care. These are strengths. Data gaps include eating habits, 3-day recall; immunizations; dates of last dental, vision, and breast exams, and Pap smear; use of alcohol and other substances including over-the-counter drugs; exercise; family and individual health history; and knowledge of labor and delivery.

The overall family strengths identified are nonconflicting values, functional communication patterns, mutual nurturance, links to society, and adequate housing and regular prenatal care.

The family nursing diagnoses are:

1. Potential stress related to role change.
2. Potential for sibling rivalry related to new baby.
3. Potential economic concern related to loss of income.
4. Maintenance of family health.
5. Incomplete data base: past decision outcomes and process, relationship with extended family, family need-response, family recreation, reproduction history, sexual history, past coping and resources, and health care practices.

---

*Asterisk indicates concerns for nursing diagnoses.

Table 7-5. Analysis/synthesis of the community client: Klein's interactional framework applied to one census tract

Deliberation		Judgment			Choice
I	II	III	IV	V	VI
Data	Model application	Strengths and concerns	Relationships	Data gap	Nursing diagnoses
	A. Community as a social system				
Paper boy delivery of PM papers; television antennas on most homes; posters in grocery window; neighborhood newsletter in store; several elderly women in store	1. Communication Formal and informal	Strength		Places where people meet: bars, drug stores, restaurants; effectiveness of communication	
Two elected representatives to Priority Board	2. Decision making			Identified leaders; effectiveness of leadership	
Parochial school next to Catholic Church; senior citizen's center in church	3. System linkage			Transportation; nonchurch relationships and support to community	
Railroad on two sides; freeway on one and industry on other side	4. Boundary maintenance Physical	Concern	Boundaries	Routes, frequency of emergency vehicles	Potential for community isolation related to boundaries.

Psychological

Potential noise pollution related to industry, railraod and freeway

Decibel level, noise abatement; zoning rules

Political and social norms

Mortality, morbidity, recreational resources, nutrition, and services for elderly

B. Population and environment

1. Demographic data

Age	0-4	5-14	15-44	45-64	65+
Census tract	20	60	100	200	640
Males	11	40	20	75	140
Females	9	20	80	125	500*

Income:
Below $5,000   800*
$5-15,000   90
$15-24,000   None
$25-49,000   None

2. Physical environment

Frame houses, 30-40 yr old, peeling paint.

Many windows boarded.

Small yards, chain link fences.

Large fertilizer industry on north boundary; no sidewalks; no health resources, facilities, or personnel.

Size of census tract, emission and zoning enforcement — Concern

Lack of health resources — Concern

Safety concerns related to lack of sidewalks, peeling paint, and boarded buildings — Concern

Potential air pollution related to industry and freeway — Concern

3. Psychological environment
Values and beliefs

Community history, culture, religion, orientation to past, future, and plans — Concern

*Asterisk indicates concerns for nursing diagnoses.

Community

Analysis/synthesis: Klein's interactional framework

Klein's theoretical perspective of a community[9] includes (1) the community as a social system; components of this category are communication, decision making, system linkage, and boundary maintenance. (2) The population and environment; components include demographic data and the physical and psychological environment. Community data from one census tract are applied to this framework.

In the *community as a social system* category, *communication* includes formal and informal methods. Data observations include paper boy delivering evening paper, television antennas on most homes, and posters in neighborhood grocery window. A neighborhood newsletter was also available in the grocery, which is where people meet. The data gap includes other places where people meet, such as drug stores, bars, and restaurants. From the limited data there appear to be adequate methods of communication, but the effectiveness is unknown.

Decision making in this census tract is directly related to the two elected neighborhood representatives to a regional Priority Board. Data gaps include identification of neighborhood leaders and effectiveness of leadership.

System linkage refers to interdependence among groups and organizations within the census tract. The Catholic school that houses a senior citizen's center is an example of system linkage. Data gaps include transportation, nonchurch relationships, and support to the community.

Boundary maintenance is indicated in this census tract physically by its boundaries of railroad tracks on two sides, an industry on one side, and a freeway on the other. This suggests a potential concern of isolation, especially with regard to emergency vehicles coming into the neighborhood.* Data gaps include routes and frequency of emergency vehicle use. There is also a potential noise concern with the two railroads and the freeway.* Data gaps include decibel level and noise abatement, zoning rules, and political and social norms.

The second theoretical perspective of a community is the *population and environment. Demographic characteristics* are:

Age and sex distribution

Age	0-4	5-14	15-44	45-64	65+
Census tract	20	60	100	200	640
Males	11	40	20	75	140
Females	9	20	80	125	500*

Income

Below $5,000	$5-15,000	$15-24,000	$25-49,000
800*	90	None	None

These data indicate that most of the population in this census tract are widowed or single women over 65 years of age with incomes of less than $5,000. There are also more boys than girls from ages 5 to 14 and more women than men from ages 15 to 64. Data gaps include mortality, morbidity, recreational resources, nutrition, and services to the elderly.*

---

*Asterisk indicates concerns for nursing diagnoses.

Data describing the *physical environment* include: frame houses approximately 30 to 40 years old, with peeling paint; many windows boarded; small yards fenced with chain link; large fertilizer industry on north boundary; no sidewalks; and no health resources, facilities, or personnel. These data indicate the following actual or potential concerns: potential air pollution related to industry, railroads, and highway*; safety problems related to lack of sidewalks, peeling paint, boarded buildings*; and lack of health services.* Data gaps include size of census tract in square miles, and emission and zoning enforcement.

The *psychological environment* includes the community's values and beliefs. Data gaps include community history, culture, religion, orientation to past and future, and plans.

The only apparent strength is community communication, although there are many data gaps.

The community nursing diagnoses are:
1. Potential for community isolation related to boundaries.
2. Potential noise pollution related to industry, railroads, and freeway.
3. Lack of health services.
4. Safety concerns related to lack of sidewalks, peeling paint, and boarded buildings.
5. Potential air pollution related to industry and freeway.
6. Incomplete data base: places where people meet, identification of neighborhood leaders and their effectiveness, transportation, non-church support of community, morbidity and mortality, nutrition and services to elderly, community history, culture, religion, and size.

SUMMARY

This chapter discussed the definition and process of analysis/synthesis. Theories, models, and concepts were related to this component of the assessment phase of the nursing process. The intellectual processes of critical thinking, decision making, and inductive and deductive reasoning were included and synthesized with guidelines. Examples for the individual, family, and community client were included in the application section.

---

*Asterisk indicates concerns for nursing diagnoses.

REFERENCES

1 Bates, B.: A guide to physical examination, ed. 2, Philadelphia, 1979, J.B. Lippincott Co.
2 Bower, F.L., and Bevis, E.O.: Fundamentals of nursing practice: concepts, roles, and functions, St. Louis, 1979, The C.V. Mosby Co.
3 Braden, C.J., and Herban, N.L.: Community health: a systems approach, New York, 1976, Appleton-Century-Crofts.
4 Durand, M., and Prince, R.: Nursing diagnosis: process and decisions. In Marriner, A.: The nursing process: a scientific approach to nursing care, ed. 2, St. Louis, 1979, The C.V. Mosby Co.
5 Duvall, E.M.: Marriage and family development, ed. 5, Philadelphia, 1977, J.B. Lippincott Co.
6 Erikson, E.H.: Childhood and society, New York, 1963, W.W. Norton & Co., Inc.
7 Friedman, M.M.: Family nursing: theories and assessment, New York, 1981, Appleton-Century-Crofts.
8 Haber, J., and others: Comprehensive psychiatric nursing, New York, 1978, McGraw-Hill Book Co.
9 Klein, D.: Community dynamics and mental health, New York, 1968, John Wiley & Sons, Inc.
10 La Monica, E.L.: The nursing process: a humanistic approach, Reading, Mass., 1979, Addison-Wesley Publishing Co., Inc.
11 Little, D.E., and Carnevali, D.L.: Nursing care planning, ed. 2, Philadelphia, 1976, J.B. Lippincott Co.

12 Malasanos, L., and others: Health assessment, St. Louis, 1977, The C.V. Mosby Co.

13 Maslow, A.H.: Motivation and personality, ed. 2, New York, 1970, Harper & Row, Publishers, Inc.

14 Masters, W.H., and Johnson, V.E.: Human sexual response, Boston, 1966, Little, Brown & Co.

15 National Commission on Community Health Services: Health is a community affair, Cambridge, Mass., 1967, Harvard University Press.

16 Parsons, T., Bales, R., and Shills, E.A.: Working papers on the theory of action, New York, 1953, The Free Press.

17 Roy, Sr. C.: Introduction to nursing: an adaptation model, Englewood Cliffs, N.J., 1976, Prentice-Hall, Inc.

18 Satir, V.: Peoplemaking, Palo Alto, Calif., 1972, Science and Behavior Books.

19 Shortridge, L.M., and Lee, E.J.: Introduction to nursing practice, New York, 1980, McGraw-Hill Book Co.

20 Stevenson, J.S.: Issues and crises during middlescence, New York, 1977, Appleton-Century-Crofts.

21 Williams, S.R.: Essentials of nutrition and diet therapy, ed. 2, St. Louis, 1978, The C.V. Mosby Co.

22 Yura, H., and Walsh, M.B.: The nursing process, ed. 3, New York, 1978, Appleton-Century-Crofts.

BIBLIOGRAPHY

Bailey, J.T., and Claus, K.E.: Decision making in nursing: tools for change, St. Louis, 1975, The C.V. Mosby Co.

Black, M.: Critical thinking, Englewood Cliffs, N.J., 1952, Prentice-Hall, Inc.

Bloch, D.: Some crucial terms in nursing: what do they mean? Nurs. Outlook **22:**689, 1974.

Burgess, A.W.: Nursing: levels of health intervention, Englewood Cliffs, N.J., 1978, Prentice-Hall, Inc.

Campbell, C.: Nursing diagnosis and intervention in nursing practice, New York, 1979, John Wiley & Sons, Inc.

Ford, J.A.G., Trygstad-Durland, L.N., and Nelms, B.C.: Applied decision making for nurses, St. Louis, 1979, The C.V. Mosby Co.

Mitchell, P.: Concepts basic to nursing, New York, 1973, McGraw-Hill Book Co.

Murray, M.: Fundamentals of nursing, Englewood Cliffs, N.J., 1976, Prentice-Hall, Inc.

The Nursing Theories Conference Group: Nursing theories: a base for professional nursing, Englewood Cliffs, N.J., 1980, Prentice-Hall, Inc.

Rogers, M.E.: An introduction to theoretical basis of nursing, Philadelphia, 1970, F.A. Davis Co.

Schaefer, J.: The interrelatedness of decision making and the nursing process, Am. J. Nurs. **74:**1852, 1974.

Tinkham, C.W., and Voorhies, E.F.: Community health nursing: evolution and process, New York, 1977, Appleton-Century-Crofts.

Nursing diagnosis

PHYLLIS BAKER ANDREWS

GENERAL CONSIDERATIONS
Definition

A nursing diagnosis is a clear, concise, and definitive statement of the client's health status and concerns that can be affected by nursing intervention. It is derived from inferences of assessed validated data and from perceptions. It follows a careful investigation of the data and results in a decision or opinion.

Nursing is not the only profession that makes diagnoses. Workers in other professions and trades, such as auto mechanics, television repairers, social workers, and physicians make diagnoses. Nursing's responsibility is to diagnose human responses to health-related issues and concerns, and the effects of these concerns on activities of daily living.

There are many definitions of nursing diagnosis in nursing literature. Some of the writers who have defined nursing diagnosis are Campbell,[5] Gebbie,[8] Gordon and Sweeney,[11] Little and Carnevali,[15] Mundinger and Jauron,[18] and Yura and Walsh.[26] Their definitions include process, structure, and competency. The First National Conference on the Classification of Nursing Diagnosis[8] (1973) accepted a process definition: nursing diagnosis "is the judgment or conclusion which occurs as a result of nursing assessment." The importance of nursing diagnosis is indicated by the definition of nursing adopted by the American Nurses' Association[2] convention in 1976 and refined in 1980 to read "Nursing is the diagnosis and treatment of human responses to actual or potential health problems."

Nursing diagnosis is probably the least understood, most controversial, and weakest link in the nursing process. It has been identified as an essential component that requires a high level of intellectual skill. It is the basis for planning, intervention, and evaluation of the client's health concerns.

There are several reasons for writing nursing diagnoses. Nursing diagnoses make it possible to give clients comprehensive health care by identifying, validating, and responding to specific health concerns. Nursing diagnoses provide a common language within the nursing profession. Use of a common language enhances communication among peers and other health professionals, improves continuity of care, and represents an organized body of clinical science in nursing. According to Gordon and Sweeney,[11] nursing diagnoses can help formulate expected outcomes in quality assurance, assist

111

in measuring cost effective nursing care, help in making staff assignments, provide the focus of the "clinical science" in nursing education, and constitute the emphasis of clinical nursing research.

Many nurses are hesitant to write nursing diagnoses. They fear the risk of making a judgment that others can read. Some fear ridicule or criticism; others fear making an error or not being "perfect." These fears are usually ill founded, as most peers are willing to participate and contribute assistance if asked. Nurses have been making diagnoses for years by identifying client concerns, but now professionals are being held accountable for their critical thinking and inferences. Only through practice does writing nursing diagnoses become easier. Although most diagnoses reflect a probability rather than a certainty, it is better to state a strong possibility than not to decide anything. Indecision may indicate lack of knowledge, self-confidence, or courage.

This chapter reviews historical developments and discusses misconceptions related to nursing diagnoses. Guidelines are suggested for writing a nursing diagnosis. The last section of the chapter cites nursing diagnoses for the individual, family, and community clients related to frameworks and models.

Historical perspectives
The term "nursing diagnosis" evolved in the 1960s with increased use of the nursing process. The American Nurses' Association[1] included nursing diagnosis as an integral part of the nursing process in the publication of the Generic Standards of Nursing Practice in 1973. Several states also include the term in their recently revised nurse practice acts. It is also included in the revised state board examinations. Nursing diagnoses are being used in studies to determine their feasibility as a means of structuring nursing care and measuring resources in an experimental reimbursement system.[19]

Nursing judgments regarding client concerns have been made for years. Recently nurses began to collaborate in identifying and categorizing these judgments. A national task force of nursing professionals has been working on a typology or taxonomy of nursing diagnoses since 1973, when the First Conference on Nursing Diagnosis[9] was sponsored by St. Louis University. In developing a standard classification system, the Fourth Conference identified approximately 42 diagnostic categories in 1980. These are shown in the list on p. 113. These categories are recognized by nurses from all geographic areas of the United States and Canada as concerns they treat in their clinical nursing practice. Additional work is needed to increase the list and to validate the present list; however, these nursing diagnoses are the beginning of a scientific basis for nursing practice and are the most current and acceptable list.

Accepted nursing diagnoses*

Airway clearance, ineffective
Bowel elimination, alterations in:
    Constipation
    Diarrhea
    Incontinence
Breathing patterns, ineffective
Cardiac output, alterations in: decreased
Comfort, alterations in: pain
Communication, impaired verbal
Coping, ineffective individual
Coping, ineffective family:
    Compromised
    Disabling
Coping, family: potential for growth
Diversional activity, deficit
Fear
Fluid volume deficit:
    Actual
    Potential
Gas exchange, impaired
Grieving:
    Anticipatory
    Dysfunctional
Home maintenance management, impaired
Injury, potential for
Knowledge deficit (specify)
Mobility, impaired physical
Non-compliance (specify)
Nutrition, alterations in:
    Less than body requirements
    More than body requirements
    Potential for more than body requirements
Parenting, alterations in:
    Actual
    Potential
Rape-trauma syndrome
Self-care deficit (specify level: feeding, bathing/hygiene, dressing/grooming,
    toileting)
Self-concept, disturbance in
Sensory perceptual alterations
Sexual dysfunction
Skin integrity, impairment of:
    Actual
    Potential
Sleep pattern disturbance
Spiritual distress (distress of human spirit)
Thought processes, alterations in
Tissue perfusion, alterations in
Urinary elimination, alteration in patterns of
Violence, potential for

---

*From Classifications of nursing diagnosis: procedures of the Fourth National Conference, New York, 1982, McGraw-Hill Book Co.

MISCONCEPTIONS
One of the most frequent problems in accepting the term "nursing diagnosis" is the misunderstanding brought about by confusion with the medical diagnosis. The medical diagnosis identifies and labels the precise pathological disease. It is made to prescribe treatment, to cure the disease, or to reduce the injury. If the disorder cannot be identified, frequently the signs and symptoms are treated. The medical diagnosis describes a disease, syndrome, or specific set of observations that is classified as one of the 999 medical diagnoses listed in the International Classification of Diseases. The nursing diagnosis describes the effects of these symptoms and pathological conditions on the client's activities and life-style. It is the statement of the client's behavioral response to the condition or situation, such as "anxiety related to diagnostic tests" or "inability to perform self-care related to fractured right arm."

The medical diagnosis is an important component of the client's total condition and cannot be ignored. There are independent nursing actions that can be made in response to the medical diagnosis. For example, a medical diagnosis with many nursing implications is diabetes. One nursing diagnosis could be "alterations in the metabolic system related to diabetes." Independent nursing actions include assessment of the client's knowledge of the disease and its complications; the client's compliance with diet, medications, and skin care; and effects on the individual and family life-style and coping mechanisms. After all these areas have been assessed, additional nursing diagnoses may be written, such as "impaired skin integrity of both feet related to lack of knowledge, lack of care, or impaired circulation," and "alterations in nutrition related to inadequate income, lack of knowledge, or eating habits." Another medical diagnosis with many nursing implications is hypertension. The nursing diagnosis may be "alterations in the circulatory system related to hypertension." Independent nursing strategies include observation of extremities for edema, warmth, and color; measurement of the vital signs, pedal pulses, and ankle circumference; assessment of the client's knowledge of hypertension, diet, medication, and exercise; and health teaching. Related nursing diagnoses include "noncompliance with dietary regimen related to lack of knowledge," "noncompliance with medication regimen related to lack of motivation," and "decreased mobility related to edematous extremities."

The nursing diagnosis is not a restatement of the medical diagnosis or the diagnostic test, the medical treatment, or the equipment. The nursing diagnosis reflects the specific effects of the medical diagnosis, the diagnostic test, medical treatment, or equipment on the client and daily living. It includes the client's response to these things. Table 8-1 shows examples of incorrect and correct nursing diagnostic statements.

A nursing diagnosis is not just a single conceptual label such as obesity, immobilization, or constipation. These labels are too general and do not define the specific concern or show necessary relationships that are needed to develop meaningful individualized nursing orders. Examples of more definitive nursing diagnoses are "alterations in nutrition related to eating habits," "impaired mobility related to weakness," and "constipation related to lack of fluids."

Another misconception is that the nursing diagnosis is a statement of the nurse's problem with the client; but it is not a nursing problem or goal.

Table 8-1. Nursing diagnoses in response to medical diagnoses, diagnostic tests, medical treatment, or equipment

Incorrect	Correct
1. Schizophrenia	1. Alterations in identity related to schizophrenia or Difficulty in continuing independent living related to schizophrenia
2. Cardiac catheterization	2. Anxiety related to cardiac catheterization or Fear related to lack of knowledge of cardiac catheterization
3. Radiation therapy	3. Alterations in nutrition (decreased) related to radiation therapy or Depression related to daily radiation treatments
4. Nasogastric tube	4. Impaired skin integrity of nares related to nasogastric tube or Restlessness related to presence of nasogastric tube

"Provision of adequate fluids" is a nursing goal statement, not a nursing diagnosis. Occasionally nurses and clients develop interpersonal or communication conflicts that result in the nurse's labeling the client as "difficult," "demanding," or "impossible." The problem is really the nurse's and may actually interfere with the client's adjustment to the health concern. There is a need to differentiate between the client's situation and coping deficits and the staff's problem in coping with the client. Examples of *incorrect* nursing diagnoses are "uses inappropriate language with staff," "uncooperative," or "constantly complains."

GUIDELINES FOR WRITING A NURSING DIAGNOSIS

These guidelines are a map to help write nursing diagnoses. They are not meant to be the *only* way to do it; they are *one* way to do it. They are also not intended to be a "cookbook" approach. They suggest a path to follow that will help define the client's health status.

There are two categories into which the guidelines are grouped. The first category is process, which provides a method for arriving at the nursing diagnosis. The second category is structure, which clarifies terminology and types of diagnostic statements.

Process guidelines

According to Henderson, the process of determining the nursing diagnosis must include the following elements: a situation with one or more clients; thorough subjective and objective data collection; a nursing conceptual framework; an existing or potential health concern; an appropriate cause, condition, or situation; and a requirement for intervention "within the professional domain of nursing."[14]

The diagnostic process is never complete as long as there is nurse-client contact. Nursing diagnoses made after initial data collection are usually tentative and may require further assessment or validation. As long as the client has a health concern, there will be continued adaptation and change in response to it. The nurse needs to assess these changes and adapt the nursing diagnoses and interventions to them. For example, the nursing diagnosis may change from "anxiety related to impending surgery" to "fear related to the possibility of cancer."

The process of determining a nursing diagnosis includes assessing and analyzing/synthesizing. These process guidelines continue with identifying client concerns, writing the diagnostic statement, validating, and arranging diagnoses according to priority.

The first step in determining a nursing diagnosis is to identify the client's health status and concern. Sometimes there is confusion in differentiating need from concern; needs must be gratified for the normal functioning of an individual. Maslow[16] identified basic needs as physiological, safety, love and belonging, social esteem and recognition, and self-actualization. A concern or problem exists when an individual cannot provide need gratification. According to Bower,[4] "a problem is an interruption in the individual's ability to meet a need; it is a difficulty or perplexity that requires resolution." Rather than stating the individual's nursing diagnosis as "need for sex" or "need for fluid," it could be stated as "sexual deprivation related to debilitated state or medication effects" or "fluid imbalance related to difficulty in swallowing or to diarrhea." An incorrect family diagnosis is "need to improve communication." A correct one is "decreased family communication related to television habits or schedules." An incorrect community diagnosis is "need for citizen participation," which could be stated correctly as "limited citizen participation related to apathy or political control."

There are various types of client concerns that are identified. There are clients with no concerns and those with actual (recognized and unrecognized), potential, or possible concerns.

1. *The client with no concerns:* If the client, with or without a medical diagnosis, is coping adequately and does not perceive any concerns, then the nursing diagnoses are written in relation to maintaining, preserving, or protecting the client's health status. Diagnoses are stated as "maintaining homeostasis or equilibrium" or "maintaining health status." The independent nursing actions include support, praise, encouragement, and providing health information or health alternatives. The nurse's definition of health influences the wording of the diagnostic statement.

2. *The client with actual and recognized concerns:* These concerns are existing conditions. They relate to a medical diagnosis, a situation, or a state. They are stated in terms of the client's response to these factors and can be expressed in relation to a stressor,[15] a deficit,[20] or maladaptive behavior.[22] Examples of nursing diagnoses for individuals are (1) "inadequate bowel elimination related to inactivity or to inadequate fluid intake" and (2) "impaired skin integrity of right foot related to decreased circulation." Sample family diagnoses are (1) "role reversal related to wife's chronic disease" and (2) "decreased

communication related to use of blaming or withdrawal." Community concerns may be stated as (1) "high infant mortality rate related to inadequate prenatal services, inadequate nutrition, or lack of motivation for care in high-risk populations," and (2) "inadequate health services for seniors related to inadequate funds or lack of planning."

3. *The client with an actual but unrecognized concern:* These concerns are existing conditions identified by the nurse but not acknowledged by the client. The client may deny the concern or acknowledge the concern but refuse to do anything about it. Respecting the client's autonomy, the nurse lists the concern on the health status list but notes it as unresolved.

4. *The client with a potential concern:* Potential concerns are those that are high risk or probable. Henderson states that "a potential health problem is the presence of significant risk factors that can be modified to prevent the occurrence of disease or disability."[13] If a client has the medical diagnosis of arthritis but has no existing concerns, the nursing diagnosis should be "potential for alterations in musculoskeletal system related to arthritis." The independent nursing actions would include assessment of mobility and pain, as well as preventive or maintenance nursing actions. Another example is the client who smokes two packages of cigarettes daily. The nursing diagnosis could be "potential for respiratory impairment related to cigarette smoking." The nursing activities then include assessment of the client's knowledge of the effects of smoking and the desire to decrease the habit, as well as the provision of health information. Examples of family nursing diagnoses are "potential for social isolation related to institutionalization" and "potential for decreased communication related to family schedule." A community nursing diagnosis is "potential for impaired health care related to inadequate compensation of health care workers."

5. *The client with a possible concern:* A possible concern is one that has not been verified or validated. The nurse may need more data to clarify the related factors. This is similar to a hypothesis that needs to be accepted or not accepted; it is the nurse's impression, which is a "vague notion or feeling retained from the encounter and [connoting] a tentative conclusion."[17] It may be stated as "impression of confusion: source undetermined" or "possible depression."

6. *The client with strengths:* Most clients have strengths and assets that aid them in coping. Strengths are identified and noted in the conclusion of the analysis/synthesis. They may be used and reinforced in nursing actions. It is difficult to list them as a nursing diagnosis, since they may apply to all the health concerns. Another reason for not listing them as a diagnosis is that nursing plans flow from the list. The plans for each strength would be important to include in health care. Strengths that could be noted are adequate coping mechanisms, numerous situational supports, adequate finances, and thorough knowledge and acceptance of condition. Community strengths include enthusiastic leaders in community, well-organized community, and adequate representation. Family role acceptance and family cohesiveness are examples of family strengths.

The second step is to write a nursing diagnosis. This is a concluding or summary statement regarding each health concern. The structure of the statement is discussed later in this chapter.

The third step is to validate the nursing diagnosis. There are two steps in validating nursing diagnoses. The first relates to the cluster or pattern of signs and symptoms that defines the diagnosis. This validation involves reviewing the data that led to the judgment, and verifying their sufficiency and accuracy. The nurse also evaluates the scientific rationale on which the diagnosis is based to reinforce the reasonable degree of probability.

The second validation is one of the most important aspects of nursing diagnosis and may be the one most frequently omitted. This second phase of validation is collaborating with the client in the confirmation of the nursing diagnosis. Collaboration is an essential component of successful change for three reasons: first, working together is the basis of a trusting relationship, which is more likely to provide accurate and valid data; second, the trusting relationship provides the client with an anchor and support for risking and for changing behaviors. Last, the collaborative relationship indicates mutual influence. According to Orlando,[21] if there is no mutual validation, the nurse is engaging in a nontherapeutic activity.

In presenting the perception and interpretations to the client, one approach is to state something like: "After looking at the information you gave me, it seems to me that there are a few areas we may be able to help you with. You told me that _____ was bothering you. I was wondering if you also saw _____ as something we could work on. Here are some other areas I would like you to tell me about. _____ What do you think about this one?"

The client's acceptance of the diagnostic statements usually indicates mutuality. If the client does not perceive the nursing diagnosis as accurately indicating a health concern, there is no mutuality and even the most comprehensive and sensitive nursing plans will be meaningless. Nursing care cannot exist in a vacuum, striving for written perfection without client participation. When the client refuses to acknowledge an actual health concern, the nurse may record the diagnosis as inactive, which indicates it is still a concern but unacknowledged by the client.

Client involvement from the beginning establishes a participatory relationship and encourages the self-care concept. The only exceptions to this second step of validation would be an emergency or an unconscious client.

The fourth step is to arrange the nursing diagnoses in order of priority. After the client and nurse are in agreement with the list of health concerns, they must rank them according to client need for nursing intervention. Setting priorities provides a logical approach to a multiplicity of concerns and is discussed in the following chapter.

Structure guidelines

The structure of the diagnostic statement is the way the data are translated into words that precisely state the client's situation and health concerns. The guidelines are criteria relating to the format of the diagnostic statement. Guidelines are discussed in terms of clarity (including appropriate use of terms), specificity, descriptive and etiological statements, direction for nursing intervention, implementation, and the health status list.

1. *The nursing diagnosis is concise and clear.* For example, there is no need to write "client" or "patient," as such terms are implicit. Clarity and conciseness facilitate communication among health team members, since a concise, clearly stated diagnosis will be read and understood, as opposed to a lengthy paragraph that takes time to read and unravel. Until a taxonomy is available it will be necessary for nurses to think and communicate concisely without loss of accuracy. Examples of nursing diagnostic categories are given by Campbell,[5] Shortridge and Lee,[24] and the Fourth National Conference on Classification of Nursing Diagnosis (see list on p. 113).

When lists of diagnostic categories are not available, nurses may compose their own nursing diagnostic statements. The following terms are helpful in writing the diagnosis. The client's response to the condition, state, or situation may be expressed as:

Alteration in	Insufficient	Unresolved
Potential for	Inability to	Difficulty in
Impairment of	Failure to	Noncompliance with
Lack of	Interruption of	Nonparticipation in
Inadequate	Depletion of	Inappropriate
Deficit in	Disturbance in	Maintaining
Diminished		Reduced

Adjectives that may be helpful in clarifying are:

Acute	Complete	Minimum
Chronic	Partial	Occasional
Full	Maximum	Sporadic
Intermittent	Mild	Moderate
Severe		

An example of a lengthy and vague nursing diagnosis is "client has open area on foot and complains of pain." This could be restated as "impairment of skin integrity of right small toe" and "pain related to skin impairment of right small toe." Examples of individual, family, and community nursing diagnoses are given later.

2. *The nursing diagnosis is client centered, specific, and accurate.* Client-centered diagnoses are stated in terms of the client's response to intrapersonal, interpersonal, and environmental stressors. The nursing diagnosis is not stated in terms of the environment, such as "television interfering with sleep." A client-centered diagnosis is "diminished sleep related to loud television."

The statement must be a precise identification of the client's actual or potential health concern, rather than a general concept or categorization. This precision is necessary for accurate and appropriate nursing interventions to be planned and implemented. If an incorrect conclusion is stated, the goals, interventions, and evaluation will be inappropriate and ineffective.

3. *The nursing diagnosis may be a descriptive statement.* The descriptive statement is used when there are inadequate data to determine the possible contributing factors or causes. It must be clinically useful and not just a list of signs and symptoms. It is the statement of the client's response to an "actual, or potential disturbance in life processes, patterns, functions or development."[10] Examples of descriptive statements for the individual are "inability to sleep, lack of knowledge of condition, noncompliance with medication regimen, increased alterations in nutrition, lack of self-esteem, and physiological (such as cardiac) crisis." Family descriptive statements are

"family communications deficit, family hostility, and developmental lag." Descriptive community statements are "inadequate funds for health services, inadequate health services, deficient garbage collections, and unresolved anger."

4. *The nursing diagnosis may be expressed as an etiological statement.* This statement is more definitive, including the client response (the descriptive statement) as well as the statement of contributing or influencing factors. The latter is the part in which nursing may intervene to help alleviate or change the client response. This part of the statement indicates the nurse's perception of the probable causative factors and must allow for flexibility and exploration. For example, one health concern may be related to several causative factors, including environmental, sociological, spiritual, physiological, or psychological factors. The nursing diagnosis may be "inability to sleep related to loneliness, fear of impending surgery, noisy environment, and pain."

The descriptive statement is joined to the etiological component by the words "related to," which indicate only relationship; they are not as legally or causally defining as "due to."

5. *The nursing diagnosis provides direction for nursing interventions.* The descriptive statement usually implies the need for additional data and indicates the need for plans to further assess particular areas. The etiological clause is the basis for planning client-centered goals and nursing actions. Nursing strategies will vary according to the etiological factors. The goal is to improve or maintain the client response by applying nursing strategies related to the contributing factors. An example of a nursing diagnosis that provides direction for nursing intervention is "potential for respiratory impairment related to inactivity." The nursing strategies would be methods of increasing the client's activity individualized according to the client's condition, situation, and developmental level.

6. *The nursing diagnosis can be implemented by nursing interventions.* Nursing interventions are activities of health promotion and education, disease prevention, nursing treatment (restoration or maintenance), and referral. The nurse identifies all areas of health concerns, including those for which others' expertise is needed. The independent nursing action for those concerns must be referred to the appropriate resource. For example, if a nursing diagnosis is "anxiety related to inadequate finances," the nursing action is referral of the client to the social worker, welfare department, or Social Security office. Since anxiety can affect the client's ability to respond to nursing interventions for other nursing diagnoses, it must also be considered.

7. *The list of nursing diagnoses reflects the client's current health status.* It is a compilation of client health concerns that is responsive to changing conditions. The list may be called the problem list, but it is not the nursing or medical problem list. It is the *client's* health concern list. The list should include all actual, potential, and possible health concerns. It should include resolved, active, and inactive concerns and provide a capsule view of the client's health status. Anyone who looks at the list should immediately discern a comprehensive thumbnail sketch of the client. It may also include a statement of "incomplete data base" with a listing of categories or patterns still needing initial assessment. The nursing diagnosis of "incomplete data base" meets this criterion; it indicates a concern affecting the client's health

status and allows for comprehensiveness. The client goal is to participate as a partner in providing necessary information. The nursing strategy is to assess or obtain the data.

Another diagnostic statement that is appropriate is in relation to termination or discharge planning. Diagnoses can be stated as "potential for dependency" or "potential for nonacceptance of termination." Plans are then included in the client record and are not forgotten or done at the last minute. This diagnosis can also include plans for establishing trust and other strategies for interpersonal communications with the client.

The next part of the chapter applies these guidelines to individuals, families, and communities, using frameworks and models.

APPLICATION OF MODELS TO NURSING DIAGNOSIS
Individuals

Diagnostic statements are influenced by the assessment tool used, the framework or model applied in assessment or analysis, and the diagnostic classification system. Table 8-2 provides examples of nursing diagnoses for a few categories of theoretical models according to the guidelines. Models identified in the first column are biopsychosocial systems, Henderson's,[13] Maslow's,[16] and crisis.

The second column in the format is used for an adjective to clarify the diagnostic statement.

The third column is the statement of the client's response to the situation, state, or condition. These words usually indicate a change from normal expectations.

The fourth column is the system, category, or function affected by the change. The words in this column depend on the theoretical model used. When conceptual words are used as a client response and clarified by the etiological clause, this column may not be necessary. The response column and the system, category, or function column together form a descriptive nursing diagnostic statement.

The fifth column is the etiological clause in the diagnostic statement. This category may include contributing factors, causes, situation, medical diagnoses, or symptoms. Stressors are identified here.

These examples show nurses how to write their own diagnostic statements. Although this format focuses on the components and terminology, the result is a nursing diagnosis that identifies a pattern and is understandable by other nurses.

Families

Whether nursing diagnoses of the family are stated functionally, structurally, or developmentally depends on the theoretical model used. They may be from one framework exclusively or from a combination. As with nursing diagnoses of individuals, those related to the family may deal with actual or potential dysfunctions or with promoting and maintaining positive family practice.

Major concepts of Beavers' structural family systems theory[3] that may be used as diagnostic categories are family power structure, degree of family individualism, acceptance of separation and loss, perception of reality,

Table 8-2. Nursing diagnoses for individual health concerns based on theoretical models

I Theoretical model	II Description	III Response	IV System, category, or function	V Related to
A. Biopsychosocial systems				
1. Biological	Severe	Impairment of	Integument rt great toe	Ill-fitting shoes or poor circulation
	Acute or chronic	Alterations in	Circulatory system	Hypertension or congestive heart failure
	Temporary, intermittent, or frequent	Noncompliance with	Hypertension regimen or diabetic diet	Lack of knowledge, motivation, or finances
	Temporary or chronic	Inadequate	Oxygenation	Obstructed airway, emphysema, or low hemoglobin
		Impaired	Vision	Myopia or cataracts
	Mild or generalized	Weakness of	Musculoskeletal system	Prolonged bed rest or multiple sclerosis
	Potential for	Alterations in	Oral integrity	Poor hygiene or edentulous condition
	Possible	Increased	Susceptibility to infection	Source undetermined
2. Psychological	Anticipatory or acute	Anxiety		Loss of job or spouse, or hospitalization
		Anger		Loss of body part, alteration in body image, or hospitalization
	Acute or chronic	Depression		Loss of body functioning or financial problems
		Fear		Impending surgery, inadequate knowledge, or previous hospitalization
	Delayed	Grieving		Inadequate leisure, acute illness, or loss of job
	Temporary	Alterations in identity		Edema from rhinoplasty, or recent divorce
3. Sociological		Inadequate	Income	Lack of knowledge of resources, insufficient job training, minimum budgeting knowledge, or chronic illness
		Impaired	Written communication	Lack of education or motivation or untreated hearing deficit

Table 8-2. Nursing diagnoses for individual health concerns based on theoretical models—cont'd

I Theoretical model	II Description	III Response	IV System, category, or function	V Related to
		Decreased	Socialization	Withdrawal, physical impairment, or language barrier
4. Spiritual		Alterations in	Faith	Death of mother or child or loss of job
	Complete	Hopelessness		Terminal illness or lack of control of body functions
		Diminished	Self-worth	Physical abuse, mental illness, or recent divorce
5. Developmental (Erikson)		Lack of	Trust	Multiple caregivers or frequent moves
		Avoidance of	Intimacy	Change of body image, terminal illness, or alcoholism
		Lack of	Initiative	Peer association or position in family
B. Henderson		Alteration in	Breathing	Obstruction or pneumonia
		Alteration in	Nutrition (eating and drinking)	Eating habits, lack of motivation to change, or lack of knowledge
		Inadequate	Bowel elimination	Lack of exercise, inadequate fluids, or lack of fiber in diet
		Impaired	Mobility (movement and posture)	Fractured rt leg, stroke, or weakness
		Inadequate	Sleep and rest	Anxiety of hospitalization, pain, or hunger
		Inability to	Dress and undress	Confusion, burns on left arm or hand, or disinterest
C. Maslow		Decreased	Self-esteem	Divorce or unemployment
		Decreased	Safety	Throw rugs or inadequate heating or lighting
D. Crisis		Inadequate	Coping mechanisms	Stressors of accident
		Alteration in	Perceptions	Hysteria, cultural influences, or lack of information
		Decreased	Situational supports	Unemployment or lack of family, friends, income, or insurance

and affect. Examples of a few of these categories are given in Table 8-3. Beavers' complete model is in Appendix C.

Functional areas for assessing families are family conflict or harmony, bonding, decision making and task allocation, roles and rules, and communication. Satir[23] is an example of a theorist in this category. Her four assessment areas are communication, rules, self-worth, and societal linkages. Examples of three of these areas are given in Table 8-3.

Duvall[6] and Stevenson[25] are examples of developmental theorists who list tasks and stages that can be used as diagnostic categories.

Hart and Herriott's systems theory categories[12] are processes of adaptation to the environment, integration of the parts, and decisions regarding the first two processes. Other theoretical models may also be applied to this format for writing nursing diagnoses.

The purpose in writing family nursing diagnoses is to help the family achieve or maintain equilibrium and functioning.

Table 8-3. Nursing diagnoses for families based on theoretical models

I Theoretical model	II Description	III Response	IV System, category, or function	V Related to
A. Beavers		Alteration in	Family power structure	Illness of breadwinner or inadequate problem solving
	Minimum	Acceptance of	Family individualism	Anger or beliefs
		Inadequate	Acceptance of loss	Youngest child leaving home, or divorce
B. Satir		Inflexible	Rules	Misunderstanding or authoritarian values
		Decreased	Self-worth	Inability to share feelings, altered body image, or confusion from medication
		Inadequate	Recreation	Closed societal links
C. Functional		Decreased	Bonding	Prematurity of infant, cesarean section, or absence of role model
	Potential for	Impaired	Parenting	Inconsistent discipline or lack of knowledge
		Reversal of	Roles	Chronic illness or absence of extended family
	Temporary	Alteration in	Family transaction	Recent divorce, death of spouse, decreased communication, or discovery of homosexuality
D. Developmental		Inability to accomplish	Stage-specific developmental tasks	Dysfunctional communication or lack of knowledge
E. Systems		Deprivation of	System input	Institutionalization
		Impaired	Decision making	Confusion from medication or crisis
		Decreased	Safety in environment	Physical abuse or alcoholic mate
		Maintaining	Equilibrium	Adequate coping or open communications

Communities   Community nursing diagnoses may be stated according to structure or process. Structural diagnoses include those related to demographic characteristics, aggregates (groups with similar characteristics), or systems. Systems include sociocultural, political, recreational, housing and transportation, educational, religious, environmental, economic, and health care systems. Process diagnoses include communication, decision making, participation, and leadership. Examples are given for structure and process in Table 8-4.

Nurses can identify health concerns and affect change in many areas with intervention usually pertaining to health maintenance, health promotion, health education, consultation, and disease prevention. Many community health nurses are also using the concepts of partnership, participation, and community development. It is the nurse's responsibility to work with the community in identifying the concerns and resources.

Table 8-4. Nursing diagnoses for community health concerns based on theoretical models

I Theoretical model	II Description	III Response	IV System, category, or function	V Related to
A. Structure				
1. Demographic characteristics		Increased	Respiratory diseases	Air pollution, overcrowded conditions, or inadequate ventilation
		Increased	Dog bites	Packs of roaming dogs, inadequate code enforcement, or inadequate personnel and facilities
		Increased	Infant mortality rate	Cause unknown, inadequate nutrition, or increased teenage pregnancies
2. Aggregates		Inadequate	Prenatal facilities	Lack of funds or planning
		Increased	Lead poisoning in toddlers	Substandard housing or lack of prevention or knowledge
		Increased	Dental caries in school-age children	Poor hygiene or lack of knowledge
		Increased	Child abuse	Cause unknown
		Inadequate	Programs for substance abuse	Lack of funds or priority
		Lack of	Genetic counseling	Lack of personnel or knowledge of need
		Lack of	Gerontological services	Lack of planning or funds
3. Systems		Substandard	Housing	Economic recession, lack of funds for improvement, or high unemployment
		Inadequate	Transportation	Lack of state or federal funds or interest
		Decreased maintenance of	Sewers	Lack of information, personnel or leadership
B. Process		Decreased	Communication	Political associations, sectionalism, or anger
		Lack of	Neighborhood participation	Apathy, lack of information, or cultural beliefs

SUMMARY   The nursing diagnosis is a clear, concise, definitive statement of the client's health status and concerns. The concern identified must be able to be affected by nursing interventions. Nursing diagnoses also reflect the client's response to medical diagnoses.

Nursing diagnoses may be stated in descriptive or etiological statements; the etiological form is preferred, since it gives direction for nursing plans.

REFERENCES

1 American Nurses' Association: Standards: nursing practice, Kansas City, 1973, The Association.
2 American Nurses' Association: Nursing: a social policy statement, ANA Publication Code: NP-63, 35M, Dec. 1980.
3 Beavers, W.R.: Psychotherapy and growth: a family systems perspective, New York, 1977, Brunner/Mazel, Inc.
4 Bower, F.L.: Nursing process: roles and functions of the nurse. In Bower, F.L., and Bevis, E.O.: Fundamentals of nursing practice: concepts, roles, and functions, St. Louis, 1979, The C.V. Mosby Co.
5 Campbell, C.: Nursing diagnosis and intervention in nursing practice, New York, 1978, John Wiley & Sons.
6 Duvall, E.M.: Marriage and family development, ed. 5, Philadelphia, 1977, J.B. Lippincott Co.
7 Erikson, E.H.: Childhood and society, New York, 1950, W.W. Norton & Co., Inc.
8 Gebbie, K.M., and Lavin, M.A., editors: Classification of nursing diagnosis, St. Louis, 1975, The C.V. Mosby Co.
9 Gebbie, K.M.: Development of a taxonomy of nursing diagnosis. In Walter, J.B., and others: Dynamics of problem-oriented approaches: patient care and documentation, Philadelphia, 1976, J.B. Lippincott Co.
10 Gordon, M.: Nursing diagnoses and the diagnostic process, Am. J. Nurs. **76:**1298, 1976.
11 Gordon, M., and Sweeney, M.A.: Methodological problems and issues in identifying and standardizing nursing diagnoses, Adv. Nurs. Sci. **2:**1, 1979.
12 Hart, S.K., and Herriott, P.R.: Components of practice. In Hall, J., and Weaver, B., editors: Distributive nursing practice: a systems approach to community health, Philadelphia, 1977, J.B. Lippincott Co.
13 Henderson, B.: Nursing diagnosis: theory and practice, Adv. Nurs. Sci. **1:**75, 1978.
14 Henderson, V.: The nature of nursing: a definition and its implication for practice, research and education, New York, 1966, Macmillan, Inc.
15 Little, D., and Carnevali, D.: The diagnostic statement: the problem defined. In Walter, J.B., and others: Dynamics of problem-oriented approaches: patient care and documentation, Philadelphia, 1976, J.B. Lippincott Co.
16 Maslow, A.H.: Motivation and personality, New York, 1970, Harper & Row, Publishers, Inc.
17 Mitchell, P.: Concepts basic to nursing, New York, 1977, McGraw-Hill Book Co.
18 Mundinger, M.O., and Jauron, G.D.: Developing a nursing diagnosis, Nurs. Outlook **23:**94, 1975.
19 N.J. works toward new reimbursement model, Nurs. Outlook **28:**652, 1980.
20 Orem, D.E.: Nursing: concepts of practice, New York, 1980, McGraw-Hill Book Co.
21 Orlando, I.J.: The dynamic nurse-patient relationship, New York, 1961, G.P. Putnam's Sons.
22 Roy, Sr. C.: Introduction to nursing: an adaptation model, Englewood Cliffs, N.J., 1976, Prentice-Hall, Inc.
23 Satir, V.: Peoplemaking, Palo Alto, Calif., 1972, Science and Behavior Books.
24 Shortridge, L.M., and Lee, E.J.: Introduction to nursing practice, New York, 1980, McGraw-Hill Book Co.
25 Stevenson, J.S.: Issues and crises during middlescence, New York, 1977, Appleton-Century-Crofts.
26 Yura, H., and Walsh, M.B.: The nursing process, ed. 3, New York, 1978, Appleton-Century-Crofts.

BIBLIOGRAPHY

Abdellah, F., and others: Patient-centered approaches to nursing, New York, 1961, Macmillan, Inc.
Aspinall, M.J.: Nursing diagnosis: the weak link, Nurs. Outlook **24:**433, 1976.
Avant, K.: Nursing diagnosis: maternal attachment, Adv. Nurs. Sci. **2:**45,Oct. 1979.
Block, D.: Some crucial terms in nursing: what do they mean? Nurs. Outlook **22:**689, 1974.
Carrieri, V.K., and Sitzman, J.: Components of the nursing process, Nurs. Clin. North Am. **6:**115, 1971.
Clinical panel: Dorothy del Bueno, Barbara Demers, Charlotte Isler, Carol Kushner, Mary R. Price, Peggy Stevens, Margaret Van Meter, Karin Williamson: What's your diagnosis? R.N. **43:**63, 1980.
Fromer, M.J.: Community health care and the nursing process, St. Louis, 1979, The C.V. Mosby Co.
Gebbie, K., and Lavin, M.A.: Classifying nursing diagnosis, Am. J. Nurs. **74:**250, 1974.
Hymovich, D.P., and Barnard, M.U.: Family health care, New York, 1979, McGraw-Hill Book Co.
Kelly, K.: Clinical inference in nursing, Nurs. Res. **15:**23, 1966.

Knight, J.H.: Applying nursing process in the community, Nurs. Outlook **22:**711, 1974.

MacVicar, M.G., and Archbold, P.: A framework for family assessment in chronic illness, Nurs. Forum **15:**180, 1976.

Murray, M.: Fundamentals of nursing, Englewood Cliffs, N.J., 1976, Prentice-Hall, Inc.

The Nursing Theories Conference Group: Nursing theories: the base for professional nursing practice, Englewood Cliffs, N.J., 1980, Prentice-Hall, Inc.

Price, M.R.: Nursing diagnosis: making a concept come alive, Am. J. Nurs. **80:**668, 1980.

Rogers, M.E.: An introduction to the theoretical basis of nursing, Philadelphia, 1970, F.A. Davis Co.

Rothberg, J.S.: Why nursing diagnosis? Am. J. Nurs. **67:**1040, 1967.

Ryan, B.J.: Nursing care plans: a systems approach to developing criteria for planned evaluation, J. Nurs. Adm. **3:**50, 1973.

Shoemaker, J.: How nursing diagnosis helps focus your care, R.N., August, 1979, pp. 56-61.

Thomas, M.D., and Coombs, R.P.: Nursing diagnosis: process and decision. In Marriner, A.: The nursing process: a scientific approach to nursing care, ed. 2, St. Louis, 1979, The C.V. Mosby Co.

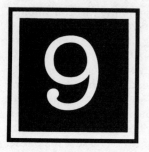

Goals and objectives

PAULA J. CHRISTENSEN

The planning phase of the nursing process is the act of determining what can be done to assist the client in restoring, maintaining, or promoting health. This phase involves judging priorities, establishing goals, developing objectives, and identifying specific strategies or techniques for implementation.

Traditionally, planning for client care was done *by* the nurse *for* the client. It was usually based on the medical diagnoses. The client was a passive person and followed what the nurse recommended without question. The client viewed the physician and nurse as "knowing best" and accepted treatment accordingly. As clients' knowledge of health and illness increased and nurses assumed responsibility and accountability for care given, the traditional bases for care were no longer valid. Nurses assess their clients' health status and formulate individual plans for care *with* their clients. Plans still reflect the client's medical concerns, but now equally address other health concerns, such as anxiety, economic difficulties, family conflict, environment, and socialization.

The planning phase is based on assessment and diagnosis of the client's health status and concerns. The planning phase is initiated after a comprehensive assessment and judgment of the client's concerns.

This chapter discusses the first three elements of the planning phase: judging priorities, establishing goals, and developing objectives. All elements of the planning phase are necessary to give direction for quality nursing care.

**JUDGING
PRIORITIES**

The process of judging priorities begins with the list of nursing diagnoses. Arranging these diagnoses in priority involves deciding a preferential order in the concerns of the client. Making this choice, however, does not mean that one concern must be totally resolved before another is considered. Usually several diagnoses are focused on concurrently.

The act of choosing one diagnosis as the most important is based on several factors. Diagnoses that involve life-threatening concerns, such as severe impairment or loss of cardiac and circulatory, respiratory, or neurological function, should be considered first. An actual or imminent life-threatening situation takes precedence over an actual or potential health-threatening situation.

Judging priorities is facilitated through the use of theories, concepts, models, and principles. One model often used to evaluate the relative priority of diagnoses is that by Maslow,[8] who speaks of what prevents people from self-actualization, or being. He identifies deficit (basic) needs that all people share: air, food, safety, and love. Growth needs are those that are not necessary for sustaining life; for example, self-esteem and self-actualization. Deficit needs are more important than growth needs; the individual must have deficit needs met before focusing on growth needs. Using this model with a client who has both deficit and growth needs unmet, the nurse would first develop and implement plans for the unmet deficit needs.

Physiological principles are also helpful in judging concerns of clients. Consideration of these principles guides the nurse in giving immediate attention to life-threatening concerns. Actual or potential health-threatening concerns are dealt with once biophysical health is stabilized. For example:

1. Knowledge that increased intracranial pressure can lead to changes in vital signs and to possible brain damage takes precedence over needs for personal hygiene.
2. Knowledge that high blood pressure poses a threat to circulatory and cardiac status takes precedence over learning needs about borderline diabetes.

Isolated data and patterns of data give cues to the nurse that aid in judging precedence. Examples of isolated cues that lead to immediate plans and interventions include vital sign readings significantly above or below general or client norms and sudden changes in client behavior. Examples of patterns of data observed over time that indicate current needs for plans and interventions include gradual changes in vital signs and subtle changes in the client's relatedness to others.

The client's involvement is also an important part of arranging concerns in order of importance. Since one of nursing's goals is to work mutually with clients, the nurse must consider the client's (1) understanding of the current situation, including values, thoughts, and feelings about resolving health concerns; (2) general state of health; and (3) ability to solve problems. The client must gain adequate knowledge regarding the current situation and problem solving to make informed decisions. The nurse is responsible for assessing the client's knowledge level and implementing accordingly. The client's values, thoughts, and feelings about resolving health concerns have an impact on the client's cooperation with certain interventions. For example, a client smokes two packs of cigarettes per day and knows the health-related hazards but chooses to continue to smoke. Plans to help the client quit smoking would be unsuccessful as long as the client did not *value* health promotion or *thought* that no number of facts would influence the decision to smoke. The client's general state of health influences the client's ability to be involved in judging health concerns. A client who is psychotic or unconscious will have little involvement compared with the client who is awake and oriented. In the former situation, the client and client's family should be informed of the priorities set by the nurse. If it is appropriate, the client's family is included in setting priorities for concerns.

Table 9-1. Example of appropriate sequence of priorities

Nursing diagnosis	Sequence of priorities	Rationale
Inadequate nutrition related to lack of knowledge of balanced diet	3	Latent health concern that can be dealt with somewhat concurrently with 2
Alteration in circulatory status related to high blood pressure	1	Most life-threatening concern at this time
Increased anxiety related to first pregnancy and fear of the unknown	2	Threatening mental health and potential threat to physical health

Specific guidelines for setting priorities for health concerns and goals are given below:

1. Actual or imminent life-threatening concerns.
2. Actual or potential health-threatening concerns.
3. Client's perception of the health concerns.

Table 9-1 provides an example of how to judge the priority of health concerns, using this rationale.

ESTABLISHING GOALS

Once priorities have been determined, the nurse establishes goals. Goals set the direction to alleviate the concern indicated by the diagnosis. A goal is a statement describing a broad or abstract intent, state, or condition that reflects an outcome.[6] If the nursing diagnoses reflect specific client concerns, then only one goal is needed per diagnosis. Diagnoses stated in broad terms require more than one goal.

Examples

Nursing diagnosis (specific): Inadequate knowledge of healthful exericse.

Goal: The client will increase knowledge of healthful exercises within 1 month.

Nursing diagnosis (general): Alteration in metabolism related to diabetes.

Goal: The client will stabilize metabolism within 1 week.

Goal: The client will decrease susceptibility to altered metabolism within 1 month.

Nature of goals

The nature of the goal depends on the diagnosis; goals reflect health restoration, maintenance, or promotion. *Health restoration* goals are appropriate when a client's internal or external resources are inadequate or diminished.

Example

Nursing diagnosis: Depleted nutritional state related to anorexia.

Goal: The client will develop an adequate nutritional state within 1 month.

Health maintenance goals are appropriate when the client should increase the existing internal or external resources or continue using those resources.

Example

Nursing diagnosis: Decreased use of open communication skills related to busy schedule.

Goal: The client will increase use of open communication skills within 2 weeks.

Health promotion goals reflect a desire to function at a higher level of health, to grow beyond merely maintaining health.

Example

Nursing diagnosis: Increased concern regarding lack of knowledge of parenting skills for adolescence.

Goal: The client will increase knowledge of parenting skills for adolescence within 3 weeks.

Differences and similarities between client goals and nurse-expected goals must be considered. The nurse may have a greater knowledge base than the client, which could help the client understand the nature of the identified diagnoses; the client can help the nurse understand the client's own concerns and motivations. The nurse is responsible for establishing congruent nurse-client goals.

Relationship to theories, concepts, models, and principles

The approaches used in the analysis/synthesis of data provide direction for establishing goals. They describe health norms and determine the rationale for the goal.

Satir,[9] for example, discusses healthy communication, describing the concepts of functional and dysfunctional communication in detail. Such information as this assists the nurse in establishing a goal for a client with dysfunctional communication.

Example

Nursing diagnosis: Dysfunctional interpersonal communication.

Goal: The client will develop functional communication with family within 3 months.

Immobility is an example of a physiological concept that gives direction to goal development. Most nursing texts elaborate on the concept of immobility and its effects on body functions as well as on the psyche. That baseline of knowledge about the concept guides the client and nurse in planning to lessen the effects of immobility.

Example

Nursing diagnosis: Potential hazards of immobility related to recent surgery.

Goal: The client will decrease susceptibility to hazards of immobility within 6 days.

Any reliable source that describes norms of behavior can be used to assist the nurse in developing client goals. Table 9-2 gives example of goals for

Table 9-2. Examples of goals with different theoretical bases

Client	Nursing diagnoses	Goals	Theoretical bases
Individual	Inadequate exercise related to low motivation	The client will exercise adequately within 1 month	Diekelmann[2]
Family	Lack of individuation related to lack of awareness of need	The family will develop individuation of family members within 6 months	Lewis and Beavers[5]
Community	Inadequate decision making related to use of coercion	The client will develop a democratic form of decision making within 1 year	Hart and Herriott[3]

different clients and shows how a variety of sources are used in establishing the goals.

DEVELOPING OBJECTIVES

Once goals are established for the appropriate diagnoses, objectives are developed to specify client performances or behavior. An objective describes an intended *result* of a particular action, not the process of the action itself.[7] Usually three to six objectives are needed for each goal.

Robert Mager[7] states three reasons that are applicable to nursing for developing objectives. First, objectives *give direction* for selecting or designing nursing strategies and orders. Next, a properly stated objective *implies the content* of, potential materials needed for, and method of the strategy or order. Last, objectives provide a *means* for the nurse and client to *organize effort*. Objectives are therefore useful tools in the design, implementation, and evaluation of client care.

Characteristics of objectives

Three characteristics of objectives that help communicate their intent have been identified as performance, conditions, and criterion.[7]

Performance

A performance is any activity engaged in by the client. It can be an activity that is directly observable or not directly observable but assessable. Overt performances are those that can be visibly or audibly directly observed. Verbs that indicate overt performances, which are directly observable behaviors, include recite, list, sort, verbalize, demonstrate, name, select, and state.

Covert performances are mental, invisible, cognitive, or internal, but have a direct way of being assessed. Verbs that indicate covert performances include identify, solve, use, compare, and determine. Whenever the performance stated in an objective is covert (such as identify), an indicator behavior (such as state) needs to be added to the objective or clarified in the evaluation phase of the nursing process as a criteria statement (see Chapter 11).

	Examples
Overt verb:	The client will demonstrate proper insulin administration according to the American Diabetic Association within 1 week.
Covert verb (with indicator behavior):	The client will identify (state) three complications of bed rest within 2 days.

The objective should create a picture of what is expected of the client, communicating its intent to the client and those reading it. Each important outcome or performance needs to be written in a separate objective. Therefore, each objective should contain only one performance verb.

Conditions

An objective may indicate the conditions under which the client is to complete the performance. Conditions may include the experiences the client is expected to have had before completing the objective, the resources available for use during the performance of the objective, or the environmental conditions under which the client will carry out the performance.[4] The conditions need to be included if they are essential to meeting the objective. Conditions need not be included if the performance clearly states what is expected.

	Example
Objective with clear expectations:	The client will state three barriers to effective communication within 1 week.

Below are examples of the three ways that conditions may be stated in an objective.

Condition	**Example**
1. The experiences before completing the objective.	*After attending* two group sessions of diabetic classes, the client will name two major types of diabetes.
2. The resources available during the performance of the objective.	*Given a menu* of a variety of foods, the client will circle the foods composing a 2000-calorie intake for one day.
3. The environmental conditions during the performance.	*When at home* the client will maintain a 2000-calorie diet according to the American Diabetic Association.

Criterion

The criterion is the standard by which a performance is evaluated.[7] Criteria within the objective may be stated in one of four ways:
1. *Speed:* Set a time limit that is reasonable given the client's health state and the client's and nurse's capabilities and limitations.
2. *Accuracy:* Identify a specific degree of performance quantitatively.
3. *Quality:* Indicate the standard that is expected in terms of given acceptable procedures.
4. *Criterion-referenced:* Use a book, pamphlet, or other resources as a guide. Criteria give direction to plans for meeting the objective. They also provide a measure to evaluate the achievement of the objective.

Below are examples of the four ways of stating criteria in objectives.

Criterion	Example
1. Speed	The client will name four complications of bed rest *within 3 days*.
2. Accuracy	The client will list *four out of five* symptoms of high blood sugar.
3. Quality	The client will catheterize self using *aseptic technique*.
4. Criterion-referenced	The client will describe (state) three components of the self-breast exam *according to* the American Cancer Society.

Domains of objectives

Objectives can be classified into three domains, which provide direction for selecting the strategies and orders. The three identified domains are cognitive, affective, and psychomotor.[1] *Cognitive* objectives are associated with changes in knowledge or intellectual abilities and skills; *affective* with changes in interests, attitudes, values, or feelings; and *psychomotor* with developing the ability to perform a manipulative or motor skill. After objectives are developed, the nurse identifies which domain each belongs in. This identification gives direction to selecting strategies and orders, such as teaching and learning (cognitive), demonstration and practice (psychomotor), or therapeutic communication (affective). Below are lists of verbs that represent the three domains.

Psychomotor	Affective	Cognitive
Administer	Listen	Inform
Demonstrate	Touch	Tell
Practice	Relate	Explore
Show	Ignore	Discuss
Assist	Regard	List
Inject	Share	Evaluate

More than one domain may be involved in the achievement of one objective or goal. Below are examples of objectives in three domains meeting one goal.

Nursing diagnosis:	Inadequate nutrition.
Goal:	The client will develop adequate nutrition intake following the recommended daily allowances of the four basic food groups within 3 weeks.
Objectives:	1. The client will state the four food groups and recommended servings within 3 days (cognitive).
	2. The client will identify (state) the importance of a balanced diet within 1 week (affective and cognitive).
	3. The client will incorporate the recommended American Diabetic Association diet into eating patterns within 2 weeks (psychomotor and cognitive).

Relationship to theories, concepts, models, and principles

The specific performances included in objectives are based on the same theories, concepts, models, and principles used in establishing goals. When objectives are developed, an in-depth understanding of the approach is necessary. The following example shows how the nurse's knowledge of the concept of immobility, related principles, hazards, and ways to prevent complications influences the development of objectives.

Nursing diagnosis: Increased susceptibility to hazards of immobility related to decreased mobility.

Goal: The client will decrease susceptibility to hazards of immobility while hospitalized.

Objectives:
1. The client will participate in four preventive measures four times a day within 1 day.
2. The client will verbalize four hazards of immobility within 2 days.
3. The client will identify (state) one way to decrease susceptibility to each hazard within 2 days.
4. The client will incorporate at least three preventive measures into daily routine four times a day within 4 days on client's own volition.

The specifics of range of motion, skin care, deep breathing, and turning could be included in the objectives themselves or referred to in the criteria statement of the evaluation phase.

Below is another example of a goal and objectives, based on Satir's model.[9] This example demonstrates the use of specific information about the importance of functional communication, barriers to it, and techniques of it. The examples of objectives show varying degrees of specificity.

Nursing diagnosis: Dysfunctional communication related to the use of blaming and projecting.

Goal: The client will increase functional communication within 1 month.

Objectives:
1. The client will describe why functional communication is important, according to Satir, within 2 days.
2. The client will state three barriers to functional communication within 1 week.
3. The client will identify (state) two verbal and three nonverbal functional communication techniques within 1 week.
4. The client will use three functional communication techniques while talking to family within 3 weeks.

GUIDELINES FOR WRITING GOALS AND OBJECTIVES

1. *Goals and objectives are client focused and reflect mutuality with the client.* The goals and objectives need to be worded in *client* terms, not nurse terms. Beginning each goal with the terms "the client will" facilitates its being client focused. Mutuality is attained through communication with the client and involved persons about identified health concerns and strengths. The nurse needs to discuss nursing diagnoses and related goals with the client to determine if the client also recognizes the strength or concern and if the client is willing to direct energy toward supporting, diminishing, or alleviating the conditions identified by the diagnoses.

Situations do arise when individual clients are unable to agree with goals and objectives because of an alteration in health status or age. The nurse is then responsible for including the client's family in decision making. The goals and objectives still need to be worded in client terms.

Example

Nursing diagnosis:	Decreased consciousness related to brain damage.
Goal:	The client will maintain or improve present level of consciousness indefinitely.
Objectives:	1. The client will participate in the assessment of level of consciousness daily.
	2. The client will accept auditory and tactile stimuli provided by the nurse at least every 2 hours.

2. *Goals are appropriate to their respective diagnosis, and objectives are appropriate to their respective goal.* The nursing diagnosis is the basis for each respective goal. Therefore, goals should clearly relate to the nursing diagnosis. Completion of the goal should support the strengths or diminish or alleviate the concerns identified by the nursing diagnosis.

Example

Nursing diagnosis:	Decreased nutrition related to inadequate food intake.
Goal:	The client will develop adequate nutritional intake within 1 month (goal clearly relates to diagnosis).
Goal:	The client will learn about adequate nutrition within 1 month (goal has limited relationship to diagnosis).

Learning about adequate nutrition does not necessarily lead to better nutrition. The first goal clearly states that the client will develop adequate nutritional intake. The goal is the basis for its respective objectives. Achievement of the objectives should be sufficient for the attainment of the goal.

3. *Goals and objectives are realistic, reflecting the capabilities and limitations of the client.* The client must perceive the goals and objectives as realistic in order to be motivated to achieve them. Being realistic involves developing goals and objectives that reflect the client's capabilities and limitations of internal and external resources. Examples of external resources to consider include time, money, family support, social agencies, and equipment. Examples of internal resources to consider include biophysical status, mental health, and coping mechanisms.

Since health is a relative term, not all goals will reflect a maximum health state. Each client has an optimum potential for health that should be reflected in the goals.

Example

1. *Client:*   40-year-old recently divorced male.
   Nursing diagnosis: Lack of socialization related to recent divorce.
   Goal: The client will develop a social support system within 6 months.

2. *Client:*   20-year-old single, mentally retarded female.
   Nursing diagnosis: Lack of socialization related to overprotection from family.
   Goal: The client will increase participation in activities involving people other than family within 3 months.

4. *Goals include broad or abstract indicators of performance.* Since a goal is broad or abstract by nature, the use of verbs such as improve, decrease, increase, maintain, promote, develop, and restore is appropriate. General criteria can be included in a goal to give more direction to further plans for implementation.

Example

Nursing diagnosis: Decrease in neighborhood safety.

Goal: The client will increase neighborhood safety within 6 months (goal without general criterion).

Goal: The client will improve neighborhood safety by increasing street lights and patrols within 6 months (goal with general criterion).

Either way is correct; both are client focused and give a general direction for further plans.

Another aspect of stating goals is their reference to a time element. Because of their breadth, goals tend to be relatively long term. The length of time is determined by considering the client's health status and available resources. The resources include both the client's and nurse's capabilities and limitations.

5. *Objectives include specific indicators of performance.* Objectives need to be more specific than goals, referring to observable and measurable performances to meet the goal. Each objective should include the person, the performance, and a specific criterion. Conditions may be added to clarify the meaning. The performance needs to be assessable, and the criterion for assessment can be stated in terms of time, accuracy, quality, or reference. Time is usually included in all objectives, since it gives the client and nurse a guideline for pacing activities realistically. Refer to p. 134 for examples of objectives with a variety of specific performances and criteria. Additional criteria statements may be cited in the evaluation component of the nursing process.

6. *Objectives are numbered in the appropriate sequence to achieve the goal.* Proper sequencing, or time ordering, of objectives gives direction and understanding of what is expected. Communicating this sequencing helps the client recognize success in movement toward goal achievement.

SUMMARY

The planning phase of the nursing process is based on a sound assessment of the client's health status. Judging priorities, establishing goals, and developing objectives constitute the first three elements of planning for implementation. Goals are broad, abstract, and long term in nature, but objectives reflect specific performances and a shorter time for achievement.

Each element of planning is based on the nurse's knowledge of theories, concepts, models, and principles. Any source describing norms of behavior can serve as a reference for planning. Guidelines for writing goals and objectives include their being client focused and mutual, appropriate to the diagnoses and goals, and realistic; they should indicate performances the client needs to exhibit to achieve the goal and objective.

REFERENCES

1 Bloom, B., editor: Taxonomy of educational objectives: the classification of educational goals, handbooks I and II, New York, 1956, David McKay Co., Inc.
2 Diekelmann, N.: Primary health care of the well adult, New York, 1977, McGraw-Hill Book Co.
3 Hart, S.K., and Herriott, P.R.: Components of practice. In Hall, J., and Weaver, B., editors: Distributive nursing practice: a systems approach to community health, Philadelphia, 1977, J.B. Lippincott Co.
4 Jones, P., and Oertel, W.: Developing patient teaching objectives and techniques: a self-instructional program, Nurse Educ. **2:**3, Sept.-Oct. 1977.
5 Lewis, J.M., and Beavers, W.R.: No single thread: psychological health in family systems, New York, 1976, Brunner/Mazel, Inc.
6 Mager, R.: Goal analysis, Belmont, Calif., 1972, Fearon-Pitman Publishers, Inc.
7 Mager, R.: Preparing instructional objectives, ed. 2, Belmont, Calif., 1975, Fearon-Pitman Publishers, Inc.
8 Maslow, A.H.: Toward a psychology of being, New York, 1968, D. Van Nostrand Co.
9 Satir, V.: Conjoint family therapy, rev. ed., Palo Alto, Calif., 1967, Science and Behavior Books.

BIBLIOGRAPHY

Atkinson, L., and Murray, M.: Understanding the nursing process, New York, 1980, Macmillan, Inc.
Conley, V.: Curriculum and instruction in nursing, Boston, 1973, Little, Brown & Co.
Curtin, L.: Six step model for analyzing ethical problems. In Freebairn, J., and Gwinup, K.: Ethics, values, and health, Irvine, Calif., 1980, Concept Media.
Little, D., and Carnevali, D.: Nursing care planning, ed. 2, New York, 1976, J.B. Lippincott Co.
Maslow, A.H.: Motivation and personality, ed. 2, New York, 1970, Harper & Row, Publishers, Inc.
Peplau, H.E.: Interpersonal relations in nursing, New York, 1952, G.P. Putnam's Sons.
Reilly, D.: Behavioral objectives in nursing: evaluation in nursing, ed. 2, New York, 1980, Appleton-Century-Crofts.

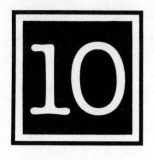

Plans, implementation, and scientific rationale

JOANNE RENAUD CROSS
GRACE MURABITO THOMAS

GENERAL CONSIDERATIONS

The nursing plan for implementation is viewed as the core or focus of the nursing process: what the nursing process is really all about. The plan directs nursing action, which assists the client in relieving a concern or meeting a need.

Historically, the community health nurse was accustomed to writing a logical plan of care for the individual, family, or community client. Given the nurse's independent practice and case load strategies, it was a logical sequence of events to carefully plan for consistency and continuity of care.

Ann Leino[3] was one of the first nurse authors to publish an article describing a method for planning client care. According to her, the information is recorded on 2×8-inch file cards under the headings of problems and approaches. Eventually plans were translated and became the Kardex. Eleanor Lambertsen[2] identified the plan as a means of communication within the team concept that was evaluated daily and revised as the need arose.

This chapter deals specifically with the nursing care plan and the guidelines for writing these plans. Before we proceed to the specifics of the plan, some broad concepts inherent in developing the plan are considered. These elements are the what, why, who, and how of planning.

BROAD CONCEPTS IN PLANNING

What is a plan?

The nursing plan begins with the nursing diagnostic statement and progresses to the goal and objectives. Once these are identified, unique nursing actions—nursing orders—are selected to help the client achieve the goals and objectives. This is the core of nursing management, the independent prescriptive role of writing nursing orders. The term "nursing order" is used synonymously with nursing plan in this text.

Nursing orders are different from "standard care" orders, such as routine procedures or common orders for all clients. Nursing orders are individually tailored to meet the specific needs of the client; the standard care plans are useful as a point of reference. Nursing care plans are not delegated medical orders or functions. Although nurses are still involved in implementing these functions and orders, the nursing order is separate and is explicitly a nursing action. The nursing order complements the medical order with related activities such as teaching, discussion, demonstration, or methods of illness prevention and health maintenance or promotion.

Example

Medical diagnosis:	Chronic obstructive lung disease.
Medical order:	Withhold all cigarettes from client; no smoking.
Nursing diagnosis:	Alterations in oxygen transport related to cigarette smoking.
Goal:	The client will improve oxygen transport within 2 weeks.
Objective 1:	The client will verbalize three harmful effects of cigarette smoking by *(specific date).*
Plan:	1. The nurse and client will explore the client's knowledge of the harmful effects of smoking.
	2. The nurse will use value clarification techniques to help the client express feelings about the cessation of smoking.
	3. The nurse will teach basic knowledge regarding the harmful effects of smoking, using pamphlets from the American Heart Association, pictures, and charts.
Objective 2:	The client will refrain from smoking beginning *(specific date).*
Plan:	1. Behavior modification strategies will be used to assist the client in refraining from smoking; a reward system will be mutually established.
	2. The client will discuss the feasibility of enrolling in a "smoke enders" program.

Why develop a nursing care plan?

A well-written plan gives direction, guidance, and meaning to nursing care. It is a central source of information to all who are involved in the care of a given client. It is the primary means of communicating, synchronizing, and organizing the actions of *all* nursing staff. The nursing care plan provides for *continuity of care* through primary nurses, constantly changing nursing staff, shift reports, and nursing rounds.

Current updating of nursing actions with new assessment data assures continuous quality of care. Adequate communication of this information, in both written and verbal form, is a mark of the professional nurse.

Who develops the plan?

The nurse and client work together to form the plan of care. The client, the family, and significant others bring their uniqueness to the situation. The nurse brings knowledge and expertise of nursing care to the client. Together, sharing this information, the client and nurse optimize the writing of the plan.

The principal facilitators in developing the plan are the primary nurse, the client, the client's family, other nurses involved in direct care, and selected resource people. Complex client concerns require additional assistance. Resource people include the clinical nurse specialist, dietitian, physical therapist, occupational therapist, social worker, chaplain, and physician. An interdisciplinary health team conference is a vehicle for getting resource assistance. Frequently the exercise of the group process produces highly creative and diverse solutions to assist clients in achieving health goals.

After conferring, consulting, and communicating with others, the primary nurse is responsible for developing and overseeing the final plan. This is the unique independent function of the professional nurse that demonstrates accountability to the client and to the profession.

Nursing care plans written with the client take on the quality of client power. The probability of the plan's success is enhanced when the client and family are consulted and take an active role. Client concerns often require some change of behavior for family members. For example, the obese client who needs to change eating habits needs family support regarding eating habits and food preparation.

How is the nursing plan developed?

The client-family situation is complex. Therefore, nursing decisions and plans are based on the nurse's awareness of the client's and family's knowledge, abilities, and skills. The nurse uses this information to consider many variables in client situations. For example, when the nurse is working with a recently diagnosed diabetic client, the nursing order may read: "Teach the client the American Diabetic Association diabetic diet and the method of administering insulin." Before implementing this order, the nurse considers the following variables:

1. Are there ethnic or cultural attitudes influencing the client's eating habits?
2. What are the client's attitudes toward health care in general?
3. To what extent does the client know about the diabetic condition?
4. To what extent does the nurse know teaching and learning principles?
5. Can the client learn about the diabetic condition in 2 days, or will it require 2 weeks?
6. Is the client capable of administering the insulin or would it be preferable for another member of the family to do this?
7. Does the client have the necessary equipment and other resources for diet and medications?
8. Does the client have support persons to assist with this diet and medication administration?
9. Does the client need to be referred to a community health nurse for follow-up in diet and medications?

A variety of possible plans are developed after these variables have been considered. The nurse chooses the most appropriate plan for the client situation. There are many ways to achieve the same objectives and goal.

The nurse's philosophy about individuals, health, society, and nursing directly influences the plans. Nurses' beliefs affect the choice of theoretical approaches. Awareness of beliefs facilitates careful selection of appropriate approaches and plans for client care.

GUIDELINES FOR WRITING PLANS FOR IMPLEMENTATION

The following guidelines are suggested for writing plans for implementation.

1. *The plan is dated and contains the signature of the responsible nurse.* The date is important, since the nursing orders are reviewed and updated periodically. The date the plan is written is used as a point of reference for evaluation and future planning. The time span for reviewing the plan depends on the client, setting, and specific circumstances.

The signature of the nurse writing the plan demonstrates accountability—both ethical and legal. This accountability is not only to the client and family for nursing care but also to the profession, since the effectiveness of nursing actions can be evaluated through review.

2. *Implementation strategies and nursing orders are appropriate to their respective objectives.* A nursing strategy is defined as an overall plan or tactic that serves as a guide for individual nursing orders. Clearly defined objectives provide a sound basis for selecting nursing strategies. Strategies are derived from theories, frameworks, models, and principles—any source that provides a plan or tactic for working with clients. Examples of strategies include role play, problem solving, basic nursing care, and therapeutic use of self.

Selection of nursing strategies and orders is based on the domain of the objective. Strategies in the cognitive domain include teaching and learning, problem solving, and decision making. The psychomotor domain requires such strategies as demonstration, practice, and teaching and learning. Strategies included for the affective domain are role playing, therapeutic use of self, and value clarification. The successful outcome of nursing actions depends on selecting strategies relevent to their respective objectives.

Plans should be flexible and subject to revision if the approaches are to be effective. However, the rightness or wrongness of any nursing action is not determined solely by the apparent client outcome. The objectives and nursing action might be sound, but, since the client's uniqueness is the variable in a given situation, the nursing action may need to be revised or altered. There are many ways to achieve the same goal.

3. *Plans are written in terms of client and nursing behaviors sufficient to achieve goals and objectives.* Nursing plans define the types of nurse and client actions. In some plans, such as crutch walking, the client takes over the action completely; in other plans the nurse assumes the dominant role. The ultimate goal, however, is for the client to do as much as possible to maintain a sense of personal control over the situation.

On an average, two to six plans are needed to achieve a given objective. The actions indicated are directly related to the objective.

4. *The nursing plans are stated in specific terms, giving direction to the behavior of the nurse and client.* The nursing orders need to be specific. What does the client need to do to achieve the objectives and goal? What does the nurse need to do? Who is the person best suited to assist the client? For example, if the statement of the objective directs the client to ambulate four times daily and the goal is to decrease the hazards of immobility, where do the client and nurse begin? Considering the assessment data and nursing diagnosis, do they begin with range of motion exercises, passive or active? When is the best time to do this? How much can the client tolerate? For how many

days should this be done? How far should the client ambulate the first time? How should the client be prepared for the activity? What does the nurse need to do to prepare for the activity? Is the assistance of a third person needed to ambulate the client? All these aspects must be considered in planning. Nursing orders are frequently limited in scope in that they are not precise and specific as to what the implementor should do.

Nursing plans begin with action verbs indicating the behavior that the implementation will involve. The words are specific, and modifiers may be used to make them even more precise. Some examples of specific plans include the following:

1. *Ask* the client to *list* three hazards.
2. *Encourage* the client to *ambulate* three times daily.
3. *Demonstrate* the use of insulin equipment in giving injections within the next 2 days.
4. *Role play* the use of assertiveness with the client.

Using the word "teach" is not sufficient. The writer should state exactly how one teaches and use such words as demonstrate or discuss, or provide practice experiences.

Resources and references used in implementing nursing actions need to be specific and appropriate to the objectives set forth. Books or pamphlets appropriate to the comprehension level of the client are to be used; if the client cannot read, filmstrips, films, pictures, videotapes, or other means can be used. For the client who speaks a foreign language, other sources need to be used. When the nurse is working with a client from a different culture, various factors must be considered to achieve the objectives.

For example, consider teaching a client about basic nutrition. First, the nurse would assess the client's knowledge of nutrition and daily diet. The latter can be assessed by asking the client to write a 3-day nutritional recall of what has been eaten. If the client cannot or does not wish to write it, a verbal recall can be done. The nurse and client would then consider the nutritional needs of the client according to age, height, weight, exercise patterns, and prescribed dietary patterns. Food budgets, cultural food preferences, and consumer shopping for nutritional foods would be discussed. The last step involves having the client plan nutritional menus for 1 or 2 days.

The time element is another aspect to be considered. It is stated in relation to:

Precise hourly time, such as 9 AM or 9 PM.

Specific nursing actions, such as when to give a back massage or morning care.

Specific client response, such as when the client becomes agitated or the client's temperature rises above 102 degrees.[4]

Client's preference, such as choice of time for bath.

5. *The plan includes preventive, promotional, and rehabilitative aspects of care.* All three aspects of care—prevention, promotion, and rehabilitation—are included in the plans for each client. The client's general state of health, identified health concerns and strengths, and the situation dictate which aspect is the focus. At times, all three aspects are dealt with concurrently. The following are examples of preventive, promotional, and rehabilitative nursing actions:

Examples

Preventive	Turn client every 2 hours during the day and night, maintaining proper body alignment of the client.
Promotional	Teach client basic nutrition patterns, explaining the basic food groups with the use of pamphlets and pictures; use the dietician or nutritionist as a resource person.
Rehabilitative	Assist client with range of motion exercises for the affected right leg and hand every 2 hours during the day; maintain the limb in a position of use and in good alignment during the night by using pillows and splints.

6. *The nursing plan includes collaborating and coordinating activities.* Collaboration and coordination are essential components of nursing leadership that are intrinsic to the nursing care plan. With whom do you need to collaborate to assist the client in achieving the objective: the physical therapist, nutritionist, community health nurse, or agency that can supply information, materials, finances, consultation, equipment, or appliances to the client?

Coordination and collaboration begin the first day, when the client and nurse enter into a contract for care. These activities must be thoughtfully planned. For instance, a referral to the community health nurse is appropriate for a client who lives alone and has had a stroke. This referral should be initiated and facilitated by the nurse well before the day the client will be discharged.

7. *The plans are placed in an appropriate sequential order based on priority.* The nurse needs to establish the sequence of events in order to achieve the objective. What is the most important action to take first? When the objectives have been arranged in order of priority, the nursing orders should follow accordingly.

Some strategies provide a specific sequence of steps. For example, the problem-solving strategy has a defined sequence. The strategy of therapeutic use of self stresses the importance of gaining rapport before dealing with certain issues with clients. The following is an example of a family situation with specific nursing orders in the appropriate sequence:

Example

Nursing diagnosis:	Maternal overprotection of child, resulting in the child's overdependence.
Goal:	The client (mother) will promote the child's independent behaviors within 1 month.
Objective:	The mother will encourage her child to dress herself by April 18.

Plan	**Rationale for priority**
1. The nurse will explore the mother's feelings about her child doing things for herself (child's general dependent behavior) by April 5.	The nurse must first reach the feeling level of the mother and assess her awareness of the situation.[7]
2. The nurse and mother will discuss the developmental needs of a 4-year-old child by April 8.	The nurse supplements the mother's knowledge before determining which behaviors to change.[8]

Plan	Rationale for priority
3. The mother will decide on the method to help her child become independent by April 10.	The nurse and client establish the plan before implementing it.[4]
4. The nurse will assist the mother in setting up a realistic time schedule for the child's dressing of herself, allowing for frustrations and obstacles, by April 10.	
5. The nurse and mother will explore the mother's feelings toward her child's progress in dressing herself by April 17.	Evaluation of changes occurs after the plans have been implemented.[8]

8. *The plan incorporates the autonomy and individuality of the client.* The plan is individually tailored to the unique characteristics of the client. Autonomy and individuality can be encouraged by giving the client the choice in setting the times for care as well as in selecting the methods to be used. For instance, if the client had a sleepless night, the morning care could be postponed. When it is appropriate, the client can decide how far to ambulate, or choose between having warm milk at bedtime to promote sleep and taking a sleeping medication. The client should have as much control of the plan as possible, since people tend to lose control over what happens to them in health care settings. Control by the client is important to preserve a sense of power, to maintain self-esteem, and to prevent regression.

9. *Plans are kept current and revised and include alternate plans when indicated.* For a plan to remain current, it must be flexible. The nurse must modify goals and approaches as situations change. The client's situation may change from moment to moment or from day to day or may remain the same for weeks, months, or longer. Current plans only describe what is happening with the client at a given moment. Frequent assessments are necessary and the plan should be revised as needed.

10. *Plans for the client's future are included.* The two major concepts in the area of future planning are the termination of the nurse-client relationship and discharge. The nurse-client relationship terminates when the client no longer needs professional nursing care. The last phase of the interpersonal process is resolution.[7] The client's needs have been met by the collaborative efforts of the nurse and client, but dependency needs continue on a psychological level even when the physiological needs have been met. The final resolution may be difficult for both the client and nurse if this phase is not successfully completed.

Plans for termination begin with the initial contact between the nurse and client. The first step clarifies the length of time the nurse will be with the client. The client is kept informed about the number of meetings or visits remaining. The final step of the termination plan is an evaluation of the professional relationship by both the client and nurse. If it is necessary, a referral to another nurse or agency for follow-up is part of the termination plan.

Discharge planning is broad in scope, including an educational process for both the client and the client's family and frequently a referral to an outside agency. Education includes providing information about diet, activity, medications, and treatments. Discharge planning and teaching begin during the hospital stay in an environment conducive to learning. They should not be postponed until the day the client is going home.

IMPLEMENTATION OF THE NURSING PLAN

Implementation is the execution of the nursing plan. The nurse considers three major phases when implementing the nursing order: preparation, implementation itself, and post-implementation.

Preparation consists of the nurse's being aware of the nursing orders; having the knowledge to implement them; being cognizant of the legal and ethical aspects; and knowing the possible side effects and complications, as well as what technical skills and resources are needed. Preparation also includes arranging a suitable environment in which the client and nurse may implement the plan. A quiet environment free of distractions enhances learning.

The physical and psychological comfort of the client is the main concern of the nurse during the implementation of the plan. Excellence, safety, and competence are the criteria the nurse uses while performing the nursing interventions.

During the post-implementation phase, the nurse's actions and the client's reactions are communicated to other health team members through recording them in the client's record. The client is left in a comfortable, safe environment, and resources are returned to their original places.

Evaluation is the follow-up step of the post-implementation phase. The effectiveness of the strategies used and the achievement of the objectives and goals are evaluated.

SCIENTIFIC RATIONALE

Knowledge is the basis for prescribing and implementing nursing orders. A scientific rationale describes and explains the basis for nursing orders. For example, consider the scientific rationale relevant to the following questions:

Why do we restrict fluids at certain times for clients who have problems of the circulatory or excretory system?

Why should the nurse assess learning needs before teaching?

Why must clients learn to take their pulses before leaving the hospital for home if they will be taking digoxin at home?

Why do we encourage clients to cough to loosen bronchial secretions if we know that deep breathing will produce coughing?

Why do we avoid arguing with a delusional client?

The rationale in each case is based on theories, models, frameworks, and scientific principles from nursing, the natural and behavioral sciences, and the humanities. The principle, concept, or theory that supports each step of the plan is stated.

The rationale for the steps of the plan is usually not written into the nursing orders, but it must be known by the nurse. In some instances the rationale is written into the plan to ensure effective communication. For example, if a client is asked to change a complicated dressing alone, it may be necessary to include a written rationale. Otherwise, another care provider may do it for the client, not realizing that the client needs to learn how to change the dressing alone.

The following guidelines are suggested for writing a scientific rationale:

1. *The scientific rationale addresses the identified topic and strategy and the individuality of the client and family.*
   a. *Topic* refers to the content of the plan or nursing order, such as nutrition, personal hygiene, exercise, communication, family planning, values, and assertiveness; and their appropriate theory base. Updated readings and research are valuable sources for the rationale.
   b. *Strategy* specifies the methods through which the implementation is accomplished, such as demonstration, discussion, or practice. The rationale centers on the theories, conceptual frameworks, and other knowledge needed by the nurse for successful implementation. For example, if the client is learning about a new medication, the teaching and learning principles require active involvement and participation by the learner. Research may also be used to provide rationale for new approaches.
   c. *Individuality* reflects the life-style and the developmental, sociocultural, biophysical, spiritual, and psychological aspects of the client. For example, a young child facing surgery may apply a dressing to a doll's abdomen as psychological preparation for the child's abdominal surgery.
2. *The scientific rationale cites appropriate research findings and current literature.*

Research findings are a scientific basis for nursing actions. Which approach is best for a specific nursing diagnosis and the ensuing goals and objectives? For example, nurses have done research on different ways decubitus ulcers can be healed; the use of such nursing research studies is a guide to planning care. Other sources to be used include interviews with experts, textbooks, journal articles, and reference books. Any reliable writings or persons may be considered appropriate. The resource is cited for each supporting scientific rationale.

Following are three examples of scientific rationale for plans concerning an individual client, a family client, and a community client.

Example of an individual plan and scientific rationale

Situation: The client is a 75-year-old woman with decreased vision who lives alone in her apartment. The client and nurse agree that a need exists to increase the safety of the client in her home because of potential hazards in the environment.

Nursing diagnosis: Decreased safety in the home related to sensory (visual) deprivation.

Goal   Client will increase the level of safety in her home.

Objective   Client will verbalize three ways to increase her safety by *(specific date).*

Plan	**Rationale**
1 The client and nurse will walk together through the client's home to identify the safety hazards.	Effective learning requires active participation by the learner (teaching and learning *strategy* by Pohl).[8]
	Since the client has decreased vision, safety hazards need to be identified *(topic).*
2 The nurse and client will discuss the hazard of throw rugs.	Older adults are at high risk for falls *(individuality).*[10]
3 The nurse and client will discuss the needs related to hazards involved in taking a bath.	Participation by the learner enhances learning *(strategy).*[8]
There is a need for a nonslip mat in the tub.	Older adults are at high risk for falls *(individuality).*
4 The nurse and client will discuss the importance of keeping a flashlight at the bedside in case the client wakes at night to use the bathroom.	Many accidents occur at night when the elderly person wakes up and moves in the dark *(topic).* Concept development aids learning *(strategy).*[8] Older persons' eyes adapt to darkness less rapidly *(individuality).*[10]
5 The nurse and client will discuss the importance of keeping a list of legible emergency numbers by the phone: physician, ambulance, neighbors, and relatives.	Immediate accessibility of phone numbers aids in decreasing the time needed to obtain help *(topic).*[10] Recent memory may be altered with age *(individuality).*[10]

(More objectives are needed to achieve the goal.)

Example of a family plan and scientific rationale

Situation: This family is an extended one, with various members living in three different homes on the same street. Family members feel responsible for the welfare of other members. One member is elderly and has diabetes. The diabetic client is able to give herself insulin, but the nurse, on assessing the situation, learned that the client had been giving herself insulin in the thighs only. The nurse recognized the need for family members to learn about and use other areas appropriate for insulin injections.

Nursing diagnosis: Inadequate knowledge of insulin injection sites.

Goal   The family will demonstrate increased knowledge of insulin injection sites *(specific date).*

Objective 1   The family members will verbalize three appropriate sites for insulin administration for the diabetic client by *(specific date).*

Plan	Rationale
1 The family will state the present injection site by *(specific date).*	New learning is based on previous knowledge and experience.[8] It is necessary to learn what the family knows and proceed from its current knowledge to new knowledge *(strategy).*
2 The nurse will discuss with family reasons for rotating insulin injection sites by *(specific date).*	Development of concepts is a part of learning.[8] Insulin, if given in the same site over a period of time, causes fibrosis and scarring and increases lipotropic tissue. This decreases the absorption of insulin *(topic).*[12]
3 The nurse will discuss with the family alternate sites for injections and show charts and pictures of alternate injection sites.	Teaching requires effective communication *(strategy).*[8] The use of charts and pictures aids in communicating what is being taught.

Objective 2   Family members will demonstrate administration of insulin at various sites by *(specific date).*

Plan	Rationale
1 The family members will demonstrate on each other the present insulin injection method without puncturing the skin by *(specific date).*	Effective learning requires active participation by the learner *(strategy).*[8] The family members' knowledge of procedures assists the client *(topic).*
2 The nurse will demonstrate other sites for insulin injection: abdomen, arms, and buttocks.	Learning occurs through imitation *(strategy).*[8] (Individuality not directly addressed)

**Example of a community plan
and scientific rationale**

Situation: The school nurse discerned that a group of third graders had inadequate nutrition. When the nurse asked the students what they ate for breakfast, some said "nothing," and others identified foods that did not provide adequate nutrition according to the American Dietetic Association. The third graders wanted to learn about the basic four food groups and learn to use them in their daily breakfast.

Nursing diagnosis: Inadequate knowledge of the basic four food groups, leading to an inadequate breakfast.

Goal	The third graders will increase their knowledge of the basic four food groups and improve nutritional intake at breakfast.
Objective 1	The third graders will identify the four basic food groups.

Plan	**Rationale**
1 The nurse will assess the students' knowledge of the food groups.	Learning is based on previous knowledge *(strategy).*[8]
2 The students and nurse will discuss the need for the four food groups for growth.	The American Dietetic Association recommends minimum daily requirements in the four basic food groups as needed for growth *(topic).*[13]
3 The nurse will use charts for teaching the four food groups.	Audiovisual aids enhance learning *(strategy).*[9]
	Age-appropriate materials facilitate learning *(individuality).*[9]

Objective 2	The third graders will identify their own individual nutritional needs.

Plan	**Rationale**
1 Each student will write a 3-day nutritional recall.	Active participation enhances learning *(strategy).*[5]
2 The students will compare their own nutritional recalls with the daily nutritional needs of a third grader.	Analysis of food habits increases knowledge of adequate nutritional intake, which promotes growth and development *(topic).*[13]
	Nutritional needs vary according to different age groups *(individuality).*[13]

Objective 3 The third graders will plan a balanced breakfast including the basic four food groups.

Plan	Rationale
1 The students will verbalize what they could eat for a nutritional breakfast.	Discussion reinforces learning *(strategy).*[8]
2 Students will write four different menus for breakfast.	Planning a nutritional breakfast increases knowledge *(topic).*[13]

Objective 4 The third graders will prepare a balanced breakfast with the help of an adult at home.

Plan	Rationale
1 The nurse will send a letter to the parents asking for their participation in the project.	Active participation will enhance learning *(strategy).*[8]
	Collaboration with parents will make the project more effective *(topic).*[1]
	The third grader is a member of a family *(individuality).*[5]
2 The student will prepare a balanced breakfast at home.	Active participation enhances learning *(strategy).*[8]
	A nutritional breakfast provides energy for the morning *(topic).*[11]

Objective 5 Each third grader will eat a nutritious breakfast for 1 week, keeping a list of what was eaten each day.

Plan	Rationale
1 Each student will list what was eaten.	Evaluation is an integral part of learning *(strategy).*[8]
2 Each student will bring the list to school for a group discussion.	Evaluation of a nutritious breakfast increases learning *(topic).*[13]
	Discussion reinforces learning *(strategy).*[8]
	School-age children strive for approval and are interested in learning *(topic).*[6]

SUMMARY

The plan for implementation communicates the nursing orders to other health team members. Based on theories, concepts, and scientific knowledge, plans are developed with the client. They are based on assessment data, analysis, nursing diagnosis, goals, and objectives. The client's individuality gives direction to the plan. Suitable strategies are selected to achieve the objectives and goals. Nursing orders or actions are stated specifically as to *who* does *what* and *when* it is done. These nursing orders give direction to the nurse and the client. Preventive, promotional, and rehabilitative aspects of client health care guide development of the plan. Establishing priorities for nursing actions are included, along with revisions and alternate plans. Collaboration and coordination are written into the nursing orders. Written communication and implementation of the nursing orders are essential. The final steps of the plan include implementation and evaluation. When these steps are performed, the client is ensured quality nursing care.

REFERENCES

1 Hall, J.E., and Weaver, B.: Distributive nursing practice: a systems approach to community health, Philadelphia, 1977, J.B. Lippincott Co.
2 Lambertssen, E.C.: Nursing team, organization and functioning, New York, 1953, Teachers College, Columbia University.
3 Leino, A.: Planning patient-centered care, Am. J. Nurs. **52:**324, 1952.
4 Little, D.E., and Carnevali, D.L.: Nursing care planning, Philadelphia, 1976, J.B. Lippincott Co.
5 Murray, R.B., and Zentner, J.P.: Nursing assessment and health promotion through the life span, ed. 2, Englewood Cliffs, N.J., 1979, Prentice-Hall, Inc.
6 Murray, R.B., and Zentner, J.P.: Nursing concepts for health promotion, ed. 2, Englewood Cliffs, N.J., 1979, Prentice-Hall, Inc.
7 Peplau, H.E.: Interpersonal relations in nursing, New York, 1952, G.P. Putnam's Sons.
8 Pohl, M.L.: The teaching function of the nursing practitioner, ed. 2, Dubuque, Iowa, 1973, Wm C. Brown Co., Publishers.
9 Redman, B.K.: The process of patient teaching in nursing, ed. 4, St. Louis, 1980, The C.V. Mosby Co.
10 Reinhardt, A.M., and Quinn, M.D., editors: Curent practice in gerontological nursing, vol. 1, St. Louis, 1979, The C.V. Mosby Co.
11 Waechter, E.H., and Blake, F.G.: Nursing care of children, ed. 9, Philadelphia, 1976, J.B. Lippincott Co.
12 Watson, J.E.: Medical-surgical nursing and related physiology, Philadelphia, 1979, W.B. Saunders Co.
13 Williams, S.R.: Essentials of nutrition and diet therapy, ed. 2, St. Louis, 1978, The C.V. Mosby Co.

BIBLIOGRAPHY

Bloom, B.S., editor: Taxonomy of educational objectives: the classification of educational goals, handbooks I and II, New York, 1956, David McKay Co., Inc.
Carlson, S.: Practical approach to the nursing process, Am. J. Nurs. **72:**1589, 1972.
Cornell, S., and Carrick, A.G.: Computerized schedules and care plans, Nurs. Outlook **21:**781, 1973.
Forman, M.: Building a better nursing care plan, Am. J. Nurs. **79:**1086, 1979.
Jones, P., and Oertel, W.: Developing patient teaching objectives and techniques, Nurse Educator **77:**3, Sept.-Oct. 1977.
Kramer, M.: Standard 4: nursing care plans . . . power to the patient, J. Nurs. Adm. **2:**29, Sept.-Oct. 1972.
La Monica, E.L.: The nursing process: a humanistic approach, Reading, Mass., 1979, Addison-Wesley Publishing Co., Inc.
Lewis, L.: Planning patient care, ed. 2, Dubuque, Iowa, 1976, Wm. C. Brown Co., Publishers.
Mager, R.S.: Preparing instructional objectives, Belmont, Calif., 1975, Fearon-Pitman Publishers, Inc.
McCloskey, J.C.: The problem-oriented record vs the nursing care plan: a proposal, Nurs. Outlook **23:**493, 1975.
The Nursing Theories Conference Group: Nursing theories: the base for professional nursing practice, Englewood Cliffs, N.J., 1980, Prentice-Hall, Inc.
Standevan, M.: The relevant "who" of problem solving, Nurs. Forum **10:**166, 1971.
Stevens, B.J.: Why won't nurses write nursing care plans? J. Nurs. Adm. **2:**6, 1972.
Stryker, R.: Rehabilitative aspects of acute and chronic nursing care, Philadelphia, 1977, W.B. Saunders Co.
Stuart, M.: The nursing care plan: a communication system that really works, Nurs. 78 **78:**28, Aug. 1978.
Wagner, B.M.: Care plans, right, reasonable and reachable, Am. J. Nurs. **69:**986, 1969.
Yura, H., and Walsh, M.B.: The nursing process, ed. 3, New York, 1978, Appleton-Century-Crofts.

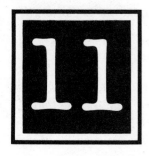

Nursing evaluation

JANET W. GRIFFITH

JANET W. GRIFFITH

GENERAL CONSIDERATIONS

Evaluation is a planned, systematic comparison of the client's health status with defined objectives and goals. It is an ongoing, deliberate activity involving the client, nurse, and other health care team members. It requires a knowledge of health, pathophysiology, and evaluation strategies.

Evaluation serves several purposes. One major purpose is to determine the client's progress in meeting stated goals. Evaluation judges the effectiveness of the nursing plans, strategies, and care.

Evaluation is frequently the most neglected part of the nursing process. Nursing literature is confusing and describes evaluation in many different ways. Ideally, evaluation is an integral part of each component of the nursing process, beginning with the initial assessment. The client's initial assessment is later compared with present behavioral patterns to determine progress. The goals and objectives, formulated in the planning stage, serve as the evaluation standards against which the client's progress is to be measured. During implementation, the nurse appraises the client's response to nursing actions and decides whether the plans are assisting the client's progress. Considering the client's response, the nurse may reorder, modify, maintain, or change priorities in the care plan.

Evaluation examines such questions as: Was the health care effective? Were the goals and objectives met to the degree specified? Were the changes in the client's behavior in the direction expected? If so, which nursing strategies were effective? If not, what was lacking in the nursing care? By measuring the client's progress toward meeting the objectives, the nurse judges the effectiveness of nursing actions; thus nurses are able to judge the quality of their care and determine ways to improve it. This demonstrates accountability for their actions. Accountability implies responsibility for one's behavior; it requires the ability to define, explain, and measure the results of nursing actions. Evaluation identifies those effective nursing strategies and may promote nursing research.

This chapter begins with a brief history of developments in the concept of evaluation. Different aspects of evaluation are discussed, such as structure, process, and outcome. Establishing criteria and standards is explained, and the general characteristics of evaluation are described. Last, guidelines and examples for implementing evaluation are presented.

153

HISTORICAL PERSPECTIVES

In the last two decades, evaluation of health care delivery has changed hands and focus. These changes were sparked by the concerns of consumers and the government over increasing costs and inadequate services. In health care agencies client evaluation was formerly the prerogative of physicians. With new legislation and interest among all health care providers, evaluation is now performed by each profession. Recently the federal government created professional standard review organizations to monitor costs of health services, and the Joint Commission on the Accreditation of Hospitals[4] developed guidelines to evaluate hospital services.

Traditionally nurses were evaluated by their supervisors. Characteristics such as clinical skills, organization, leadership, dependability, and punctuality were judged. These evaluations did not consider the effectiveness of nursing care or improvement in the client's health status. As the responsibility for evaluation was dispersed among health care professionals and agencies, nurses recognized the need to change their focus and improve their methods. Currently, professional nurses are establishing standards of quality care and measuring their ability to meet those standards. This involves evaluating delivery of nursing care to both individual clients and agencies. Agency evaluation is usually called quality assurance and may involve nursing audits with standard guidelines.

Evaluation of nursing care is a complex task, since it is extremely difficult to separate the unique contributions of nurses to client care from the overlapping functions of other team members. This difficulty in distinguishing nurses' unique activities makes it hard to evaluate the results of nursing actions. The activities unique to nursing need to be identified and the results of nursing interventions evaluated. These are problems the profession must continue to address.

FORMS OF EVALUATION

Evaluation may be conceptualized in three forms: structure, process, and outcome. Process and outcome evaluation can both be subdivided into two categories, concurrent (present) and retrospective (past), as shown in Table 11-1. Each form will be discussed separately.

Structure

The focus of structure evaluation is on the physical facilities, equipment, and organizational pattern of the agency. Examples of structure evaluation are the nursing audit of the Association of Operating Room Nurses and the Joint Commission on the Accreditation of Hospitals[5] form. Most hospitals have established guidelines for evaluation of structure.

Process

Process evaluation focuses on the activities of the nurse. The nurses' activities are judged by observing the nurse's performance, asking clients what the nurse did, or reviewing the nurse's notes in the chart. This form of evaluation, concentrating on whether procedures are properly performed, asks such questions as: Does the nurse identify the client when giving medications? Is the consent form signed before surgery? Are procedures explained to the client? Standards for evaluating the quality of nursing care have been developed but require further refinement.

Concurrent process evaluation examines nursing performance when it takes place. Examples include judging the nurse's ability to teach insulin administration and noting if neurological checks are performed accurately and on time. The Slater Nursing Competencies Rating Scale[7] and the Quality Patient Care Scale[8] are examples of tools for concurrent process evaluation. Also, the chart may be reviewed for evidence of appropriate nursing actions while the client is receiving the nurse's care.

Table 11-1. Evaluation forms

Structure	Process	Outcome
Purpose		
Structure evaluation measures the existence and adequacy of the facilities, equipment, procedures, policies, and staffing to meet the client's needs	Process evaluation measures the adequacy of the nurse's actions and activities in implementing each component of the nursing process	Outcome evaluation measures the changes in the client's behavior in comparison with the expected response or the client's written goals and objectives
Tools or instruments		
Joint Commission on the Accreditation of Hospitals (JCAH) form	Slater Nursing Competencies Rating Scale	Wisconsin system JCAH performance evaluation procedure (PEP) partially
Association of Operating Room Nurses nursing audit	Quality Patient Care Scale Nursing Audit	
Sources of data		
Procedure manuals	*Concurrent*	*Concurrent*
Policy statements	Nurse demonstrates knowledge and performance of skills	Client demonstrates new knowledge, skills, and physiological and psychosocial improvement in health status
Position descriptions		
Nursing care plans		
Orientation plans and in-service programs	Chart contains evidence of nursing actions performed	
Staff educational level		
Facilities and equipment available	*Retrospective*	*Retrospective*
Charting and Kardex	Chart cites nursing procedures implemented, such as checking of vital signs and teaching	Chart cites evidence of changes in client's behavior, skills, and knowledge

Table 11-2. Methods of process and outcome evaluation

Process (evaluation of nurse)	Outcome (evaluation of client)
Concurrent	
Client: Ask the client about the actions performed by the nurse. *Nurse:* Observe the nurse administering care, teaching, and examining client. *Chart:* Audit the client's chart for documentation of appropriate nursing action, plans, and evaluation while client is receiving service.	*Client:* Observe the client for changes toward improved health status through new knowledge, skills, or abilities. Observe the client's physiological status or psychosocial affects and behaviors for signs of improvement.
Retrospective	
Chart audit: Look for documentation of nursing actions: nursing history, client goals and objectives, nursing plans, and actions implemented, such as vital signs, medications given, and teaching performed, after client has been discharged from the health service.	*Chart audit:* Look for documentation of changes in the client's health status, knowledge, abilities, or skills. Physiological and psychosocial behavioral changes toward improved health would also be appropriate evidence, after the client has been discharged from the health service.

Retrospective process evaluation is implemented after the client has been discharged. Nursing actions are evaluated after the fact. Criteria and standards for the chart review are usually developed in cooperation with the nursing personnel. Chart reviews or audits show that specific procedures were implemented, such as the admission nursing history, recording of intake and output, and ambulation of the client as ordered. This audit is usually performed by trained clerks. Examples of tools for retrospective process evaluation include the Nursing Audit by Phaneuf[3] and Monitoring Quality of Nursing Care forms developed by Jelinek and others.[6] The specific differences between concurrent and retrospective evaluation are shown in Table 11-2.

Outcome

Outcome evaluation focuses on changes in the client's behavior and health status. The nurse looks for evidence of improved health status resulting from nursing intervention; for example, that the client is free from signs of infection, or that the client accurately states the correct dose of and time to take medication.

Concurrent outcome evaluation judges the client's ability to demonstrate behavioral and measurable progress in health status, knowledge, or abilities. Examples of relevant behaviors include the client's demonstrating crutch walking, preparing and administering insulin accurately, or planning a low sodium diet. The chart may be examined for documentation of the client's progress, knowledge, and abilities. Examples of client outcomes that can be found in the chart include evidence of wound healing, stable temperature, or fluid intake equivalent to the amount expected. Hover and Zimmer reported on the Wisconsin system,[2] which describes a method of concurrent and retrospective outcome evaluation.

Retrospective outcome evaluation examines the chart after the client has been discharged. The chart is reviewed for evidence of the client's progress resulting from nursing intervention. Examples include documentation that the client performed activities of daily living, demonstrated positive attitudinal change, or planned a daily diabetic menu. The Joint Commission on the Accreditation of Hospitals[5] incorporated some aspects of retrospective outcome evaluation in their guidelines. Outcome evaluation is the most difficult to write and is the least developed form in the nursing profession, but it is the most meaningful way to judge the effectiveness of nursing interventions. Eventually, the profession will develop a taxonomy of relevant outcome criteria for evaluating nursing actions.

CRITERIA AND STANDARDS

The concepts of criteria and standards are often used interchangeably in evaluation, but they are different. Criteria are measurable qualities, attributes, or characteristics that specify skills, knowledge, or health status. They describe acceptable levels of performance by stating the expected behaviors of the nurse or client.

In process evaluation, criteria are used to define the level of nursing care; they state the specific level of acceptable performance. In outcome evaluation, criteria statements can be the client objectives or specific behavioral outcomes. They state the client's desirable response or performance. In written criteria or behavioral outcomes for clients, the following categories may be included:

1. The client's *physiological responses*, such as normal temperature, wound healing, blood pressure within normal range, or appropriate responses to stimuli.
2. The *skill* a client will demonstrate, such as crutch walking or administering insulin accurately.
3. The client's level of *knowledge* about the illness, including treatment measures and medications.
4. The client's level of *adaptive behaviors*, such as the ability to perform activities of daily living, to exercise, or to resolve grief.

Standards represent acceptable, expected levels of performance by the nursing staff or other health team members. They are established by authority, custom, or general consent. Professions develop standards to improve the levels of practice. In 1973 the American Nurses' Association[1] established the Standards of Nursing Practice, which describe the steps in the nursing process. These standards have been modified and adopted by each clinical specialty. The standards provide a frame of reference for judging quality nursing care.

GENERAL CHARACTERISTICS OF EVALUATION

Several factors influence the evaluation process and need to be considered before defining the steps in evaluation. This section examines who evaluates what and when it is done. It also discusses the differences between formative and summative evaluation.

Who, what, and when of evaluation

Who determines what is evaluated? The Standards of Nursing Practice address this question, stating: "The client/patient's progress or lack of progress toward goal achievement is determined by the client/patient and the nurse."[1] This statement means that the client and nurse mutually evaluate the client's progress. Other health team members who have worked with the client may also participate, but the nurse is responsible for writing the evaluation data in the client's chart.

What is evaluated? In the nursing process, the client is the focus and the client goals and objectives define what is evaluated. The objectives may be further specified by criteria that are used to describe what client behaviors are evaluated.

When does the nurse evaluate? Evaluation is an ongoing process. It begins with the initial assessment to collect baseline information and continues during interactions with the client. Some nurses prefer periodic evaluation of the plan and objectives. The frequency depends on the health status of the client, the type of changes expected, and the objectives. For example, the unconscious client may need to be checked every 15 minutes for signs of change, but the client with gradual changes from a chronic disability may need to be evaluated at greater intervals. When implementing nursing care, the nurse should evaluate the effect of the interventions in achieving the plan and the client's progress toward the objectives and goals.

Formative and summative evaluation

Evaluation is both formative and summative. Formative evaluation is ongoing, judging each step in the plan as it is carried out to measure the client's progress toward meeting the objectives. As the plan is implemented, the nurse evaluates the client's response to determine the effectiveness of the plan or the need for change. For example, the plan may state, "The client will discuss dietary likes and dislikes." The evaluation might read, "Mr. X said he likes red meat and chicken, but won't eat liver or seafood." Formative evaluation judges the steps in the plan and the objectives as a basis for continuing or changing the plans.

Summative evaluation describes the client's progress or lack of progress toward the goal. It is written after several objectives have been accomplished. Sometimes the objectives are inadequate or the resources are not available, and although the objectives have been met, the client has not achieved the goal. As an example of summative evaluation, the goal may state, "The client will modify his diet to lose weight." After achieving several objectives toward this goal, the nurse's evaluation might state, "The client can explain the reasons for weight loss and plan appropriate menus, but lacks motivation to stay on the diet. Further counseling is needed." The summative evaluation describes how well or to what extent the client has achieved the goal.

GUIDELINES FOR EVALUATION

The guidelines describe the steps in evaluation. They presuppose the achievement of the preceding components in the nursing process.

1. *Evaluation criteria are given if the objectives lack specificity.* Evaluation criteria are indicators of the *expected* client behaviors. They are written like objectives but clarify the behaviors more specifically. When criteria are written, it is important to remember that they are:

Appropriate to the objective, client's situation, capabilities, and limitations, and resources.

Observable and measurable, distinguishing satisfactory from unsatisfactory performance.

Realistic and attainable within the time and resources available.

Relevant to the domain (cognitive, psychomotor, or affective) stated in the objective.

Types of criteria were described previously as physiological responses, skills, knowledge, and adaptive behaviors of the client.

2. *The formative evaluation describes whether and to what extent the client and nurse have achieved the stated plans and objectives.* During each interaction, the nurse observes and compares the client's behavior with the criteria for the objectives. The effectiveness of the plan is determined by changes in the client's behavior. The client's statements and behaviors, such as signs and symptoms, skills, knowledge, and abilities are written in the chart. The responses related to each criterion and step in the plans are recorded in the evaluation column of the nursing care plan. The nurse may also record appropriate information from the family and other health care team members.

3. *The summative evaluation describes the client's progress or lack of progress in achieving the goals.* The nurse evaluates the client's response in meeting the objectives and judges whether the client's behavior shows progress toward goal achievement. Is the client's response in the expected direction and safe, desirable, and reasonable, considering the time and situation? Have the client's needs, concerns, or potential concerns been resolved, and if so, to what extent? The nurse may gather evaluation data from the family, team members, and chart. The client's response toward goal achievement is recorded in the chart and in the nursing care plan.

4. *The nursing care plan indicates revisions if the goals and objectives have not been adequately met.* Modification of the plans, criteria, objectives, or goals is the last step in the evaluation process. During ongoing evaluation, the nurse may judge that the plans or objectives are ineffective in achieving the goal. The client's behavior may show little or no change, or change in the wrong direction. Now the nurse examines possible reasons for the client's lack of progress. Some reasons for modifying the plan are:

The plans were unrealistic in time or resources.

The plans overestimated or underestimated the client's capabilities.

More data became available, which altered the concern.

New concerns appeared or old concerns were resolved.

New resources became available.

The nurse determines the possible reasons the plans, objectives, or goals were ineffective and then decides to reassess the client or revise the care plan. New goals, objectives, criteria, or plans are mutually established by the client and nurse and written in the Kardex or chart and the nursing care plan.

Examples of individual, family, and community evaluation follow. These reflect only partial evaluations.

Example of individual evaluation

Nursing diagnosis: Inadequate knowledge of diabetic diet.

Client goal   The client will apply the American Diabetic Association (ADA) diabetic diet in menu planning and daily nutritional intake.

Objective   The client will accurately plan his diabetic meals for 3 days by April 10, 1982.

Plans	Evaluation—formative
1 The nutritionist will meet with the client and explain the ADA diabetic diet by 3/20/82.	On 3/18/82 Miss S., the nutritionist, met with Mr. G. and explained the diabetic diet. Mr. G. was receptive, asked relevant questions, and took notes.
2 The nutritionist or nurse will provide the following literature on diabetic diets by 3/24/82. (List names of diabetic booklets.)	On 3/19/82 Mr. G. was given three booklets on the diabetic diet. He read and underlined in them that evening.
3 The client and nurse will discuss the ADA diabetic diet by 3/22/82 to determine:	
a Client's comprehension.	Mr. G. correctly stated carbohydrate (CHO), protein, and fat intake for his diet.
b Client's food preference.	Mr. G. stated that he will give up sweets, but will miss his ice cream.
c Need for more teaching.	Mr. G. seemed unsure of how to calculate CHO intake.
d Need for family involvement.	Mr. G. asked if we would explain his diet to his daughter, who cooks for him.
4 The client will write three daily menu plans that meet the ADA diabetic standards for him by 3/24/82.	Mr. G. wrote three daily menu plans, which included snacks. These plans were accurate in fat and protein, but excessive in CHO on 2 days.
5 The client and nurse will discuss the client's three written menus by 3/26/82 in relation to:	On 3/26/82 the client and nurse discussed Mr. G.'s three menu plans.
a Accuracy.	Mr. G. recognized his excess CHO intake and was able to correct it.
b Preparation.	Mr. G. described how he or his daughter would prepare his diet.
c Food preference.	Mr. G.'s three menus reflected his personal food preferences.

Summative evaluation: Mr. G. has shown some movement toward goal achievement by writing three accurate daily diabetic menus. Continued supervision will be necessary. It is recommended that he continue writing menu plans and that his daughter meet with the nutritionist to receive instruction in diabetic menu planning. More objectives are needed to reach the goal.

Example of family evaluation

Nursing diagnosis: Inadequate safety precautions in the home.

Family goal   The family will eliminate safety hazards to children from their home (mutually established).

Objective 1   The family will identify ways to remove safety hazards from their home by 6/5/82.

Plans	Evaluation—formative
1 The nurse will write a checklist of safety factors that homes with small children should have.	On 4/30/82 the nurse, after consultation with the health department, wrote a safety checklist.
2 The family and nurse will discuss the checklist and the family will complete the list by 5/15/82.	On 5/5/82 Mr. and Mrs. T. seemed enthusiastic in reading the checklist and agreed to fill it in during the next week. On 5/7/82 the nurse visited the family, but they had not completed the safety list. They promised to work on it.
3 The family and nurse will discuss the results of the safety checklist by 5/20/82.	On 5/15/82 the checklist was completed and discussed with the family. Four areas were deficient, and the family agreed to work on improving safety in those areas.
4 The family and nurse will explore ways to eliminate safety hazards in four areas by 5/25/82.	On 5/20/82 the family and nurse discussed several ways to remove each safety hazard.

Objective 2   The family will remove safety hazards from their home by 6/30/82.

Plans	Evaluation—formative
1 The family will decide the best way to eliminate safety hazards in their home by 6/1/82.	The family discussed alternatives for eliminating each safety hazard and decided on a specific measure for each on 6/1/82.
2 The family will implement each safety precaution they previously decided on by 6/21/82.	On 6/7/82 the family agreed to take the necessary measures but had not had time to do so yet. On 6/14/82, the family showed the nurse how they had corrected each safety hazard. The family seemed pleased by their action.
3 The family and nurse will evaluate the results of their safety precautions by 6/30/82.	On 6/21/82 the family and nurse discussed the family's feelings about precautions, and the family expressed relief and gratitude to the nurse.

Summative evaluation: This family was able to identify and correct four safety hazards to their children in its home. The family took appropriate measures to eliminate safety hazards and maintained these measures. The family goal was effectively met; no further action is deemed necessary at this time.

Example of community evaluation

Nursing diagnosis: Increased incidence of venereal disease among teenagers in the community.

Community goal   The community will reduce the incidence of venereal disease among teenagers by 9/30/82.

Objective   Appropriate community officials will develop strategies to reduce venereal disease by 7/30/82.

Plans

1 The nurse will meet with the public health department, county board of health, and high school personnel to discuss (1) the increased incidence of venereal disease, (2) complications of venereal disease, and (3) venereal disease control strategies by 6/30/82.

2 The nurse will develop a list of strategies for improving teenagers' knowledge of prevention and treatment of venereal disease from suggestions of community health members by 6/30/82.

Evaluation—formative

On 6/5/82 the nurse and public health officials met and discussed plans 1-3. Three of five members expressed an interest in developing improved educational services.

On 6/10/82 the nurse and 10 members of the county board of health met to discuss plans 1-3. The board moved to increase educational services and publicity to reduce the incidence of venereal disease among teenagers.

On 6/18/82 the nurse met with six high school personnel to discuss plans 1-3. They suggested having a special assembly program on venereal disease.

The nurse developed the following list of strategies from suggestions of community members contacted above:
 Radio and television messages.
 Venereal disease pamphlets distributed in high school.
 High school assembly on venereal disease.
 Posters with information on signs and treatment clinics.

Summative evaluation: Community members from the public health department, the county board of health, and the high school met with the nurse during June 1982 to discuss the increased incidence of venereal disease among teenagers and to suggest strategies to reduce the incidence. Each group demonstrated an interest in reducing this community concern and offered several suggestions for improving education about venereal disease and trying to reduce the incidence. Community members are aware of the problem, but the nurse will follow up and facilitate community action to improve educational services and clinic information. Some progress has been made toward goal achievement, but follow-up is necessary. More objectives are needed to achieve the goal.

SUMMARY Evaluation is an ongoing, systematic, planned process of comparing the client's health status with the objectives and goals. It takes place primarily during nurse-client interactions. Evaluation involves comparing the client's present responses with previous responses to determine the client's progress in achieving the objectives and goals. Judgments about the client's progress are made from observations, interactions, and measurements by the nurse, client, family, and team members. If there is insufficient progress toward objectives and goals, the client and nurse will revise the plan of care.

REFERENCES

1 American Nurses' Association: Standards of nursing practice, Amer. Nurse **6**:11, July 1974.
2 Hover, J., and Zimmer, M.: Nursing quality assurance: the Wisconsin system, Nurs. Outlook **26**:242, 1978.
3 Jelinek, R.C., and others: A methodology for monitoring quality of nursing care, HEW Publication (HRA) 74-25, 1974.
4 Joint Commission on the Accreditation of Hospitals: Accreditation manual for hospitals, Chicago, 1980, The Commission.
5 Joint Commission on the Accreditation of Hospitals: Procedure for retrospective patient care audit in hospitals, nursing edition, Chicago, 1973, The Commission.
6 Phaneuf, M.: The Nursing Audit: profile for excellence, New York, 1972, Appleton-Century-Crofts.
7 Wandelt, M.A., and Ager, J.W.: Quality Patient Care Scale, New York, 1974, Appleton-Century-Crofts.
8 Wandelt, M.A., and Stewart, D.S.: Slater Nursing Competencies Rating Scale, New York, 1975, Appleton-Century-Crofts.

BIBLIOGRAPHY

Barba, M., Bennet, B., and Shaw, W.J.: The evaluation of patient care through use of ANA's standards of nursing practice, Superv. Nurse **9**:42, Jan. 1978.
Block, D.: Evaluation of nursing care in terms of process and outcome: issues in research and quality assurance, Nurs. Res. **24**:256, 1975.
Davis, A.I.: Measuring quality: development of a blueprint for a quality assurance program, Superv. Nurse **8**:17, Feb. 1977.
Deets, C., and Schmidt, A.: Process criteria based on standards, AORN J. **26**:685, 1977.
Deets, C., and Schmidt, A.: Outcome criteria based on standards, AORN J. **27**:657, 1978.
Diddle, P.J.: Quality assurance: a general hospital meets the challenge, J. Nurs. Adm. **6**:7, July-Aug. 1976.
Dracup, K.: Improving clinical evaluation, Superv. Nurse **10**:24, June 1979.
La Monica, E.L.: The nursing process: a humanistic approach, Reading, Mass., 1979, Addison-Wesley Publishing Co., Inc.
Lang, N.M.: Quality assurance in nursing, AORN J. **22**:180, 1975.
Mager, R.F.: Preparing instructional objectives, Belmont, Calif., 1978, Fearon-Pitman Publishers, Inc.
Marriner, A.: The nursing process: a scientific approach to nursing care, St. Louis, 1975, The C.V. Mosby Co.
Munley, M.J.: An evaluation of nursing care by direct observation, Superv. Nurse **4**:28, Apr. 1973.
Nichols, M.E.: Quality control in patient care, Am. J. Nurs. **74**:456, 1974.
Passos, J.Y.: Accountability: myth or mandate, J. of Nurs. Adm. **6**:26, Oct. 1976.
Phaneuf, M.: The nursing audit for evaluation of patient care, Nurs. Outlook **14**:51, June 1966.
Ramey, I.G.: Setting nursing standards and evaluating care, J. Nurs. Adm. **3**:27, May-June 1973.
Ramphal, M.: Peer review, Am. J. Nurs. **74**:63, 1974.
Roeder, M.A.: Patient care plans and the evaluation of nursing process, Superv. Nurse **11**:57, June 1980.
Ryan, B.J.: Nursing care plans: a systems approach to developing criteria for planning and evaluation, J. Nurs. Adm. **3**:50, May-June 1973.
Schmidt, A., and Deets, C.: Writing measurable nursing audit criteria, AORN J. **26**:495, 1977.
Schmidt, A., and Deets, C.: Responsibilities for audit criteria, AORN J. **27**:657, 1978.
Tucker, S.M., and others: Patient care standards, ed. 2, St. Louis, 1975, The C.V. Mosby Co.
Watson, A., and Mayers, M.: Evaluating the quality of patient care through retrospective chart review, J. Nurs. Adm. **6**:17, Mar.-Apr. 1976.
World Health Organization: Summary report of a working group on the evaluation of inpatient practice, J. Adv. Nurs. **3**:413, 1978.
Yura, H., and Walsh, M.B.: The nursing process: assessing, planning, implementing, evaluating, ed. 3, New York, 1978, Appleton-Century-Crofts.
Zimmer, M.J.: Quality assurance for outcomes of patient care, Nurs. Clin. North Am. **9**:305, 1974.
Zimmer, M.J.: Guidelines for development of outcome criteria, Nurs. Clin. North Am. **9**:317, 1974.

III

Application of the NURSING PROCESS to practice

NURSING PROCESS
of the individual client

PAULA J. CHRISTENSEN

Orem's concepts of practice[7] are used as the overall guide for this case study. The eight universal self-care requisites are incorporated throughout the nursing process. Orem's concepts of the nursing system and health-deviation self-care are also applied. For a review of Orem's conceptual framework, see Chapter 2.

The individual client in this case study is a 15-year-old female, C.K., who injured her right knee in a trampoline accident 4 years ago. She is on the track team at school, and her knee has become progressively weaker and painful to the point that she has stopped running and is now timekeeper for the team. She will have surgery on her right knee. The nursing process reflects 3 consecutive days of contact with the client, ranging from the first preoperative day to the second postoperative day.

A complete nursing process is shown in the left-hand columns of this chapter. A critique of the process appears in the right-hand column, adjacent to the respective topic. The critique points out strengths and areas needing improvement based on the guidelines described in Chapters 3 through 11. The application of theoretical approaches and the use of standards and norms are also critiqued. The abbreviations "O" for observations, "I" for interactions, and "M" for measurements are used to guide the reader to the point in the nursing process that is being critiqued.

The nursing process is organized into three sections. First the nursing assessment and analysis/synthesis for each of the 3 consecutive days are presented. Then, the list of nursing diagnoses is presented. Last, the nursing plans, which include the goals, objectives, plans for implementation, scientific rationale, and evaluation, are presented and critiqued. Although the nursing plans are placed last, they are written after the initial assessment and are implemented and updated with each successive visit. The dates of each implementation are identified in the objectives, plans, and evaluations. The nursing plans—goals through evaluation—are written consecutively to show their interrelationship and sequence. They are placed at the end of the nursing process because they are ongoing and subject to revision and because they demonstrate the continuity of the care plan.

Data collection. The data appear in the order they were obtained.

Analysis/synthesis of data. Orem's conceptual framework guides the multifocal analysis/synthesis. Supplemental resources are used to identify standards and norms. The focus of this component is biophysical because of C.K.'s surgery. C.K.'s reactions to health concerns are included as well.

Nursing diagnosis. The nursing diagnoses are worded using Orem's concepts.

Plans for implementation. The plans—including goals, objectives, nursing orders, and scientific rationale—are given for four nursing diagnoses. Plans are implemented in visits 1, 2, and 3. Data indicating implementations are shown in the data collection column of their respective day.

Evaluation. Evaluation data indicating nursing implementations are in the evaluation column. When plans have not been implemented, questions are given to guide evaluation of future plans. The critique is based on the guidelines.

DATA COLLECTION—day 1

Observations	Interactions	Measurements	Critique
1-14-81			
From chart:		From chart:	Health history not obtained on admission.
1. Client's initials: C.K.		1. Age: 15 yr	Data gap.
2. Reason for admission: rt medial menisectomy and release and advancement of vastus medialis 1/15.		2. Urinalysis: Color: yellow Clarity: clear Specific gravity: 1.031 pH: 5.0	
3. Trampoline accident 4 years ago.		Protein: neg	
4. Injuries of subluxation of rt knee.		Glucose: neg	
5. Lives with parents.		Acetone: neg Hb: neg	
6. Religious preference: protestant.		WBC: none RBC: none	
7. Insurance: Blue Cross–Blue Shield		3. Complete blood count:	Statement of norms should be given in analysis/synthesis, not data collection (M 3).
8. Surgical consent signed by mother.		WBC: 8.0 RBC: 5.67	
9. Regular diet.		Hb: 17.1 HcT: 50.8	Biographical information obtained from chart (O 1-10).
10. NPO after midnight.		MCV: 90 MCH: 30.2 MCHC: 33.7 (All within hospital norms)	
From client 1/14 evening:	1/14/81 evening:		
11. Eye contact with nurse; smiles.	1. Hi, yeah, I'm C.K.	4. Chest x-ray: normal	"Normal" is subjective. Cite data from x-ray reading (M 4).
12. Lying supine in bed with head of bed up.	2. Oh, pretty good.	5. Admission blood pressure: 110/70	

DATA COLLECTION—day 1—cont'd

Observations	Interactions	Measurements	Critique
13. Reaches to rt knee with rt hand and rubs it.	3. Well, my right knee hurts some—but that's nothing new. 4. Oh, it's been bothering me a lot for about 6 months. 5. It hurt a little most of the time, but then it started going out on me when I ran.	6. Admission TPR: 98.4°, 90, 20 7. Height: 5'3" Weight: 115 lb 8. Preop medications: Demerol 75 mg Vistaril 25 mg IM together on call	Baseline physical data obtained from chart (M 1-7). Data presented objectively—facts given from chart (M 1-8).
14. Head resting on pillow.	6. Yeah, I really like running. I like sports in general. 7. I swim and bicycle, too. Then I like to watch football and basketball games with friends.		
15. Looks down toward bed.	8. It has been hard not being able to run. . . . I don't really feel a part of the team anymore.		To be more systematic, physical assessment should have been done at this time.
16. Looks toward nurse.	9. I sure hope I'll be able to run again after the surgery.		Pattern of "normalcy" addressed in I 6-9; data also relate to "social interaction."
17. Flat facial expression.	10. No, I'm not too sure what's going to happen tonight or tomorrow.		Rapid topic change (I 9-10). Could have obtained more data about her concerns. This limited multifocal data collection.
18. Maintains eye contact with nurse.	11. Oh, O.K. 12. No, I think I understand now.		
19. Uncovers legs.	13. Sure—what do you want me to do?		Pattern of "air intake" addressed in I 14, O 20-21, M 3-6.
20. Both legs warm to touch.	14. No, they don't tingle or anything [her feet and legs].		"Rapid" (O 21) is rather subjective. Need to measure number of seconds.
21. Toes on both feet have rapid capillary return when blanched.			
		From client:	
22. Looks at rt knee when moving it.	15. Yeah, it hurts too much if I try to go any further.	9. Flexes lt knee 0°-135°	Objective measurements (M 9, 10).
23. Smiles at nurse.	16. OK, I'll see you tomorrow night. 17. Thanks, bye.	10. Flexes rt knee 30°-90°	Pattern of "activity" addressed in I 6-9 and M 9-10. Objective quotations cited from client (I 1-17). The client and chart were the only sources used for data collection. Data collection tools are used appropriately. Format is systematic. Data are recorded appropriately.

Analysis/synthesis	Critique

When Orem's concepts related to self-care are used, each universal self-care requisite is addressed and appropriate data are referred to. Supporting theories and concepts are included when appropriate.

Critique: Named nursing model to be used as general multifocal guide for analysis/synthesis.

1. Maintenance of sufficient intake of air: Some data obtained about this pattern (O 20, 21; I 14; M 4-7). The data indicate adequate circulation to C.K.'s legs. Malasanos[5] cites normal ranges for (a) blood pressure: systolic 95-140, diastolic 60-90 mm Hg; (b) pulse for a person over 4 years old: 60-100 beats per minute; (c) respiration: 16-20 per minute; and (d) temperature: 97°-99.6° F (orally). When these norms are compared with C.K.'s vital signs, a tentative inference can be made regarding adequate intake of air. More readings of vital signs, other circulatory data, and her history of smoking are data needed for a conclusion to be made. Datum O 2 indicates that C.K. may have an inadequate intake of air in the future because of surgery.

Critique: Need to summarize data relevant to pattern of intake of air rather than just referring to data by number.
Cited source for norms given. Specific norms given for each vital sign.
What data gaps are present regarding intake of air?
Not clear. Need to elaborate on this regarding why there is a potential threat to intake of air.
Need to cite data, not just reference numbers.

2. Maintenance of sufficient intake of water: Minimum data (M 2, 3) refer to hydration of the client. A very tentative inference can be made of adequate water intake. More data are needed, such as observations of the skin and mucous membrane condition. Datum O 10 indicates that C.K. may have an inadequate intake of water in the future.

Critique: Data gap identified. Also need measurement data of usual fluid intake.
A physiology or physical assessment text is needed for norms of adequate fluid intake.

3. Maintenance of sufficient intake of food: No data were collected about C.K.'s eating habits. She is on a regular diet now and will be NPO after midnight, which will alter food intake (O 9, 10). Her height and weight (M 7) fall within the norms given by Malasanos for her age (M 1). (Height range: 59.5-68.1 inches; weight range: 89.5-150.5 lb.) The sources of her nutrition are data gaps at this time.

Critique: A nutrition text will be needed to analyze "sufficient" intake of food when more data are obtained.
Cite C.K.'s height and weight.
Data gap: 3-day nutritional recall. This is not a priority at this time because of impending surgery.

4. Adequate elimination processes and excrements: Minimum data (M 2) were obtained. The values of the urinalysis did fall within the norms given by the hospital. Urinary excretion can be considered adequate, but data gaps exist about patterns of excretion as to difficulties experienced previously and bowel output.

Critique: Cite data, not just reference number.
Norms should be cited here and a source given. The hospital's norms and a physiology or physical assessment text will be needed.
An admission health history is useful to obtain these kinds of data.

5. Maintenance of balance between activity and rest: According to Diekelmann,[1] the young adult should exercise at least four times per week for approximately 20 minutes in an activity that increases heart rate and respirations. Data collected (O 2-4; I 4-9; M 9, 10) indicate that the client had regular exercise before her knee injuries, but for the last 6 months has not been able to participate as before. Malasanos indicates that the normal range of motion of the knee is 0°-135° flexion. According to data M 9, 10, C.K. has a right knee flexion deformity of 30° with further flexion to 90°. Data gaps exist regarding frequency of exercise, sustained pulse and respirations, and alternative modes of exercise. A tentative inference of inadequate exercise can be made at this time, especially in anticipation of upcoming surgery (O 2). No data were obtained regarding rest and sleep patterns.

Critique: Source and norm cited for exercise requirements of appropriate age group. Another source will be needed for norms for sleep and rest.
Good summary of data.
Good discussion regarding knee movement. Very specific conclusions can be drawn using this information. Cite data.
Data gaps mentioned are specific and give direction for further data collection.

6. Maintenance of balance between solitude and social interaction: The data obtained (I 6-9) indicate that C.K. is involved in activities with other people. Orem

Critique: Summarize data from I 6-9.

Analysis/synthesis	Critique
discusses the importance of bonds of affection, love, and friendship; social warmth and closeness; and individual autonomy. More data need to be collected regarding C.K.'s family and friends in meeting these needs. Data O 11, 18, 23 indicate friendliness and warmth toward nurse. Observations of the number of visitors, cards, and phone calls C.K. has, as well as how she responds to these, will be important data to obtain.	Appropriate use of nursing model to establish norm for needs of social interaction. Other sources will be needed for more in-depth discussion of this requisite. Data gap: No data regarding presence or absence of family on preoperative day or on admission. Does C.K. have family support?
7. Prevention of hazards to human life, functioning, and well-being: Orem describes this requisite as including awareness of potential hazards and knowledge of preventive measures to avoid or minimize their effects. Data O 2-4, 8, 13, 22; I 3, 4, 9, 10; and M 8-10 indicate that C.K. has had and will have hazards to her functioning. One specific hazard is her lack of understanding of the events surrounding her surgery.	Important to briefly define pattern that may not be self-explanatory. Need to expand on this. Merely listing data pieces does not facilitate understanding.
8. Promotion of human functioning and development within the individual's potential and desire to be normal: Orem describes the elements of this requisite as having a realistic self-concept, fostering human development, and acting to maintain and promote the integrity of human structure and function. Some data (O 2, 8) indicate that the client is striving to maintain and promote her physical integrity. Data regarding what she has done to promote and maintain her health up until this time need to be collected. Erikson[2] discusses the developmental task of this age as identity versus identity confusion. The adolescent essentially restages each of the previous stages of development in reestablishing a separate autonomy. Many data are needed from C.K. to ascertain her stage of development and sense of identity. Sundeen and others[11] describe self-concept as the aspects of the self that the individual is aware of. Self-concept includes the individual's feelings, values, and beliefs that influence behavior. Self-ideal is the standard by which one judges one's own behavior, including goals, aspirations, or values one would like to achieve. Based on limited data (I 6, 8, 9), one can tentatively infer that C.K. is not achieving her potential in the area of realistic self-concept.	Data are categorized according to patterns of self-care requisites throughout analysis. Summarize data from O 2, 8. Lengthy theoretical discussion without data to compare—no need to cite detailed norm if no data are available to discuss pattern. Good use of supporting theory, but premature. A summary of these data is needed to promote understanding of conclusion.

Considering the previous review of universal self-care requisites, the following strengths and health concerns are identified:

Strengths	**Health concerns**	
1. Adequate intake of air.	1. Potential alteration of intake of air, water, and food.	Good list of strengths and health concerns, based on discussion of each self-care requisite.
2. Adequate urinary excretion.		
3. Desire to promote human functioning.	2. Inadequate activity.	
4. Desire to be normal in relation to peer group.	3. Hazards to human functioning.	
	4. Decreased self-concept.	

Because of the concerns listed, C.K. has a therapeutic self-care demand and health-deviation self-care requisites. Her desire and ability to promote her own human functioning, plus assistance from health care professionals, place her in a supportive-educative nursing system at this time.	Orem's terms could use some explanation. Good overall summary of analysis/synthesis of data.

DATA COLLECTION—day 2

Observations	Interactions	Measurements	Critique
1/15/81 evening			
From chart:	From 7-3 report from nurse:	From chart:	
20. Postop orders: Cl liq as tolerated to soft diet. I and O. Elevate rt leg. Ice to rt knee. Bed rest. Tylenol gr. X q.4h. prn; temp 101° po Tylenol tab #3 g.4h. po pain, prn IV: D₅NS at 75 cc/hr Vital signs q.4h.	17. She's been sleeping since she got back until 1500. 18. I gave her Tylenol #3 at that time for pain. 19. Circulation checks have been OK. 20. Ice bag is on her rt knee.	10. TPR: 98.4°, 76, 18 (preop) 99°, 72, 16 (postop) 11. BP: 108/60 (preop) 110/68 (postop)	Data sources include another nurse, the chart, and the client. Pattern of "rest" addressed in I 17, 18. Appropriate use of tools (I, O, M).
21. Preop med given per order at 0700—to OR at 0730. 22. Returned from surgery at 1200. 23. Client sleeping most of time since 1200. 24. Tolerating clear liquids po sm amts. 25. IV infusing on time.	21. Vital signs are stable—next due at 1600. 22. She's been taking a little ice and 7-Up by mouth with no problem. 23. Yes, she has voided.	12. Tylenol #3: 2 tabs given at 1500 13. I and O (7-3): I: IV (surg): 500 cc IV (unit): 225 cc PO: 100 cc O: 500 cc (urine)	Pattern of "elimination" addressed in I 23, M 13. "On time" (O 25) is somewhat subjective. Should cite specific time unless not given in chart. Pattern of "intake of fluids" addressed in M 13 and I 22.
From client: 26. Lying supine in bed with head of bed (HOB) up 15°. 27. Rt leg elevated on two pillows.	From client: 24. Hi, not so good right now. I just had a couple of pain pills—they've helped some.		Systematic data collection—observed, interactive, and measured related data during one visit.
28. Compression dressing on rt leg from ankle to groin. 29. No drainage noted through dressing. 30. Rt toes warm to touch. 31. Rapid capillary return when rt toe nails blanched. 32. Wriggled rt toes when asked.	25. I had to use the bedpan a while ago and that was hard to do—but I did go. 26. Uh-huh. I can feel it. 27. OK [in response to telling C.K. to let me know if she has any tingling or numbness of rt leg].	From client: 14. Vital signs at 1600: BP: 106/66 TPR: 99°, 76, 18	Pattern of "intake of air" addressed in O, I, and M. "Rapid" (O 31) is subjective term. Pattern of "promotion of human functioning" addressed in I 27, 28 by encouraging C.K. to take part in her own care.
33. Facial skin and arms warm, dry, and pinkish. 34. Lips pink and moist. 35. Flat facial affect.	28. I see [in response to telling C.K. about the possible postop complications of decreased sensation, discomfort, and decreased circulation, as related to surgery].		Qualifying statements given to aid understanding of interaction data (I 27, 28). Nursing intervention of assessing and monitoring physical status (O 27-34, I 24-26, M 14).

DATA COLLECTION—day 2—cont'd

Observations	Interactions	Measurements	Critique
36. Eye contact with nurse.	29. Yeah, they showed me earlier [in response to nurse asking if she knew how to CDB].		Nursing intervention of initiating CDB (O 37). What is the nature of cough? Dry? Moist?
37. Took five deep breaths and coughed (CDB) when nurse requested her to do so.			
Observations of environment:	30. I'll try [in response to nurse informing C.K. about the need to CDB q.2h. while she is on bed rest to increase air intake].		
38. Mother at bedside.			
39. Call light within C.K.'s reach.	31. OK [in response to nurse encouraging her to rest now].		
40. Bedside table within reach.			
41. Glass of clear liquid and ice chips on bedside table.			Observations of environment (O 38-43) reflect pattern of "prevention of hazards."
42. Television on low volume.			
43. Roommate in bed watching television.			
(Later)	(Later)	(Later)	
44. Turned to rt side with ease when bedpan was placed under buttocks.	32. I need to use the bedpan again.		
	33. Thanks.		
45. Urine deep amber and clear.	34. I'm better now—it still hurts but not as much.	15. Voided 350 cc urine	Pattern of "elimination" (O 45, I 32, M 15).
46. IV infusing into lt hand at 75 cc/hr (D₅NS).			Observation data 46-47 are measurement data.
47. HOB up 30° for supper.	35. Oh, that's enough.		
48. Drank all of broth and juice and ate Jell-O by herself.		16. Oral intake: 575 cc (supper)	Pattern of "intake of food" addressed in O 48, M 16.
49. Pillows resituated to provide more support for rt leg.	36. That's better.		
50. New ice bag applied to rt knee.	37. When will I be able to get this thing out [referring to IV]?		Nursing interventions to prevent hazards to well-being (O 49-51).
51. CDB five times when nurse initiated.	38. Oh, OK [in response to "probably tomorrow" from nurse].		
52. Mother remained at bedside until 1900.			Pattern of "social interaction" addressed in O 52-54.
53. Minimum interactions between client and her mother.			Should note nature of interactions between C.K. and mother.
54. Mother assisted C.K. in reaching items on supper tray.			
(Later)	(Later)	(Later)	
55. Rt toes warm to touch.	39. No, no tingling or anything.		
	40. Could I have those pain pills again?		
	41. It's just a constant aching most of the time—now it's starting to pound.		Nature of pain assessed.

Continued.

DATA COLLECTION—day 2—cont'd

Observations	Interactions	Measurements	Critique
56. Swallowed pills with ease.			
57. HOB to 10° elevation.			
58. Turned to rt side—back-rub given.			Turned C.K. before allowing pain medication to work (O 56, 58)
59. Skin on back moist and warm.	42. Could I have some more 7-Up, too?	17. Vital signs at 2000:	—not systematic in assessment of skin and
60. No redness on back or hips.		BP: 110/70	lungs (O 59, 61).
61. Lung sounds clear to auscultation.		TPR: 98.6°, 72, 16	Focus on biophysical data because of recent
62. IV infusing on time.		18. Tylenol #3:	surgery (O 58-63, M 17-
63. CDB five times on request of nurse.		2 tabs given at 2000	18). Characteristics of cough? (O 63)
(Later)		(Later)	
64. C.K. lying supine with eyes closed.		19. Oral intake: 120 cc 7-Up	
65. Relaxed facial muscles.		20. I and O (3-11):	Nursing intervention of monitoring intake, out-
66. Body in alignment.		I:	put, and physical func-
67. Rt leg elevated with ice bag to rt knee.		IV: 600 cc PO: 695 cc O: 350 cc urine	tioning (O 66, 67; M 19, 20).
			Format is systematic and data are recorded appropriately. Data reflect updating.

ANALYSIS/SYNTHESIS OF DATA—day 2

Analysis/synthesis	Critique
Orem's concepts of universal self-care requisites are addressed individually.	
1. Maintenance of sufficient intake of air: Data O 20-21 indicate that C.K.'s intake of air has been threatened because of surgery and immobility. Phipps and others[8] state that the effects of both anesthesia and immobility impair adequate intake of air. According to the norms given previously by Malasanos and the implementation of preventive postoperative measures suggested by Phipps and others and Ferrell,[3] data indicate that this self-care requisite is being met now but remains a potential health concern.	A summary of these data (O 20-21) should be given. Good use of supporting texts to analyze "sufficient" intake of air. Cite these data.
2. Maintenance of sufficient intake of water: Data O 20-22 indicate that C.K.'s intake of water has been threatened because of surgery and inability to take fluids in volume by mouth. Phipps and others state that fluid volume depletion manifests itself with the following symptoms: poor skin turgor, dry mucous membranes, low blood pressure, tachycardia, increased respiration, decreased vein filling, weight loss, low urine output, and increased specific gravity. Phipps and others and	Data discussion needs elaboration. Good citing of reference observations indicating fluid volume deficit.

ANALYSIS/SYNTHESIS OF DATA—day 2—cont'd

Analysis/synthesis	Critique

Ferrell provided the rationale for plans for implementation that were initiated regarding threatened intake of water (IV replacement, clear liquid diet). According to the data, C.K. does not exhibit symptoms of fluid volume deficit and is participating in the implementation of plans to prevent inadequate intake of water, and is, therefore, maintaining a sufficient intake of water. This self-care requisite remains a potential health concern.

Nursing texts used to guide data collection and analysis of these data (as well as nursing interventions).
Cite C.K.'s data to support this statement.

Even though intake is adequate now, it is important to note whether this remains a concern because of the circumstances.

3. Maintenance of sufficient intake of food: Williams[12] states that adequate protein intake is of prime importance postoperatively because of the loss of protein from tissue breakdown and loss of plasma proteins. Essential amino acids are necessary for wound healing. The goal is to reach 100-200 gm. protein daily and a minimum of 2800 calories a day. One L of a 5% dextrose solution contains 50 gm sugar and 200 calories. According to the above information compared with the data, C.K. is not maintaining a sufficient intake of food. Progressing C.K. from a clear liquid diet to a regular diet should be done as soon as she can tolerate it. Overall eating habits remain a data gap.

Additional source cited to analyze "sufficient" intake of food.

Excellent discussion of appropriate sources of nutrition and how they are meeting C.K.'s need.
Summarize data of C.K.'s intake.
Giving direction in analysis toward future implementation helps establish the priorities of concerns.

4. Adequate elimination processes and excrements: Phipps and others state that intake of fluids will exceed output for about the first 48 hours after surgery. This is due to the loss of fluid in surgery, insensible fluid loss, vomiting, and increased secretion of antidiuretic hormone (ADH). The client should be expected to void within 6-8 hours after surgery. Data indicate that C.K. has voided within the recommended time and that her fluid intake does exceed her fluid output. According to the above data and norms for the postoperative client, C.K. is maintaining adequate urinary output. Phipps and others state that bowel patterns are altered after surgery because of the stress response, anesthesia, use of narcotics, and immobility. Even on a clear liquid diet and IV replacement, a client should have bowel movements if peristalsis is present. C.K. has not had a bowel movement at this time, which is normal. Bowel function remains a potential health concern at this time. Further data need to be obtained in regard to bowel function.

Good review of effect of surgery on elimination. Source cited.

Cite data of intake and output.

Good discussion of bowel elimination norms after surgery.

Be more specific regarding types of data needed.

5. Maintenance of balance between activity and rest: Phipps and others and Ferrell indicate that early activity and ambulation are beneficial for increasing alertness, morale, ventilation, muscle tone, and peristalsis; facilitating voiding and wound healing; and decreasing venous stasis. Adequate rest is necessary for an accurate perception of pain and events surrounding recovery from surgery. Ferrell states that quadriceps-setting exercises should start as soon as the client is awake after surgery. According to the data, C.K. has had minimum activity, has not started the quadriceps-setting exercises, and has had adequate rest. Therefore there is an imbalance between activity and rest.

"Early" is subjective—be specific as to when activity should start to achieve benefits named.

"Adequate" is a subjective term. No norm given for rest.

Cite supporting data.

Good summary.

Continued.

ANALYSIS/SYNTHESIS OF DATA—day 2—cont'd

Analysis/synthesis	Critique
6. Maintenance of balance between solitude and social interaction: Data indicate minimum interactions with others at this time because of her need for rest and her sedation from the anesthetics and analgesics. Data gaps remain concerning visitors, and cards and phone calls from friends.	Biophysical needs are a priority at this time because of recent surgery. Data should be collected regarding this pattern soon. Cite data. Data gap: Further interaction data from C.K. regarding friends and family as a support system. Summarize data more meaningfully.
7. Prevention of hazards to human life, functioning, and well-being: Data indicate that C.K. is more aware of potential hazards and is participating with preventive measures cooperatively. Because of the surgery, this remains a health concern at this time.	
8. Promotion of human functioning and development within the individual's potential and desire to be normal: Data obtained reflect biophysical health promotion at this time because of the recent surgery and actual and potential changes in biophysical health. C.K. needs assistance in promoting all aspects of human functioning.	Summarize data. Vague and too general to be useful. What does this mean?

According to the previous review of universal self-care requisites, the following strengths and health concerns are identified:

Strengths	Health concerns	
1. Adequate intake of air.	1. Potential alteration of intake of air and water.	Updated list of strengths and health concerns is based on continuous data collection and analysis.
2. Adequate intake of water.	2. Inadequate intake of food.	
3. Adequate urinary excretion.	3. Potential alteration of bowel elimination.	
4. Cooperative in actively participating in methods to decrease hazards to human functioning.	4. Inadequate activity.	
	5. Hazards to human functioning.	

In view of the concerns listed, C.K. continues to have a therapeutic self-care demand and health-deviation self-care requisites. Because of her recent surgery and inability to maintain universal self-care requisites and therapeutic self-care demands without assistance, C.K. is in a wholly compensatory nursing system.

More explanation of terms would help understanding this summary.

No incongruencies in the data were identified.

Good summary.

DATA COLLECTION—day 3

Observations	Interactions	Measurements	Critique
1/16/81 evening	From 7-3 report from nurse:	From chart:	Pattern of "intake of air" addressed in M 21.
From chart:	43. She's had a good day today.	21. Ranges of vital signs:	
68. New orders: Out of bed in chair at least t.i.d. PT to fit for crutches. Discontinue IV.	44. I started her on the quad-setting exercises and she's done them every couple of hours.	BP: 106/68-112/74 T: 98.4-99° P: 68-76 R: 12-18	Nursing interventions regarding "prevention of hazards" in O and I.
69. Tolerating soft diet well.	45. I had her try a straight leg raise, but she could not do it now.		
70. Cooperative with quad-setting.	46. Started her on a soft diet this morning and she's tolerating it well.	22. Tylenol #3: tabs 2 at 0200, 0730, 1200	
71. Circulation checks: warm rt foot, can move rt toes.	47. I tried to get her out of bed this afternoon, but it was too long after pain medica-	23. I and O: (11-7): I: 600 cc (IV) 400 cc (PO)	Patterns of "intake of water" and "elimina-tion" addressed in O and M.
72. Vital signs stable (see measurements).	tion and too soon for an-other—she had pain and and tensed up so she couldn't get into the chair.	O: 400 cc urine	
73. Washed self except for back in AM.	48. PT was notified to come and fit her for crutches.	(7-3): I: 275 cc (IV) 1005 cc (PO)	Appropriate use of data collection tools.
74. IV discontinued at 1030.	49. She had quite a few visi-tors up today, so she's pretty tired and has been sleeping off and on.	O: 450 cc urine	
From client:	From client:	From client:	
75. Looks at nurse and smiles.	50. Hi, Paula.	24. Vital signs at 1600: BP: 110/72 TPR: 98.4°, 76, 16	
	51. I'm doing OK. I had a hard time trying to get out of bed, though. Guess I didn't do well.		
	52. Yeah, I could use the pills again. Oh, OK [in response to waiting half an hour, then getting up into a chair].	25. Tylenol #3: tabs 2 at 1600.	Systematic assessment—wait until after pain medication works to move client.
76. C.K. focuses eyes on rt leg—muscle visible above compression dressing tenses and relaxes as rt foot flexes toward head.	53. Uh-huh. I've been doing these exercises about every 2 hours. OK, I'll do it again now.		Nursing intervention of "promotion of func-tioning" and "preven-tion of hazards" in O, I, and M.
77. Rt toes warm to touch.	54. I think so—aren't the exercises to keep my leg strong so I can use the crutches?		
78. Rapid capillary return when rt toenails blanched	55. Yeah, I remember some of the possible complications.		"Rapid" (O 78) is subjec-tive term.
79. Wriggles rt toes when re-quested.	56. Well—bad circulation, pneumonia, funny feeling in my leg.		
80. Rt leg elevated on two pillows.			

Continued.

DATA COLLECTION—day 3—cont'd

Observations	Interactions	Measurements	Critique
81. Ice bag to rt knee.	57. That's why you have me do all this—like breathing and coughing, and the exercises, keeping my leg up, isn't it?		
Environment:	58. OK [in response to suggestion to rest now].		
82. Two plants and one set of flowers at bedside.			
83. Several cards on bedside stand.			
(Later)	(Later)	(Later)	
	59 Oh, boy, here we go!		
	60. OK [in response to instructions on how I will support her leg while turning her body and holding rt leg for her].		
84. C.K. helped herself move rt side of bed by sliding her body across mattress with support of her arms.			
85. Nurse supported rt leg in horizontal position.	61. Yeah, I'm OK.		
86. Blank facial expression.			
87. Looked at rt leg while standing.			
88. Took a few deep breaths upon instruction.			
89. Stood on lt leg and pivoted to chair at side of bed.	62. OHHHHHH!		
90. Sat in chair using arms to support herself as she sat.			
91. Rt leg elevated on pillow on second chair.	63. Well, it's OK.		Nursing intervention of "prevention of hazards" and "activity" (O 84-91).
92. Bedside tray with supper placed in front of C.K.	64. Thanks.		
(Later)	(Later)	(Later)	
93. C.K. had eaten two thirds of food on tray.	65. I need to use the bedpan. Then I'm ready to go back to bed.	26. Oral intake: 450 cc (supper)	Pattern of "intake of food" addressed in O 92-93, M 26.
94. Lifted herself up with arms when bedpan was placed and removed.		27. Voided 500 cc urine	Pattern of "elimination" (M 27).
95. Assisted back to bed. Nurse held rt leg horizontally while C.K. stood on lt leg and pivoted.	66. It was easier this time.		
96. CDB five times on request.			

DATA COLLECTION—day 3—cont'd

Observations	Interactions	Measurements	Critique
97. Smiled at nurse.	67. The doctor told me today that I should be able to run again. 68. Sure, that makes me happy. The track team means a lot to me. 69. Oh, she said it'd be about 6 months before I could really run. 70. I'd like it to be sooner, but at least I know it'll be OK sometime. 71. I can still be the time-keeper until I can run. That way I can still be with my friends.		Systematic assessment—waited to talk to C.K. until she was more comfortable.
98. Pointed with rt hand to flowers.	72. Yeah—they gave me most of these cards—and those flowers. 73. The rest are from my relatives. 74. Maybe if I work hard at exercising I'll be able to run sooner!	30. Drank 240 cc 7-Up. 31. I and O (3-1130): I: 690 cc (PO) O: 500 cc urine	More multifocal data obtained this visit—the effect of surgery on life-style. Pattern of "social interaction" and "development" addressed (I 67-74).
99. Rt leg elevated on two pillows. 100. Ice to rt knee. 101. Rt foot warm to touch. 102. Hair groomed, own nightgown on.	75. See you later.		Nursing interventions of monitoring "prevention of hazards" (O 99-101).

ANALYSIS/SYNTHESIS OF DATA—day 3

Analysis/synthesis	Critique
Orem's concepts of universal self-care requisites are addressed individually:	
1. Maintenance of sufficient intake of air: According to data and norms given in analysis/synthesis 2, C.K. is maintaining adequate air intake. This still remains a potential health concern because of her decreased mobility.	Still need more elaboration on data. Referring to previous discussion of norms is appropriate to prevent repetition.
2. Maintenance of sufficient intake of water: According to the norms given in the last analysis/synthesis regarding intake of water, C.K. is meeting this health care requisite. This requisite also remains a potential health concern because of her surgery.	Data from this data collection should be cited. Current status of previously identified concern given.
3. Maintenance of sufficient intake of food: Data show that C.K. has started eating a soft diet and is tolerating it. According to the projected ideal intake of food and calories given in the last analysis/synthesis, C.K. has a greater chance to meet the requirements now that she is eating solid foods. Data gaps exist regarding the nutritional value of the food she is eating. This is a potential health concern.	Good discussion of intake of food. What kind of information is still needed?
4. Adequate elimination processes and excrements: C.K.'s intake still exceeds her output, which was stated as a norm for postoperative clients in the last analysis/synthesis. Bowel function remains a potential health concern and a data gap.	Give specific intake and output.
5. Maintenance of balance between activity and rest: According to the data, C.K. is beginning to get the activity she needs. The activities recommended in the discussion of analysis/synthesis 2 have been implemented. This remains a health concern until C.K. is more mobile independently.	Cite data. Stating status of previously identified health concerns is important.
6. Maintenance of balance between solitude and social interaction: Data indicate that C.K. is having more contact with friends and family. A data gap still exists with respect to the quality of these relationships and how they satisfy C.K.'s needs.	Cite or summarize data. Good recognition of data gap.
7. Prevention of hazards to human life, functioning, and well-being: Data indicate that C.K. is aware of these hazards and is cooperating in preventive measures to decrease the potential of complications developing. Continued monitoring of these measures is needed until C.K. is more mobile independently.	Cite data. Vague discussion—need more specifics.
8. Promotion of human functioning and development within the individual's potential and desire to be normal: The norms given in analysis/synthesis 1 regarding adolescent development compared with these data support C.K.'s concern with her self-concept and relation to peers. This remains a health concern—and will require greater focus—as C.K.'s role will be altered for an extended period.	Body image theory is an appropriate source to use at this time to analyze normal progression of stages of body image change. The eight self-care requisites are used consistently and multifocal and analysis/synthesis is ensured.

ANALYSIS/SYNTHESIS OF DATA—day 3—cont'd

Analysis/synthesis	Critique

The following lists represent C.K.'s strengths and health concerns at this time:

Strengths
1. Adequate intake of air.
2. Adequate intake of water.
3. Adequate urinary excretion.
4. Social interaction with significant other people.

Health concerns
1. Potential alteration of air, food, and water.
2. Potential alteration in bowel elimination.
3. Inadequate activity.
4. Hazards to human functioning.
5. Altered self-concept.

Critique:
Updated lists of strengths and health concerns reflect current health status.

Lists are multifocal, reflecting use of nursing model.

According to the concerns identified, C.K. still has a therapeutic self-care demand and health-deviation self-care requisites. Since C.K. remains dependent on others to maintain universal self-care requisites and therapeutic self-care demand, she is in a wholly compensatory nursing system.

No incongruencies in the data were identified.

Critique:
Current health status summarized using Orem's concepts.

Terms could be explained.

NURSING DIAGNOSIS

Date	Diagnoses	Priority number 1/14	1/15	1/16	Date resolved	Critique
1/14	**1.** Hazards to human functioning related to upcoming surgery and lack of knowledge concerning surgery.	1	3	5	1/16/81	All statements are client centered and specific, and four out of five are etiological.
1/14	**2.** Potential alteration of air, water, and food intake related to upcoming surgery.	2	1	2		Wording based on Orem's terms tends to make statements lengthy.
1/14	**3.** Decreased self-concept related to alteration in role of an active sportsperson.	3	4	1		Priorities established according to guidelines—the most life
1/14	**4.** Inadequate activity related to right knee injuries and upcoming surgery.	4	2	3		and health threatening first.
1/15	**5.** Potential alteration of bowel elimination.		5	4		Priority of diagnoses revised according to current health status and concerns.

(Plans for diagnoses 1, 2, 3, and 5 are given on the following pages. Initial plans for diagnosis 4 are included in diagnosis 2. A more detailed plan is needed regarding increasing C.K.'s activity and discharge planning.)

Critique:
All nursing diagnoses can be treated by means of nursing interventions.

No diagnostic statement given regarding major gaps in data collection.

PLANS FOR IMPLEMENTATION

Nursing diagnosis 1: *Hazards to human functioning related to upcoming surgery and lack of knowledge (1/14/18).*
Goal: *The client will decrease hazards to human functioning by increasing knowledge of upcoming surgery by 1/17/81.*

Objectives	Plans	Scientific rationale
1. The client will name the sequence of events leading to surgery by 1/14/81.	1a. The nurse and client will discuss previous experiences the client has had with surgery on 1/14/81.	1a. Teaching-learning strategy by Pohl.[9] Principle of learning: New learning is based on previous knowledge and experience.
	1b. On 1/14/81 the nurse will use open communication techniques such as: Open-ended questions and statements. Clarifying statements. Summary statements.	1b. Principles of teaching: Good nurse-learner rapport is important. Teaching requires effective communication.[9]
	1c. The nurse will explain the events leading to surgery on 1/14/81: Preparation of rt knee. Enema this evening. NPO after midnight. Injection in AM. To surgery ½ hr later. Return to room about 3 hr later.	1c. Increase C.K.'s sense of physical control and knowledge to promote powerfulness of client.[10]
	1d. The nurse will ask C.K. if she understands the sequence of events on 1/14/81.	1d. Evaluation is an integral part of learning.[9]
2. The client will state three of five effects of surgery on human functioning according to Ferrell by 1/17/81.	2a. The client and nurse will discuss C.K.'s knowledge of the surgery and it effects on functioning on 1/16/81 after surgery.	2a. Principles of teaching and learning.[9] New learning is based on previous knowledge and experience. Planning time for teaching and learning requires special attention. Physical and mental readiness is necessary for learning.
	2b. The nurse will review the effects of surgery on human functioning according to Ferrell on 1/16/81 (see criteria statement for effects). The nurse will state that some differences may occur because of physician's individual practice.	2b. The immobilization of the right knee joint allows for healing of traumatized tissue.[3] The exercises facilitate strengthening of muscles around traumatized tissue.[3] Knowledge of what to expect after surgery increases the client's sense of physical control and powerfulness.[10]
	2c. The nurse will ask C.K. to state the effects of surgery on human functioning on 1/17/81.	2c. Effective learning requires active participation of the learner.[9] Evaluation is an integral part of learning.[9]
	2d. The nurse and client will discuss the client's feelings about altered functioning on 1/17/81.	2d. A positive body image is particularly important to the adolescent.[10]

Evaluation	Critique
Criteria statement: 　The client will cite the following events: 　　Preparation of rt knee. 　　Enema. 　　NPO after midnight. 　　Injection in AM. 　　To surgery ½ hr later. 　　Return to room about 3 hr later.	*Goal* The goal relates directly to an expressed lack of knowledge by the client. *Objective* Time limit given because of surgery the next day. Not specific about how many of the events client should name. *Plans*
The nurse implemented plans 1a-1d 1/14/81. The client responded that she understood the sequence of events on 1/14/81 (I 12).	Another plan is needed to ask C.K. to cite the sequence of events—not just understand them. Plans are dated, specific, and sequential. Plans are health promotional. *Scientific rationale* The strategy was named (teaching-learning) but the topic and individuality are less well defined. *Evaluation*
Objective 1 met 1/14/81.	Need more documentation to show execution of plans and achievement of objective.
Criteria statement: 　The client will name the following effects: 　　Compression dressing immobilizes rt knee. 　　Use of crutches 3 days postop nonweight-bearing. 　　Walk without crutches 10 days postop when stitches removed. 　　Hospitalized 4-7 days. 　　Need for exercises such as quadsetting, straight-leg raises, weight resistive exercises (after sutures removed).	*Objective* Stated in specific, measureable terms. These objectives will achieve the stated goal. *Criteria statement* This should also include the number of items client is expected to name. *Plans* The nurse and client are the only people involved. Could include C.K.'s family, so they would be informed of events and effects as well.
1/16/81 Plans 2a-2d implemented. C.K. indicated general knowledge of needing crutches and limits on activity, and feelings about it (I 51, 54, 67-71). Objective met. Goal met 1/16/81.	*Scientific rationale* Relevant current readings were used—no research cited. Individuality addressed specifically in 2d. *Evaluation* Better. Still need more of a summary statement. Referral to actual data when client made statements reflecting plan implementation.

Continued.

PLANS FOR IMPLEMENTATION—cont'd

Nursing diagnosis 2: *Potential alteration of air, water, and food intake related to upcoming surgery (1/14/81).*
Goal: *The client will decrease the degree of alteration of air, water, and food intake by using preventive postoperative measures by 1/16/81.*

Objectives	Plans	Scientific rationale
1. The client will verbalize three possible postop occurrences on 1/14/81.	1a. The nurse will ask C.K. what she knows about possible occurrences caused by surgery on 1/14/81.	1a. Teaching-learning strategy by Pohl. Principle of learning: New learning is based on previous knowledge and experience.
	1b. On 1/14/81 the nurse will use open communication techniques to discuss postop occurrences such as: Decreased air intake and circulation. Decreased sensation. Discomfort. Decreased physical activity. Decreased food and water intake.[3]	1b. Principle of teaching: Teaching requires effective communication. These are considered possible occurrences after surgery due to the effect of anesthesia and immobility on general body systems. The possibly decrease in circulation, sensation, and discomfort in the right leg is related to swelling of tissue as a response to surgical intervention.[8]
	1c. The nurse will ask C.K. to verbalize three of the possible occurrences mentioned above on 1/14/81.	1c. Principles by Pohl: Effective learning requires active participation of the learner. Evaluation is an integral part of learning.
2. The client will name three preventive measures for possible postop occurrences on 1/14/81.	2a. The nurse will use open communication techniques to discuss preventive measures for possible postop occurrences on 1/14/81: CDB every 2 hours. Elevate rt knee on pillows. Ice bag to rt knee. Positioning for comfort and analgesics. Quad-setting (eventually straight leg raising and crutch walking). IVs and clear liquid diet as tolerated to regular diet as tolerated.[3,8] Out of bed within 24 hr.[3,8]	2a. Principle of teaching: Teaching requires effective communication.[9] To increase ventilation of lungs and facilitate removal of secretions.[8] To facilitate venous return and decrease swelling.[3] To decrease swelling and pain, and facilitate circulation.[3] To decrease pain and increase comfort.[3] To strengthen muscles around surgical area.[3] Fluid is lost during surgery and must be replaced. ADH is stimulated post trauma. GI function slowed.[8] Increases morale, alertness, ventilation, muscle tone, and peristalsis. Facilitates healing and voiding. Decreases pain and venous stasis.[8]
	2b. The nurse will ask C.K. to name three of the above preventive measures on 1/14/81.	2b. Principles by Pohl: Effective learning requires active participation of the learner. Evaluation is an integral part of learning.

Evaluation	Critique
Criteria statement:	*Goal*
The client will name three of the following possible occurrences:	The goal is broad and dated realistically.
	No signs of mutuality established at this time.
Decreased air intake and circulation.	*Objective*
Decreased sensation.	The word "state" is more specific and appropriate.
Discomfort.	*Criteria statement*
Decreased physical activity.	No need to repeat list already provided in plan 1b.
Decreased food and water intake.	*Plans*
Plans were not implemented because of nurse's lack of planning on 1/14/81.	Source given for specific information to be taught.
Objective 1 not met—to be implemented 1/15/81 and 1/16/81.	Plans are not signed.
	Plans are preventive in nature.
Plans 1a and 1c not implemented 1/15 because of C.K.'s health status.	*Scientific rationale*
	Sources cited for rationale statements.
Plan 1b was implemented 1/15. C.K.'s responses indicated she acknowledged information given to her (I 27-30).	Rationale for topic of postop occurrences given in adequate detail.
	Evaluation
Plans 1a and 1c implemented 1/16 (I 56).	Reasons for plans not being implemented according to projected dates given.
Objective met.	
Criteria statement:	*Objective*
The client will name three of the following preventive measures:	Stated in specific, measurable terms. May not be realistic because of time limits on preop day.
See list in plan 2a.	*Criteria statement*
Plans not implemented because of nurse's lack of planning on 1/14/81.	Appropriate referral to list in plan 2a.
	Plans
Objective 2 not met—to be implemented on 1/15/81 and 1/16/81.	Plans are specific, giving direction to nurse regarding what needs to be taught.
Plan 2a partially implemented 1/15. C.K. acknowledged nurse's information (I 27-30).	Sources cited for items to be taught.
	Plans are rehabilitative in nature.
Plan 2b not implemented 1/15 because of client's health status.	*Scientific rationale*
	Detailed rationale given for each preventive measure.
Plan 2b implemented 1/16. C.K. identified preventive measures (I 54, 57).	Individuality not addressed.
Objective met.	Strategies used (teaching-learning and effective communication) and topic (prevention of complications) discussed.
	Evaluation
	Need more discussion regarding achievement of objective.

Continued.

PLANS FOR IMPLEMENTATION—cont'd

Nursing diagnosis 2: *Potential alteration of air, water, and food intake related to upcoming surgery (1/14/81).*
Goal: *The client will decrease the degree of alteration of air, water, and food intake by using preventive postoperative measures by 1/16/81.*

Objectives	Plans	Scientific rationale
3. The client will participate in at least four post-op preventive measures by 1/16/81.	3a. The nurse will demonstrate the following on 1/14/81: CDB. Quadriceps setting. 3b. C.K. will demonstrate the above on 1/14/81.	3a. Learning may occur through imitation.[9] 3b. Effective learning requires active participation of the learner. Repetition strengthens learning.[9]
	3c. The nurse will provide necessary equipment and monitor their effectiveness for the following preventive measures on 1/15/81: Elevate rt leg on pillows. Ice bag to rt knee. Position rt leg for comfort. Administer analgesics per physician order as needed. IVs and clear liquid diet as tolerated to regular diet.	3c. The nurse is responsible and accountable for the client's physical safety and well-being postoperatively.[8] (See rationale for each preventive measure in objective 2.)
	3d. The nurse will monitor intake and output postoperatively 1/15/81 and as needed.	3d. Physiological changes due to surgical intervention and anesthesia interfere with usual intake and output.[8]
	3e. The nurse will initiate use of measures in 3a when appropriate.	3e. Health restoration and maintenance are the responsibility of the nurse.[8]

Evaluation	Critique
Criteria statement: 　The client will participate in at least four of the following preventive measures: 　See list in plans 3a and 3c. Plans 3a and 3b not implemented because of nurse's lack of planning on 1/14/81. (To be implemented on 1/15/81.) Plan 3a partially done 1/15 (I 29). Plan 3b done 1/16 (O 76, I 53). C.K. showed nurse how to CDB and quad-set. Plan 3c done 1/15 and 1/16. Plan 3d implemented 1/15 and 1/16. 　I and O maintained by nurse. Plan 3e implemented 1/15 and 1/16. Objective met. Goal met (needs monitoring until C.K. is more mobile) 1/16/81.	*Objective and criteria statement* Who chooses which of the preventive measures C.K. will participate in? *Plans* Demonstration is appropriate when teaching a client an activity. C.K. is old enough to learn this way. *Scientific rationale* Referring back to previous objective is appropriate to avoid repetition. *Evaluation* Short statements documenting implementations given. Important to state whether goal needs further monitoring.

Continued.

PLANS FOR IMPLEMENTATION—cont'd

Nursing diagnosis 3: *Altered self-concept related to change in role of an active sportsperson (1/14/81).*
Goal: *The client will accept a realistic self-concept considering her role change by 1/21/81.*

Objectives	Plans	Scientific rationale
1. The client will verbalize at least two feelings regarding loss of function by 1/18/81.	1a. The nurse and client will discuss C.K.'s perception of the loss of function from surgery on 1/17/81.	1a. Strategy of therapeutic communication[11] combined with the strategy of decision making.[4] The client's reaction to a temporary or permanent loss depends on the client's perception of the loss.[9]
	1b. The nurse will ask C.K. how and what she feels regarding the loss of function of her rt leg on 1/17 or 1/18.	1b. The nurse needs to facilitate ventilation of feelings regarding loss.[8] In adolescence, the body acts as a source of acceptance or rejection by others.[6] Problem identification step of decision-making process.[4]
	1c. The nurse will accept and support C.K.'s response in 1b on 1/17 and 1/18.	1c. The nurse needs to support client in all phases of body image change.[10]
	1d. The nurse will ask C.K. to think about coping methods on 1/17 to be discussed on 1/18.	1d. Active participation by the learner promotes learning.[9] Generation of options of decision making.[4]
2. The client will state three ways she can cope with altered body function by 1/20/81.	2a. The nurse and C.K. will discuss all possible ways of coping with altered body function on 1/18 and 1/19. (See criteria statement for ways taken from Phipps and others and from Roberts.)	2a. Identification of options in decision-making process.[4] The nurse is responsible for health promotion.[8] The nurse needs to participate in supporting the client with all aspects of changed body image.[10]
	2b. The nurse and client will discuss the feasibility of each possible coping measure on 1/19 and 1/20.	2b. Analyzing alternatives in decision-making process.[4] Increasing C.K.'s sense of physical, psychological, and environmental control and knowledge to promote powerfulness.[10]
	2c. C.K. will choose at least three ways she will cope with altered body function on 1/20/81.	2c. Increasing sense of powerfulness.[10] Making the decision in the decision-making process.[4] A positive body image is built or reconstructed through encouragement of movement and activities.[10]
3. The client will exhibit at least two signs of acceptance of altered body function by 1/21/81.	3a. The nurse will ask and encourage C.K. to initiate use of at least two coping measures by 1/21.	3a. Increase C.K.'s sense of physical, psychological, and environmental control and powerfulness.[10]
	3b. The nurse will monitor and evaluate the use of coping measures by 1/21.	3b. The nurse is responsible for promotion of health.[8] Evaluation is an integral part of teaching.[9]
	3c. The nurse will give positive reinforcement to C.K. for using coping measures by 1/21/81.	3c. The nurse needs to participate in and support the client with all aspects of changed body image.[10]

Evaluation	Critique
Criteria statement: The client will verbalize at least two feelings, such as sadness, anger, neutrality, frustration, pleasure, and joy on 1/17 (cognitive domain). Plans not implemented because of dates not yet occurring. Objective not met.	*Criteria statement* Specific examples given of feelings yet broad enough for individual response. *Plans* The plans will promote the client's achieving the objective. Health promotion plans are included here. *Scientific rationale* Strategies, topic, and individuality addressed adequately. *Evaluation* How did C.K. act when talking about feelings of loss of function? Was C.K. willing to discuss this? Did the nurse support C.K.'s responses?

Criteria statement:
    The client will name three of the following coping methods by 1/20/81:
      Take care of own body.
      Participate in diversional activities.
      Learn to use crutches and increase mobility to the best of her ability within limits.
      Ask family to arrange home to allow C.K.'s increased mobility.
      Ask friends to carry books for her at school.
      Plan to continue being timekeeper for track team.
      Initiate social contact with friends (cognitive domain).
Plans not implemented because of dates not yet occurring.
Objective not met.
	Criteria statement
	Stated in specific, observable terms.
	Appropriate domain identified.
	Plans
	Sources and specific examples of coping mechanisms given.
	Included client in decision making.
	Plans include significant other people in C.K.'s life—promoting individuality of the client.
	Evaluation
	How many coping mechanisms could C.K. name on her own?
	Was C.K. receptive to having others help her?
	Could C.K. identify three ways she would be comfortable with?

Criteria statement: The client will participate in at least two of the coping measures listed in criteria statement for objective 2 by 1/21/81 (psychomotor domain). Plans not implemented because of dates not yet occurring. Objective not met. Goal not met.	*Objective* Meeting this objective (plus 1 and 2) will meet goal. Appropriate domain identified. *Plans* Plans are in the appropriate sequence to meet the objectives and goal. *Evaluation* How much encouragement did C.K. need to activate coping measures? What kind of reinforcement did the nurse use?

Continued.

PLANS FOR IMPLEMENTATION—cont'd

Nursing diagnosis 5: *Potential alteration in bowel elimination related to recent surgery and immobility (1/15/81).*
Goal: *The client will resume normal pattern of bowel elimination by 1/19/81.*

Objectives	Plans	Scientific rationale
1. The client will identify (state) decreased bowel function as a possible complication of surgery and immobility on 1/17/81.	1a. The nurse will ask the client if she knows any other possible complications of surgery and immobility on 1/17. 1b. According to C.K.'s response, the nurse will explain to C.K. the possible complication of altered bowel function on 1/17/81. 1c. The nurse will ask C.K. to acknowledge information given above on 1/17/81.	1a. Teaching-learning strategy by Pohl. New learning is based on previous learning and experience.[9] 1b. Anesthesia and immobility decrease peristalsis and therefore potentially alter bowel function.[8] 1c. Evaluation is an integral part of teaching.[9]
2. The client will participate in the assessment of bowel function on 1/17.	2a. The nurse will ask C.K. if she has felt any need to defecate or any "rumbling" in lower abdomen or passed any flatus ("gas") since surgery on 1/17/81. 2b. The nurse will use the following physical assessment techniques to collect data about bowel function on 1/17/81: Inspection. Auscultation. Palpation. Percussion.[5]	2a. Subjective data are an important source regarding bowel function.[8] 2b. Physical assessment techniques used to identify distention, bowel sounds, bowel segments, and fluid, gas, and solid elements in bowel.[5]
3. The client will participate in three measures to stimulate bowel function by 1/18/81 if needed.	3a. The nurse will ask C.K. about her knowledge of measures to stimulate bowel function on 1/17/81. 3b. According to the above response, the nurse will identify measures to increase bowel activity based on Phipps and others on 1/17/81: Fluids to 2000-3000 cc per day. Maximum safe physical activity. Fruit juice intake. Mild laxative. Hypertonic enema. 3c. The nurse will encourage C.K. to participate in the first three measures above if needed on 1/17/81 and 1/18.	3a. Pohl's learning principle: New learning is based on previous learning and experience. Learning needs must be assessed.[9] 3b. The development of concepts is a part of learning.[9] These measures increase fluid volume in bowel and stimulate peristalsis.[8] 3c. The nurse is responsible for health promotion and maintenance.[8]

Evaluation	Critique
Criteria statement: The client verbally states or acknowledges with an affirmative word or gesture indicating that bowel function is a possible complication on 1/17/81 (cognitive domain). Plans not implemented because of dates not yet occurring. Objective not met.	*Goal* Goal is appropriate to diagnosis. *Criteria statement* Written in specific, observable terms. Domain of statement is given. *Plans* Plans are adequate to meet the objective. Plans are preventive in nature. *Scientific rationale* Strategy and topic are addressed, but individuality is not. *Evaluation* Could C.K. name other possible complications? Was C.K. receptive to learning about possible altered bowel function?
Criteria statement: The client will answer questions and position body to facilitate data collection of bowel function upon request on 1/17/81 (psychomotor domain). Plans not implemented because of dates not yet occurring. Objective not met.	*Criteria statement* Stated specifically to explain what "participate" means. Statement is also cognitive domain. *Plans* Plans give direction to client and nurse behaviors. Client's normal pattern not assessed. *Evaluation* Did nurse use interactions and observations in assessing bowel function? Which physical assessment methods were employed? Was C.K. cooperative?
Criteria statement: The client will participate in three of the measures listed in plan 3a on 1/17 or 1/18 (psychomotor domain). Plans not implemented because of dates not yet occurring. Objective not met. Goal not met.	*Criteria statement* Statement does not reflect plan 3c. Need to be specific about which plans client and nurse should try first. *Objective* Achievement of these objectives will not necessarily meet the goal. *Plans* Specific plans given from source to direct activity of client and nurse. *Scientific rationale* Individuality of client not included. Strategy and topic addressed. *Evaluation* Did C.K. understand progression of interventions for stimulating bowel function? What kind of encouragement did C.K. need?

REFERENCES

1 Diekelmann, N.: Primary health care of the well adult, New York, 1977, McGraw-Hill Book Co.

2 Erikson, E.H.: Identity, youth and crisis, New York, 1968, W.W. Norton & Co., Inc.

3 Ferrell, J.: Illustrated guide to orthopedic nursing, Philadelphia, 1977, J.B. Lippincott Co.

4 Ford, J.G., Trygstad-Durland, L.N., and Nelms, B.C.: Applied decision making for nurses, St. Louis, 1979, The C.V. Mosby Co.

5 Malasanos, L., and others: Health assessment, ed. 2, St. Louis, 1977, The C.V. Mosby Co.

6 Murray, R.B., and Zentner, J.P.: Nursing assessment and health promotion through the life span, Englewood Cliffs, N.J., 1979, Prentice-Hall, Inc.

7 Orem, D.E.: Nursing: concepts of practice, ed. 2, New York, 1980, McGraw-Hill Book Co.

8 Phipps, W.J., Long, B.C., and Woods, N.F.: Medical-surgical nursing: concepts and clinical practice, St. Louis, 1979, The C.V. Mosby Co.

9 Pohl, M.L.: The teaching function of the nurse practitioner, ed. 3, Dubuque, Ia., 1978, Wm. C. Brown Co., Publishers.

10 Roberts, S.L.: Behavioral concepts and nursing throughout the life span, Englewood Cliffs, N.J., 1978, Prentice-Hall, Inc.

11 Sundeen, S.J., and others: Nurse-client interaction: implementing the nursing process, ed. 2, St. Louis, 1981, The C.V. Mosby Co.

12 Williams, S.R.: Essentials of nutrition and diet therapy, ed. 2, St. Louis, 1978, The C.V. Mosby Co.

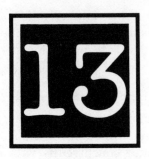

NURSING PROCESS
of the family client

JOANNE RENAUD CROSS

FRAMEWORK FOR FAMILY ASSESSMENT

Herbert Otto's framework[10] for assessing family strengths, resources, and potentials is used to gather appropriate psychosocial assessment data. This enables the nurse to identify not only those strengths of the family that are obvious, but also latent potentials or resources. Strengths identified by Otto are the following:

1. Physical, emotional, and spiritual needs of a family.
2. Child-rearing practices and discipline.
3. Communication.
4. Support, security, and encouragement.
5. Growth-producing relationships and experiences.
6. Responsible community relationships.
7. Growth with and through children.
8. Self-help and accepting help.
9. Flexibility of family functions and roles.
10. Mutual respect for individuality.
11. Crisis as a means of growth.
12. Family unit, loyalty, and intrafamily cooperation.
13. Flexibility of family strengths.

Part of Myra Levine's framework,[5] structural integrity, is used to assess biological problems. She describes nursing intervention in relation to conservation of energy and structural, personal, and social integrity. This approach is appropriate to support and promote family adaptation to changing roles and energy needs from a change in health status.

These two approaches, Otto's and Levine's, are incorporated in the plans for implementation, scientific rationale, and evaluation of the nursing process. Brief descriptions of Otto's framework and Levine's concepts can be found in Appendix C. This family nursing process reflects three visits over a 3-week period, written in detail, followed by a conclusion made after six visits over a 6-month period.

In this chapter the nursing process is shown in the left-hand columns and a critique is written in the extreme right-hand column. The critique points out strengths and areas needing improvement according to the guidelines described in this book. The application of theoretical approaches and the use of standards and norms are also critiqued. The abbreviations "O" for observations, "I" for interactions, and "M" for measurements are used to guide the reader to the point in the nursing process that is being critiqued.

The nursing process is organized in the following way. The initial assessment and analysis/synthesis is followed by the second and third assessment visits and analysis/synthesis. The list of nursing diagnoses is next. Last, the nursing plans, which include the goals, objectives, nursing orders, scientific rationale, and evaluation, are shown with the critique. Although the plans are last, they are initiated, implemented, and evaluated concurrently with the assessment visits. The plans are last because they are ongoing and subject to revision and because they demonstrate the continuity of the total nursing process.

DATA COLLECTION—preliminary information

Biographical data and initial concerns	Critique
Biographical data	
Father Jerry Davis Age 29 1 year of junior college	Biographical data are objectively stated, multifocal, and pertinent.
Mother Jenny Davis Age 28 High school graduate	
Daughter Sarah Age 8 Second grade	
Son Joey Age 5 Kindergarten	
Race: Caucasian.	
Religion: Mother and children, current Mormons; father does not attend religious services.	
Occupation: Father, foundry worker; mother, carpet salesperson (part time).	
Insurance: Major medical and life insurance.	
Language spoken: English.	
Marital status: Parents married to each other; no previous marriage for either.	
Source of referral: Home health coordinator from Poudre Memorial Hospital after mother's discharge from hospital.	The date and length of hospitalization, as well as the reason for hospitalization, should also be noted.
Initial concerns (as related by home health coordinator)	
The mother had a medical diagnosis of colitis (type not specified) made 2 years ago; she also has PVC* (origin unknown). In April 1980, hypertension and hypoglycemia were also diagnosed.	Clear, concise overview of family's health concerns.
The mother contracted measles (rubella) during the first trimester of her second pregnancy, and as a result the son is defective in two sensory areas: sight (cataracts) and hearing (deafness in one ear).	
Thus far the son's impairments have not affected his performance in kindergarten. The mother's impairments are periodically disabling and are a potential for many complications if she does not follow her prescribed medical regimen. The mother is the primary focus of nursing care in this family.	

*PVC, premature ventricular contraction.

DATA COLLECTION—phone conversation with the mother

Interactions	Observations	Measurements	Critique
Nursing goal: To establish a contract to work with the family. Date: April 28, 1980 1. Yes, I remember the home health coordinator said someone would be contacting me. 2. I've been home from the hospital for almost a month now. 3. I've had colitis in the past but it isn't so bad now. Last year I had diarrhea from March 'til December.	1. Mother's voice tone with modulations indicated strong interest in the family's wanting help with health care concerns.		Subjective statement implies judgment and inference (O 1).
4. I have hypertension and hypoglycemia. I take Apresoline with Esidrix for the hypertension and have to stay on a high protein diet for hypoglycemia. 5. I'm a born worry wart. My doctor wants me to take Valium but I don't want to take so many pills. 6. I would like to learn some relaxation techniques that I could use to help me calm down.			Data reflect the mother's priority in a future plan of care (I 6).
7. Joey is deaf in one ear and has cataracts. He doesn't wear a patch any more. That didn't work too well. I put a drop of atropine in his strong eye every morning to blur his vision so that his lazy eye has to work harder. 8. Jerry [husband] won't mind. He does whatever I ask [in answer to the question as to whether or not her husband would agree to work with the nurse to improve family health patterns].			Contract to work with the family is discussed, but the details are not firmly established (I 8). All interaction data (1-8) reflect baseline information on current health status of family.

Continued.

DATA COLLECTION—visit 1

Interactions	Observations	Measurements	Critique

TIME: May 5, 1980, 2:30 PM.

PLACE: Living room of the client family. Only Jenny is present, since husband and children are at a ball game in Detroit.

NURSING GOALS: To focus on Jenny's health care needs and those of the family, and to set up rapport and a trusting relationship with the family. Contract.

Interactions	Observations	Measurements	Critique
9. I don't drink coffee because I have PVCs; it was diagnosed 2 years ago, and I was put on Lanoxin. The PVCs went away and came back again in February. They seem worse when I am relaxing; also were getting more frequent and stronger. Better now; I am not taking Lanoxin now.	2. Light green house with aluminum siding; about 1200 sq ft.	1. BP (taken by client's mother yesterday) is 130/80.	*Patterns addressed*
	3. One shrub and tree in front yard; empty flower pots on porch. Large asphalt driveway.	2. Height: 5'11".	Levine:
		3. Weight: 220 lb.	Structural integrity.
			Personal integrity.
			Content: Multifocal.
			"Large asphalt driveway" is a subjective statement. Approximate size should be stated (O 3).
10. My new doctor had me walk around with a "Holter EKG" machine. I don't know the results yet. She is still analyzing it.	4. One station wagon and one car in driveway.		BP, height, and weight are as reported by the client in interaction—not actually validated by the nurse (M 2, 3).
11. I'm 5'11" and weigh 220 pounds. My twin brother is 6'9". I am 28 and my husband is a year older.	5. Fenced-in back yard with swing set.		Approximate size of yard should be noted (O 5).
12. My mother's boss owns a grocery and he sends me steaks and cheese every week; also fresh fruit; he is very good to me.	6. Black and white beagle dog named Snoopy.		
13. We try to balance our meals with fresh fruits, vegetables, and salads.	7. Mother wearing light green dress with cowl collar, stockings, and black heeled shoes.		
14. I had wanted twins with both pregnancies; lots of twins on both sides of the family.	8. Mother wearing light makeup; hair is shoulder length.		
15. Joey has cataracts; at first they thought it was hereditary, but now say it was due to measles which I had in my first trimester.			
16. When my health returns, I want to have more children.	9. Mother had legs crossed and was jiggling her foot during the interaction.		*Patterns addressed*
17. Jerry isn't sure about this, however.			Levine: Social integrity.
18. Both of our families live close (parents, sisters, etc.).			Otto:
			Self-help.
19. Both sets of parents are very helpful.			Individuality.
			Flexible family functions.
20. Parents helped out when I was in the hospital last month. Jerry didn't have any extra chores to do.	10. Mother speaks to nurse, smiling and maintaining eye contact.		Growth relationships. Biopsychosocial needs. Respecting individuality (I 16-17).

The mother was the only source of data on this first visit.

DATA COLLECTION—visit 1—cont'd

Interactions	Observations	Measurements	Critique
21. When Joey's eyes turned cloudy with cataracts, my neighbor took us to the hospital, since Jerry was at work and I didn't want to worry him until I found out what was happening to Joey.			Flexible family functioning (I 19-21).
22. Sarah had the chicken pox and her tonsils out.			
23. Joey has special doctors at Children's Hospital now.			
24. When Joey was 4 months old, his eyes turned white. I called Mom and then the doctor. By the time I got there, both eyes looked "milky." The doctors couldn't handle it and sent us to Ann Arbor for surgery.	11. Mother appears thoughtful—wrinkled brow.		Subjective statement (O 11); need to describe the client's facial expression in more detail.
25. We go to Ann Arbor every 6 months for a checkup.			
26. Now they treat him for a "lazy eye" and he wears glasses; sometimes he takes them off outside when he is playing. He also wore a patch over one eye for a while; he didn't like it.		4. Sighs twice.	Self-help patterns (I 23-26).

27. Jerry even wore a patch on his eye to help Joey get used to it; made a game out of it.	12. Living room has two lamps, a couch, television, stuffed chair, and desk.		Otto:
			  Responsible community relationships.
			  Meeting biopsychosocial needs.

28. Joey fell off the slide and got a skull fracture last year; it healed ok.	13. Religious pictures are on the wall of living room.		Levine: Conservation of energy.
29. Dr. Kalder is my cardiologist; he gave me Lanoxin. I changed doctors, though.	14. Carpet sample books are lying on the desk and floor.		"Religious" is a subjective statement; the pictures should be described (O 13).
30. Jerry is never sick except for colds and skin irritation. Even now he is being treated by the doctor with Mycolog two or three times a day for a skin rash.	15. Bathroom contains combination tub and shower with shower curtain. A clothes hamper is in the corner. No clothes are lying about. Clean towels are next to the sink.		Pertinent datum, but more information is needed on why doctors changed (I 29).
31. I have more energy since I got out of the hospital last month.	16. Kitchen: dishes are washed and in the drainer next to the sink. There are two windows with yellow curtains pulled to the side to allow light. The door is missing from one cupboard. There is a fresh paint smell.		Important information, but needs expansion; for example, the activities that she is doing since coming home (I 31).

Continued.

DATA COLLECTION—visit 1—cont'd

Interactions	Observations	Measurements	Critique
32. I've been working selling carpeting since a year ago last January, at a carpet outlet. I do some in-city traveling with this job. Haven't been working since I got out of the hospital.	17. General appearance of the interior, including bathroom and kitchen, is clean and neat; the family observes good hygiene practices.		Subjective statement uses judgment to make a conclusion without data to validate it (O 17).
33. The whole family goes to Dr. Jones for colds, because he gives you penicillin and you get well. Why change when you have a good thing going?			Needs clarification as to health attitudes and use of resources (I 33).
34. I've been secretary for the PTA this year, and we are busy finishing up activities for the school year.			
35. Jerry was raised general Baptist, but he never went to church with his family.			
36. Catholicism was the religion I was raised in, but now me and the children are studying to become Mormons. I had a chance to study their teachings while I was in the hospital. It has made a great change in my life.			
37. I had quite a temper when I was a kid. Then, when I got married, I held it in, or tried to, for fear the marriage wouldn't work. Then it got so pent up inside that I started screaming and cussing at everyone— mostly Jerry—for the past 2 years. Jerry doesn't do that to me as much.	18. The mother wiggles her foot when talking about Joey's skull fracture and when speaking about her temper flare-ups at home and the change in behavior since she returned from the hospital.	5. Foot wiggled 20 times a minute at 2- to 10-second intervals over a 10-minute time span.	*Patterns addressed* Levine: Personal integrity. Otto: Growth-producing relationships. Crisis as a means of growth. Pertinent datum unclear: meaning of "Jerry doesn't do that to me as much" (I 37).
38. Since I got home, I haven't screamed or cussed at Jerry. He thought something was "really wrong"; he wasn't used to the "new me."			
39. Jerry doesn't worry about the meaning of life like I do; I've thought about it since I was a kid. Sarah is like Jerry; she doesn't worry about anything either. Joey is like me: always wondering "what if" or "why."			Pertinent data relating to family relationships and growth potential (I 39).

DATA COLLECTION—visit 1—cont'd

Interactions	Observations	Measurements	Critique
40. Jerry's way is easiest, I suppose, but I couldn't do it that way.			
41. Even my friends feel hesitant toward me since I changed my behavior.	19. The client gestures with hands raised in air.		
42. I don't scream and yell any more at Jerry or the kids. And the kids don't fight as much, either.			
43. Joey will say to Sarah: "You're not supposed to be yelling at me. You might make Mommy sick again." Then *he* yells at *her!*	20. The client leans toward the nurse, gesturing with hands, and laughs.		
44. Everyone has calmed down a lot around here and it is very nice. My BP is down, too.			
45. Joey is not hyperactive. He has a lot of energy, though. He may be loud because he is deaf in one ear, or because he also hears us yelling around the house. But since I stopped screaming, he has too.	21. Smiles and appears contented.		"Appears contented" is a subjective statement; facial features should be described (O 21).
46. Jerry can "turn a switch" and can block out any unpleasantness he wants to. I can't do that.	22. Client appears thoughtful.		*Patterns addressed* Levine: Personal integrity. Otto:
47. Joey has been through so much. It made him very tough. He won't cry when he gets hurt, and in fact he seems to have a very high pain threshold. He says that he won't get sick when others do. When he got the chickenpox he said that he wasn't going to let himself get very sick and he only had a few spots.	23. Leans forward and smiles.		Individuality of family members. Growth relationships. Recreational patterns.
48. Yes, we have medical insurance. It has covered everything. We also have life insurance on both of us.			
49. I'd like us to work on some of our health problems over the next 2 months.	24. Nods head affirmatively.		
50. Usually Jerry and the kids are here at this time but today they went to a ball game at Tigers Stadium.			

Continued.

DATA COLLECTION—visit 1—cont'd

Interactions	Observations	Measurements	Critique
51. We like to do things to-gether, like bike riding, bowling, movies and, in the winter time, cross-country skiing.			
52. Come back Friday after-noon; everyone will be here. A weekday afternoon is best; you can catch us all here.			Pertinent data: contract is mutually established as to time, conveni-ence, and general con-tent (I 49, 52).
53. We always eat dinner at 4 PM. Jerry is home from work at 3:30; we eat dinner early because his lunch is at 10:30 or 11:00 in the morning.			*Summary of data collection* Data are multifocal but limited. Data are needed in all areas of activities of daily living (ADL) of all family members.
54. Yes, we almost always eat together. It's usually noisy but pretty relaxed.	25. Smiles.		Current and past health status of the family was ascertained through systematic assessment according to Levine and Otto.
55. Yes, I will be glad to fill out the health history forms; we'll talk about it next time you come?	26. Takes forms from nurse.		

ANALYSIS/SYNTHESIS OF DATA—visit 1

Analysis/synthesis	Critique

Holistic analysis April 8, 1980 (first visit)
Family

According to Otto, family strengths are those factors or forces that contribute to family unit and solidarity and that foster the development of the potentials inherent within the family. The following strengths have been identified in this family.

Physical needs are taken care of, such as taking the chil-dren or themselves to a physician when they are sick. Emo-tional needs were tended to when Jerry wore a patch over one of his eyes when his son, Joey, had to wear a patch in treatment for his lazy eye. Jenny and the children have been attending religious services since she was released from the hospital about 1 month ago. These individual data and data patterns are examples of the strengths that Otto describes as *physical, emotional, and spiritual needs of the family.*

This family has fun together, such as Jerry taking the chil-dren to the Detroit Tigers' game, and their play activities, such as bike riding, going to movies, and bowling, done to-gether as a family unit. This pattern of recreation indicates *growth-producing relationships within the family,* as stated by Otto.

Patterns addressed
Otto:
  Biopsychosociospiritual needs of family.
  Growth-producing relationships.
  Responsible community relationships.
A broad conceptual framework for analysis is stated.

There is a need to add more data regarding home furnishing, rooms in home, and space to work and play for all family members.
The spiritual values of the husband need to be addressed and explored further.

Data are categorized appropriately.

Further data are required pertaining to relation-ships outside the family.

ANALYSIS/SYNTHESIS OF DATA—visit 1—cont'd

Analysis/synthesis	Critique

The mother has accepted the community responsibility of currently being secretary for the PTA. This datum indicates her participation in *responsible community relationships.*

Otto's concept of self-help can also be described as universal self-care, described by Orem. This family fulfills the self-help criterion by practicing good food selection, hygiene, and cleanliness in their environment and by taking prescribed medications. Jenny has also verbalized how they have accepted help from relatives on both sides of their family, from friends, such as a neighbor, and from her mother's employer, who is currently sending them meat, cheese, and fresh fruit.

Orem is used as a support theorist in the concept of self-help.

There are not sufficient data to know if good food selection is present or that nutritional knowledge is adequate.

Hygiene practice was not noted in the data bank; it is not known at this time. The house's "clean" appearance is inadequate to justify the inference that the family has positive hygiene practices.

During the mother's hospitalization, both sets of grandparents filled in to help with the mother's functions rather than letting the father do it (I 10). This implies that there is not much *flexibility in family functions,* which is one of the strengths described by Otto.

It is premature to say that there is little flexibility in family functioning. There are few data to support this.

The mother states that she realizes that people have different views of life, such as her husband's lack of search for the meaning of life or for the "truth" as she does. The mother appears to be *respecting the individuality* of her husband, which is another one of Otto's strengths.

Respect for the individual has been well pointed out: pertinent datum.

The mother states that while she was recently hospitalized, she read and reflected about her own life a great deal, which has caused a great change in her life (for the better) (I 27-29). Otto would say that she has used *crisis as a means of growth.*

Data gaps still exist in some areas of Otto's framework, such as child-rearing practices and discipline; communication patterns; support, security, and encouragement; growing with and through children; family unit, loyalty, and intrafamily cooperation; and flexibility of family strengths.

Summary of data gaps.
Patterns addressed
Otto:
   Self-help.
   Flexibility in family functions.
   Respecting individuality.
   Crisis as a means of growth.

Individual

According to Levine, nursing intervention is described in relation to the conservation of energy and to structural, personal, and social integrity. The purpose of conservation is to maintain the "wholeness" or unity of the client.

Conservation of energy refers to balancing the energy output and input to avoid excessive fatigue through proper nutrition, rest, and exercise. Jenny's energy was impaired, as evidenced by her recent hospitalization because of symptoms of extreme fatigue, irritability, and tension.

Conservation of structural integrity refers to the prevention of physical breakdown and the promotion of healing. Her structural integrity may be compromised in any of the following areas: (1) the intermittent presence of PVCs and hypertension—conditions for which she is currently taking medications to assist in the restoration of balance; (2) increased weight—standard weight charts indicate that she is 65 lb overweight. Since Jenny has indicated an interest in losing weight, her motivation could be capitalized upon in a plan of care to also help reduce blood pressure; (3) Hypogly-

Patterns addressed

Levine:
   Conservation of energy.
   Structural integrity.

Good explanation of concept and application of relevant data.

Concept explanation good.
Appropriate data are cited that are relevant to the concept.

Continued.

ANALYSIS/SYNTHESIS OF DATA—visit 1—cont'd

Analysis/synthesis	Critique

cemia—she is on a strict diet (protein) for this condition, but there is no reduction of sodium or cholesterol. Jenny attests that when her hypoglycemia is not controlled she becomes irritable and that this has a great impact on the family (it has not yet been validated that hypoglycemia is the cause of her irritability).	*Patterns addressed*
	Levine:
	  Structural integrity.
	  Personal integrity.
	Pertinent point—integration of Levine's theory of structural integrity and how it impinges on family functioning.

Because of her obesity, the high sodium content in her diet, and the dietary restriction for hypoglycemia, health teaching of a therapeutic diet would be beneficial. In order to conserve her energy, the best possible use must be made of the nutrients she eats. Because of her hypoglycemic condition, she must eat a high protein diet at regular intervals as prescribed by the physician. Relaxing at home has also assisted in the restoration of energy.	There are insufficient data in assessment to support the "high sodium content" of diet. Information is needed on eating patterns, her "strict protein diet," and physician's orders. There are many data gaps here.
Personal integrity, as defined by Levine, refers to a person's self-worth and self-identity: one's own uniqueness. Jenny's self-worth is compromised, as evidenced by her internal tension and nervous habits. Jenny states that she is a "born worry wart" and would like to learn some relaxation techniques that would help her "calm down." Overt manifestations of agitation are her toe jiggling and nail biting. However, she has already started to work on her maladaptive behavior by seeking strength through her new religion. Nursing intervention could focus on some behavior modification techniques while supporting her motivation through religion.	Good explanation of concept and application of appropriate data to show a pattern. A health concern is identified.
Her *personal integrity* (individuality and autonomy) is reflected in the way she has integrated her recent experiences with depleted health and hospitalization by deriving support and strength through religion, as well as through support and cooperation of friends, physician, and family.	
Conservation of *social integrity* refers to involvement and interaction with significant others. Jenny's social integrity has been enhanced by the assistance and support of family, friends, and neighbors who helped during her hospitalization. However, Jerry seems to be "cautiously" adapting to her new behaviors since her return from the hospital.	
In conclusion, there are data to support actual and possible patterns of family strengths as defined by Otto and supported by Levine. Data exist that support possible patterns in the areas of caring for emotional needs, maintaining responsible community relationships, respecting the individuality of others, and using crisis as a means of growth. Actual patterns can be identified in the areas of care for physical and spiritual needs, growth-producing relationships within the family, and self-help.	Conclusion statement includes the integration of Otto's and Levine's theories in providing direction to nursing interventions.
However, the irritability that Jenny has when her hypoglycemia is not controlled has a negative impact on her family, whereby they too become irritable and yell at each other. If her hypoglycemia is kept under control, the decrease in irritability should have a positive effect on their family system. By using their family strengths, nursing implementations should focus on supporting Jenny's efforts to control her hypoglycemia.	

ANALYSIS/SYNTHESIS OF DATA—visit 1—cont'd

Analysis/synthesis	Critique
Also, health teaching is needed for the entire family in the areas of hypertension, hypoglycemia, obesity, and relaxation techniques. This would help increase Jenny's level of energy and minimize the effects of her chronic impairments on the other family members. Although there are no present complaints concerning PVCs and colitis, and these are not currently a concern, they remain a potential threat to the integrity of the family social system, since they have many psychosomatic manifestations.	Excellent summary: identifies actual and potential health concerns and the focus of nursing implementation. *Summary* Strengths: Data categorized according to individual and family and to the theorists Levine and Otto. Data gaps noted and identified. Patterns of behavior identified according to Levine and Otto. Both actual and potential health concerns are identified. Weakness: Limited number of supporting norms, standards, concepts, and theories used (Orem; Bates).[1,9]

DATA COLLECTION—visit 2

Interactions	Observations	Measurements	Critique
TIME: May 6, 1980, 4:00 PM. PLACE: Living room of the family home with all members present. NURSING GOALS: To complete the health history and status of the mother, Jenny, and to assess some of the family health patterns as a data base.			
Jenny speaking 56. We like to go bowling and bike riding together. In winter, sometimes we go cross-country skiing. We don't do much other exercise. Just watch TV. 57. I get car sick if we go a long distance. 58. Our parents live nearby and we visit them often. 59. My mother takes my blood pressure once a week, either here or at her house. 60. She works in a nursing home as a PN, so she is knowledgeable about hypertension and stress. She tells me about losing weight and controlling my diet. 61. We talk on the phone two or three times a week and share our problems. She needs someone to talk to.	27. The father is about 5'8" with reddish brown hair and a full beard. Eyes are "black rimmed" with carbon soot. 28. The father sat in an easy chair reading a newspaper, drinking beer, and smoking cigarettes. 29. Son (5 years old) wears braces on teeth and glasses. His pupils were almost fully dilated. 30. The mother wiggled her foot at various times. 31. The mother seemed agreeable to my contacting the doctor. 32. Although reading, the father appeared interested in what we were saying. 33. The daughter (8 years old) appeared physically and developmentally older— about 10 or 11 years old.	6. BP was 140/76 on left arm in resting (sitting) position.	*Patterns addressed* Otto: Family unity and family cooperation. Growth-producing relationships and experiences. Support, security, and encouragement. Accepting help and self-help. Judgmental and subjective statement. Her reaction should be specifically described (O 31). Unclear: describe body movements (O 32). How does he communicate his interest?

Continued.

DATA COLLECTION—visit 2—cont'd

Interactions	Observations	Measurements	Critique

62. Sure, you can talk to Dr. Jones about my health problems.
63. I would like to try the tension-release exercises—especially if it will keep my blood pressure down.
64. It doesn't seem too hard [when she was doing the tension-release exercises]. I'll probably just need to remember them.
65. We all go to bed early because Jerry gets up so early in the morning for work (5:30 AM). We usually get 8 to 10 hours of sleep.
	34. The daughter has long blond hair in two braids down her back.
	35. All the family members have blue eyes.
	36. Both mother and father smiled when speaking about the mother's changed disposition.
	37. The mother asked the father to take care of the son ["he's your son"] when he was throwing things about in his room.
	38. The son yelled for at least 10 minutes after being spanked by the father.
	39. Neither the mother nor the father paid attention to the son while he was crying in his room.
	40. The son stopped crying and emerged from his room as if nothing had happened.
		7. The mother wiggled her right foot 20 times a minute; this lasted about 5 minutes with short intervals of rest.	*Patterns addressed*
			Otto:
			  Biopsychosocial needs of family.
			  Child-rearing practices.
			  Flexibility of family functioning and roles.
			Insufficient data regarding discipline of son. Interaction information would be of benefit here (O 37).

Current health status: Jenny
Activity of daily living patterns

1. *Diet:* Currently using a diet for hypoglycemia, but not restricting sodium intake. Does not drink anything with caffeine in it because of the PVCs (also because of religious restrictions).

2. *Elimination:* Has had constipation since she was recently hospitalized in April 1980, when she had a barium enema. Has not had a normal bowel movement since, and uses plain water enema (bulb syringe) every 3 days to stimulate defecation. No concerns with urination.

3. *Hygiene:* Showers daily, brushes teeth morning and night.

4. *Substance abuse and use:* Does not use alcohol or tobacco; is currently taking Apresoline with Esidrix twice daily for hypertension, Lomotil twice daily for colitis, and Lanoxin (previously) for PVCs.

5. *Recreation and exercise:* Sews, does ceramics, and goes to garage sales. Family goes bowling, to movies, and bike riding, and visits friends as a family. During winter the family watches much television, and occasionally goes cross-country skiing.

6. *Sleep patterns:* Approximately 8 to 10 hours of sleep each night. Wakes frequently (four to five times) during the night for short periods, usually after "strange" dreams. Snacks at night before retiring.

Patterns addressed
Levine: Structural integrity.
Pertinent datum, but inadequate information. Need specific data concerning type of diet. Give details. Should include either a 3-day diet recall or a 24-hour recall.

Possible concern.

Inadequate data as to winter recreation patterns. For example, the amount of time spent watching television and the frequency of cross-country skiing should be noted.

DATA COLLECTION—visit 2—cont'd

Interactions	Critique

Health history: Jenny

Patterns addressed
Levine: Structural integrity.
Otto: Growth-producing experiences.

1. *Developmental data:* Sucked thumb until she was 13 years old; biting nails since.

Insufficient data regarding development history. Should include physical, growth, and development milestones, and social development.

2. *Promotive and preventive practices:*
   a. *Examinations:* Has been examined by different physicians since birth of second child 6 years ago. Eye exam 6 years ago. Glasses were recommended for close work. Does not wear them—allergic to metal frames—admits to much eye strain and states that she needs to get her eyes rechecked.
   b. *Immunizations:* Up to date; tetanus booster 7 years ago.

Inadequate data regarding different physicians: frequency of visits and reason for change? When was last Gyn exam? No indication of the breast self-exam.

3. *Restorative interventions:* No surgery: had a broken nose (playing croquet) and a broken toe as a child. Both healed well. Had rubella as a child (mother verified *per client*). Contracted rubella during second pregnancy (second month). Titer was checked and no antibodies were found. After "second attack," the titer was repeated and antibodies were found at this time.
4. *Allergies:* Metal (some types)—from eye glasses—skin eruption.

Inadequate data regarding type of allergy to metals and verification by a physician.

Family history

The client (Jenny) has a twin brother, another brother, and a sister. All are in good health. Both parents are alive and relatively well. All these relatives live in the immediate area. The client feels that she can call on them when she needs them.

Insufficient data. Could include health concerns of grandparents and occurrence of chronic impairments (for example, cancer and arthritis). Also include the social and emotional concerns of family, such as parental expectations and family cohesiveness.[1]

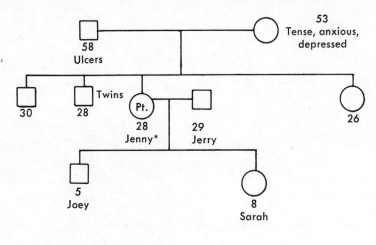

Key: Jenny's family
*Indicates patient
□ Living male
○ Living female

Continued.

DATA COLLECTION—visit 2—cont'd

Interactions	Observations	Measurements	Critique

Social history

The mother has worked as a carpet salesperson for about a year, but has worked very little since her hospitalization in April 1980. The family lives in a one-story ranch style house in Livonia, which has a bedroom for the parents and one for each of the children. Other rooms include a living and dining area, 1½ baths, and a kitchen area. (See previous data—visit 1.)

Review of systems

General state of health: No changes in height or weight; would like to lose 50 lb. Ht 5'11", wt 220 lb. No fever or chills. Not much energy, although she has more since her hospitalization.

Integumentary system:

  a. Skin:

    "I have had a hard lump on my arm for at least a year—the doctor said he would remove it if I wanted him to."

    "I also have a growth on my leg; the doctor said it was just scar tissue and did not have to be removed."

    "My skin is dry in winter." No other complaints of perspiration, pruritus, or flushing.

  b. Hair: No abnormal distribution, growth, or loss.

  c. Nails: I've been biting my nails for 14 years.

Head: Denies pain or trauma to her head except for headaches all over her head; has headaches at least once a day and thinks it could be due to eye strain or constipation. Headaches occur whenever

Observations:

Hard, red, dime-size growth on left upper arm, medial side.

"Keloid" type growth on lateral front side of upper left leg.

Dark blond, wavy hair to shoulders; normal texture.
Shiny nails with changes in texture; no ribbing.

Critique:

More information needed about life-style, home situation, immediate family, and significant others. Should list the typical day, morning, and night. Could include schooling and financial and marital status.[1]

DATA COLLECTION—visit 2—cont'd

Interactions	Observations	Measurements	Critique
crisis or stress is high—such as when Joey was being treated for cataracts. Thought it might be due to high BP, but when they were checked the headaches and BP did not correlate. So now feels it is due to tension.			
Eyes: Some visual changes that occurred just before her hospitalization—described as an object waving back and forth. During these times she felt dizzy. No symptoms other than eye strain.	Client leans forward, rolls eyes back, and gestures with right hand.		
Ears: Denies pain, discharge, hearing changes, vertigo, or ringing.			
Nose and sinuses: Denies pain, discharge, or tenderness. No obstruction, bleeding, or olfactory changes. States that deviated septum is due to broken nose when she was a child. Feels that headaches may be due to sinus flare-ups. Pain above and below eyes.	Nose appears crooked.		
Mouth and throat: Denies pain, swelling, dysphagia, bleeding, or voice changes. However, about once in a 2-week span she is hoarse in the morning when she wakes up.			Incomplete data—dental care not mentioned— last visit to dentist?
Neck: Denies swelling or enlargement. Has some pain in neck when she pulls head to the left. This also causes a headache. Because of pain, she does not have full ROM of head when pain occurs.	Client demonstrates by moving head to the left.		
Breasts: Denies any pain, discharge, or dimpling. Breast fed second child for 2 years.			Could assess her knowledge of breast self-exam.
Respiratory system: Denies pain, wheezing, coughing, dyspnea, sputum, or coughing up blood. Respirations 22 per min.	Sighs frequently.		

Continued.

DATA COLLECTION—visit 2—cont'd

Interactions	Observations	Measurements	Critique
Cardiovascular system: Denies any pain, dyspnea, palpitations, or syncope. Does have some edema characterized by swelling of hands in the morning, once every 2 weeks. Has had PVCs in the past, but they are much less frequent since her recent hospitalization in April 1980.			
Gastrointestinal system:			Incomplete data. Who diagnosed colitis, and when? Under what circumstances did the colitis occur?
· Colitis (type unspecified) was diagnosed 2 years ago. No occurrence since last hospitalization in April 1980. However, she has been constipated since then. States she has more energy since being on a high protein diet. Takes Lomotil for colitis. Triglyceride and cholesterol levels normal.			What are the specifics of her diet—exact measurement of protein, CHO, and fats?
Genitourinary system:			
a. Urinary tract: No concerns. Denies burning discharge, edema, or nocturia.			
b. Genitalia: Denies any burning, pain, lesions, or discharges. Uses contraceptive foam for birth control.			
c. Menstrual: Started menstruating at 12 years. Flows for 5 days on a 28-day cycle.			
d. Obstetrical: Two pregnancies, two living children.			
First pregnancy: Gained 72 lb during pregnancy. Nausea and vomiting during the first 4 months. Also had been spotting blood and stayed in bed "a lot" during this time. During the last 4 months had hives on thighs.			

DATA COLLECTION—visit 2—cont'd

Interactions	Observations	Measurements	Critique
Second pregnancy: Developed rubella in 2 or 3 months. In the seventh month she developed toxemia. Was placed in the hospital and told she was borderline diabetic. In seventh month she dilated 4½ cm. At full term she took castor oil to facilitate labor. Easy labor and delivery.			
Musculoskeletal system: Denies any pain, tenderness, swelling, weakness, deformities, or decreased ROM, except for neck area. Does get cramps in arches of feet. Cause unknown.			
Neurological system:			
a. General status: Denies any somnolence, convulsions, or weakness. Complains of motion sickness in car.			
b. Mental status: Denies anxiety, amnesia, phobias, or hallucinations. States there is a change in her disposition since hospitalization—"much calmer than before." Also less depressed since her hospitalization.			Incongruency in data— many symptoms of anxiety present as related in visit 1—need further assessment and exploration.
c. Motor status: Denies alteration in gait, tremors or concerns in coordination.			
d. Sensory status: Denies pain but complains of some tingling and numbness in fingertips, usually accompanied by edema of hands, once in 2 weeks.	Extends hands and looks at them.		
Hematopoietic system: Denies bleeding tendencies, lymph node enlargement, or anemia. Does bruise easily.	Holds out arm to reveal a bruise—quarter size, blue-colored contusion on lateral lower side of left arm.		

Continued.

DATA COLLECTION—visit 2—cont'd

Interactions	Observations	Measurements	Critique
Endocrine system: Denies excessive dryness of skin, perspirations, abnormal distribution of hair, changes in weight, sensitivity to temperature, polydipsia, polyuria, or anorexia. Hypoglycemia was diagnosed in April.	Skin of smooth texture, slightly pink in cheeks.		
Allergic and immunological response system: Denies pruritus, migraine, dermatitis, or urticaria. However, did develop a rash when wearing glasses.	Skin appears clear and free from blemishes.		

Data gaps

More complete information is needed on her cardiovascular system as it relates to the PVCs and her GI system as it relates to the colitis. Possibly may need to confer with physician.

Other assessment data needed are sexual history, information on "high-protein" diet, a 3-day diet recall or 24-hour recall, and spiritual and psychosocial values.

Strengths
Data comprehensive and multifocal.
The mother was the primary source of information—father nonverbally supported her.

Weakness
More information is needed in the spiritual, psychosocial, sexual, and diet areas.

ANALYSIS/SYNTHESIS OF DATA—visit 2

Analysis/synthesis	Critique

Holistic analysis May 6, 1980 (second visit)

Previous analysis is still appropriate.

According to the *conservation principles* defined by Levine, energy output should match energy input; that is, a person should get enough rest, nutrition, and exercise to build energy supply and strength to match the energy requirements of living. Exercise develops muscle tone and helps maintain circulation. Moderate, regular exercise is recommended for all adult age groups because it stimulates the health of the tissues in relation to blood supply and growth. It also lowers the blood pressure and in general improves the health status of the individual. Since there is little energy expenditure in the activities of daily living and since Jenny has never followed an established exercise routine, it would be appropriate to set up such a regimen with the support and approval of her physician.

Patterns addressed
Levine:
  Conservation of energy.
  Structural integrity.
Otto:
  Child-rearing practices.
  Communication.
  Support, security, and encouragement.
  Growth-producing relationships.
What is the reference for this?
Not clear; is this in relation to large group muscle activities or to relaxation technique activities?

ANALYSIS/SYNTHESIS OF DATA—visit 2—cont'd

Analysis/synthesis	Critique
In regard to her *structural integrity*, Jenny states that her hypertension and blood levels of cholesterol and triglycerides are within normal limits at present. However, since there is no salt restriction evident in her diet, health teaching in the area of diet and salt control is imperative. The teaching of proper nutritional habits will also aid in the resolution of weight control problems, hypertension, and hypoglycemia. Jenny has not mentioned colitis since the phone conversation. This needs to be assessed during the next visit.	"No salt restriction" was not supported in data assessment. Insufficient data to make this conclusion.
Otto has reiterated that it is considered a strength if both parents respect each other's views and decisions on *child-rearing practices* and both assume responsibility in this regard. When the son was making loud noises in his room and causing a disruption, the mother spoke to the father about it, who promptly went into the son's room and spanked him. The mother appeared pleased with this action. This datum may reflect a pattern that the parents agree about discipline.	More information needed to make a conclusion about child-rearing practices.
During the above incident, when the mother said "See to Joey, he's your son," the father understood her to mean that she wanted him to make Joey behave. This datum is an example of their *communication* technique. The father was very quiet and said very little during our interview. The mother did all the talking unless the nurse specifically asked a question of other family members. Their *communication* patterns need to be explored further to ascertain if they meet Otto's criterion as a strength.	More information needed in this area to make conclusive statements about communication.
Although not explicitly stressed by the family members, the quality of *support, security, and encouragement* (strengths identified by Otto) is implicit in their relationships as reflected in their patterns of rest and activities.	Further assessment data are needed and should be documented.
Growth-producing relationships (another strength identified by Otto) within the family may be partially ascertained in Jenny's relationship with her mother, who takes her blood pressure weekly and keeps a "watchful eye" on Jenny's condition. However, this area needs further assessment.	Insufficient data to conclude a "growth-producing" relationship with mother. The mother's "watchful eye" may impede independence and growth in Jenny and her family, thus producing tension.
Data gaps still exist in some areas of Otto's framework, such as growing with and through children and flexibility of family strength.	Data gaps: Identified but incomplete. More information is needed in family relationships, communication, and the family and social history. An increased depth of knowledge is needed in all areas.
In conclusion, there are additional data to support actual and possible patterns of family strengths as defined by Otto. Data exist that support possible patterns in the area of shared ideas about discipline and communication techniques. Actual strength patterns can be identified in the areas of family support, security, and encouragement, and in the maintenance of growth-producing relationships. The potential for complications due to the mother's chronic impairments still exists, and nursing interventions remain focused on prevention. Whether these potentials are related to lack of knowledge or lack of compliance needs to be further assessed.	Pertinent point since nursing intervention will be based on this knowledge. *Summary* Data are appropriately categorized according to Otto's framework and patterns of family behavior, and strengths and health concerns are identified.

DATA COLLECTION—visit 3

Interactions	Observations	Measurements	Critique

TIME: May 13, 1980, 4:00 PM.
PLACE: Living room of the family home with all members present.
NURSING GOALS: To further assess the family in terms of Otto's strengths, such a communication patterns, flexibility, and roles, as well as compliance to regimen (tension-release exercises and diet control) and the family's perception of the illness.

Interactions	Observations	Measurements	Critique
66. Jenny: I was told to get a thyroid test, but I haven't done it yet.	41. Jerry reading a newspaper, glanced up occasionally.		*Patterns addressed* Levine: Personal integrity. Structural integrity.
67. Jenny: I tried the tension-release exercises only four times.	42. Jenny sat, jiggling her foot rapidly.		Otto: Self-help and accepting help. Communication.
68. Jenny: I'm so busy it's hard to fit them in. (I'm not back at work yet but I do make telephone contacts about sales.) Sometimes I feel so silly doing them (the exercises).	43. Jenny appeared apologetic.		Support and encouragement. Crisis as a means of growth. May indicate lack of motivation and non-compliance. Clarification of data is needed (I 66, 68).
69. Jerry: I noticed that since she got back from the hospital, she is a lot calmer and doesn't hold her feelings inside like she did before.	44. The husband gave information only when questioned by the nurse.		Pertinent information regarding communication patterns in the family (O 44).
70. Jenny: I'm glad you asked him that, because I was wondering if he had noticed a difference. He hasn't said anything about it to me.			
71. Sarah: Yes, Mama seems a lot better since she was in the hospital. She doesn't yell as much any more.	45. The daughter sat in the room playing with a Barbie doll. She offered this information in response to the nurse's questioning.		
72. Jenny: Yes, I can do the T-R exercises for you; now? I still feel silly doing them.	46. Jenny demonstrated how she is doing the exercises—one time.		*Patterns addressed* Levine: Personal integrity. Structural integrity.
73. Jenny: I would like to have you do them with me again.	47. Jenny asked the nurse to join in doing the exercises.		Otto: Growth with children. Growth experiences. Support and encouragement.
74. Jerry: I wouldn't mind learning them, too, if it would help Jenny. In fact, it would probably help all of us.	48. Jerry agreed to do this when the nurse coaxed him into it.		Family unity and cooperation.

DATA COLLECTION—visit 3—cont'd

Interactions	Observations	Measurements	Critique
75. Sarah: Me, too; I want to learn, and then I can teach Joey.	49. Sarah dropped her doll and wanted to join in the activity.		
76. Jenny: I'll try harder next week.			
77. Jenny: Food doesn't taste good without salt. I don't watch the salt in my diet too much because I take a diuretic and that washes out the salt.			Important information regarding misconception of the relationship of diet and medication. There is a lack of knowledge regarding food preparation (I 77).
78. Jenny: I know it's important; my mother told me about strokes and eye problems from hypertention. My BP was 148/86 last week.			*Patterns addressed* Levine: Structural integrity. Otto:
79. Jenny: That would help— to have a list of foods that have a low salt content.	50. Jenny appeared eager to have the list of foods to use in preparing menus.		Flexibility of family strengths. Biosociopsychological needs of family. Support and encouragement.
80. Jenny: Maybe we can all eat the same menu, if I could prepare food without salt and still have it taste good.			Subjective statement; facial expressions and tone of voice should be described (O 50).
81. Jenny: It's easier to do (menu planning) when you have a knowledgeable person (nurse) to do it with.	51. The nurse and client sat down and prepared menus for three meals.		*Strengths* Data are multifocal and comprehensive. Varied sources of information (father, mother and daughter).
82. Jenny: I'll work on it this week; and also the exercises.			Data are pertinent to health concerns. Patterns addressed are from Levine and Otto. *Weakness* The son still was not included in the interactions.

ANALYSIS/SYNTHESIS OF DATA—visit 3

Analysis/synthesis	Critique

Holistic analysis May 13, 1980 (third visit)

Previous analyses still pertinent.

Otto described crisis as a means of growth.

In examining the process by which families define an event as a crisis, Hill and Hansen[3] identified four interrelated factors that influence the family's ability to cope with illness. Applying these criteria to this family yields the following analysis.

1. *Characteristics of the event:*
   a. Nature of the pathological conditions: The mother has hypertension controlled (in part) by a diuretic and hypoglycemia controlled by diet. For the past 2 years she has had colitis and PVCs. These last two impairments have not distressed her since her last hospitalization in April. The son has cataracts and is deaf in one ear. These are chronic concerns; while currently posing no concern to the child, they are a disability and in time will need anticipatory guidance for a productive future. The mother's impairments started with the onset of her son's concerns.
   b. Type of impairment: The mother doesn't tolerate car travel since her colitis flare-up. There are no other complications at present. Nursing intervention is designed primarily to prevent future disabilities resulting from complications related to hypertension and hypoglycemia. The son has impairments related to cataracts and nerve deafness in one ear.
   c. Prognosis: The mother's physician stated that she can control her hypoglycemia and obesity through diet, and her hypertension through diet, medication, and control of stress input. No recommendations were made regarding PVCs or colitis, since these are not current concerns.
   d. Potential for rehabilitation: The mother's energy and structural integrity should be maintained and complications prevented if she follows her physician's and nurse's counsel regarding diet and relaxation. Although the mother states that her son is not disabled, he is nonetheless permanently deaf in one ear because of nerve deafness, which in the current state of the art cannot be repaired. He wears corrective glasses in the treatment of his cataracts. He is currently in kindergarten and is assessed there for any hearing, speech, or sight alterations. So far he has not needed any special therapy in order to keep up with his peers.

Patterns addressed

All data are analyzed according to Hill and Hansen's family crisis theory, using these four criteria:

1. Characteristics of the event.
2. Perceived threat to family relationships, status, and goals.
3. Resources available to the family.
4. Past experience of similar nature.

Pertinent point relates to stress and tension as etiological factors in chronic impairments.

These concerns reinforce nursing diagnosis 1 and the need for tension-relaxation exercises.

Potential concern of deafness identified more clearly.

ANALYSIS/SYNTHESIS OF DATA—visit 3—cont'd

Analysis/synthesis	Critique
e. The family's perception of the illness: The father states that he hopes that his wife can keep her hypertension and hypoglycemia under control. He also states that he has noticed a big difference in her since her recent hospitalization, that she is a lot calmer and doesn't hold her feelings inside like she used to. Her 8-year-old daughter also stated that her mother has changed for the better since she "got sick."	
2. *Perceived threat to family relationships, status, and goals:*	
a. There has been no change in family roles; however, relations and communication patterns have changed in that the mother states that she has stopped yelling at her family. Consequently, they too have stopped yelling at each other as much as they used to.	Pertinent inference is congruent with previous data relating to communication patterns.
b. The family states that they realize the changes in their communication patterns are related to the mother's changed attitude, rather than to the illness itself.	
c. Decision-making patterns before and after the illness are characterized by seeking out and following medical advice.	
d. A data gap exists for input into individual and family "life goals" and changes in life goals secondary to the illness.	
e. The mother, father, and daughter stated that their interactions have improved since her hospitalization.	
3. *Resources available to the family:* The mother states that all of their relatives and friends support them in times of need and can be counted on to help.	
4. *Past experience with the same or similar situation:*	
a. During crises experienced prenatally (car accident, toxemia) and postnatally (child born with congenital defects, deaf in one ear and subsequent cataracts) with second child, family immediately sought medical attention and followed advice given, which resulted in corrective surgery on the baby's eyes.	
b. All family members and some friends were identified as being able to be counted on in time of crisis.	
Since the husband and wife have said very little to each other during the nurse's visits, and since the wife indicated that her husband did not communicate his pleasure in her change in behavior to her directly, it is assumed that further assessment of communication patterns should be done in future visits.	Integration of both Otto's theory and Hill and Hansen's crisis theory.

Continued.

ANALYSIS/SYNTHESIS OF DATA—visit 3—cont'd

Analysis/synthesis	Critique
Data gaps still exist in the areas of Otto's framework of flexibility of family strengths and growing with and through children.	*Strengths*
	Use of Hill and Hansen as a support theory for Otto's self-help and growth through crisis.
The mother stated that she had problems staying on a low salt diet. Intervention will be aimed at this. Tension-release exercises that she started a week ago were probably done perfunctorily. Reinforcement was done this week, and this aspect will be followed up with technique each visit.	Provides direction for nursing interventions.
	Conclusive statements are made at the end of each concept.
	Strengths and health concerns were identified as they impinge on the family.
In conclusion, the nursing implementation will remain focused on preventing potential complications in the mother due to uncontrolled hypoglycemia and hypertension, thereby reducing the amount of stress on the entire family.	Data gaps were identified.
	Data were related to appropriate concepts in frameworks to show patterns.

NURSING DIAGNOSIS

Date	Diagnoses	Critique
5/1	**1.** Loss of energy and structural integrity in the mother related to anxiety. **2.** Family tensions related to loss of energy and structural integrity in the mother. **3.** Alterations in nutrition related to the mother's lack of knowledge. **4.** Potential threat to the family's social system related to the mother's chronic impairments. **5.** Alteration in the family's adaptation related to the mother's change in values (religious beliefs). **6.** Potential family disruption related to the son's hearing impairment. **7.** Potential complications in the mother related to hypertension and hypoglycemia. **8.** Alterations in the mother's circulatory system related to hypertension.	*Summary of guidelines* 1. Each diagnosis is client centered, specific, and accurate. 2. They are clear, but tend to be wordy with the use of Levine's terminology. 3. They reflect both potential and actual concerns. 4. They relate to etiological factors. 5. The arrangement of priorities of nursing diagnoses sets the direction for nursing interventions.
5/6	Same as above.	
5/13	Same as above.	

PLANS FOR IMPLEMENTATION

Nursing diagnosis 1: *Loss of energy and structural integrity in client (mother) related to anxiety.*
Goal: *Client will increase energy level through decreasing tension by 6/6/80.*

Objectives	Nursing orders	Scientific rationale
1. Client (mother) will choose a tension-release strategy by 5/6/80.	1a. The nurse and client will discuss contractual agreement regarding the appropriate nursing interventions.	The contract must be explicit to all parties involved and the client involved in all aspects of care. Specific commitments are made so that each person is aware of the therapeutic relationship.[2]
	1b. The nurse and client will discuss the purpose and the techniques to be used.	Strategy: Teaching, learning, and discussion.[11]
	1c. The nurse and client will go through the exercises together (the nurse will first demonstrate the exercises to the client).	Strategy: Demonstration is a method of teaching skills and techniques related to nursing care that can be used with equal effectiveness for both individual and group teaching.[11]
	1d. The client will demonstrate the exercise while the nurse checks for release of tension in various muscle groups.	Reinforcement will increase the client's sense of security in knowing the sequence of movements to release tension.[11]
	1e. The nurse will give the client a set of written instructions in regard to methods of choice.	Evaluation is an integral part of learning.[11] Reinforcement is accomplished by the use of several modes of communication.[11]
2. The client (mother) will practice the selected method at least once a day for 1 week, beginning 5/6/80.	2a. The client will set times to practice these exercises for 1 week, such as: Midmorning. Before children come home from school or before dinner. Other times when she feels she is becoming "upset." Before she loses her temper. Other times she may suggest in addition to the above.	Relaxation is the "casting off" of nervous tension and anxiety.[4] "Deep muscular relaxation is almost always accompanied by mental calm." If one can release the tension, which is consuming energy, then that very energy will be released and put in action toward more constructive use.[8] Relaxation therapy may become a useful adjunct to the clinical management of hypertension.[4]

Evaluation	Critique

Contract mutually agreed upon, 5/6/80.
Criteria statement:
  The client will cite the following information:
  1. The benefit of tension-release exercises on muscle groups.
  2. The effects of tension-release exercises on hypertension.
  3. The technique of tension-release of various muscle groups.
The nurse implemented plans 1a through 1e, 5/6/80.
The client proceeded through the exercise with the nurse.
The client demonstrated the exercises with some degree of accuracy, 5/6/80.
Objective 1 met, 5/6/80.
	Goals
	Broadly stated, client focused.
	Mutually established, dated.
	Appropriate to nursing diagnosis.
	Objectives
	Client focused and specific.
	Appropriate to goals.
	Indicative of specific behavior outcomes.
	Objective 1 sounds as though it were nurse initiated rather than client initiated.
	Nursing orders
	Sequential order based on priority.
	Specific terms.
	Alternate ways to relieve tension not explored with client (not clear that client had a choice).
	Scientific rationale
	Scientific basis for nursing actions cited.
	The word "discussion" opposite plan 1b needs clarifying.
	Evaluation
	Criteria statements are adequate and appropriate.
	Summative statement needs expanding—need more client behaviors cited in order to state that objective 1 is met.

The client set up times to do tension-release exercises.
Times were:
  Early morning—9 AM.
  Before dinner—3PM.
  (Week of 5/6 to 5/13.)
The client did the exercises only four times that week; objective partially met.
	Objectives
	Specific, client focused.
	Dated, agreed on in first visit.
	Realistic, achievable.
	Nursing orders
	Dated.
	Appropriate to goal, objectives, and assessment data.
	Can achieve the objectives.
	Preventive in nature.
	Considerate of individuality of client.
	Scientific rationale
	Involves research to support nursing actions.
	Evaluation
	Criteria statements are not clearly defined as to expected behavior.
	Client behaviors cited, however, are specific and appropriate to objectives and nursing orders.

Continued.

PLANS FOR IMPLEMENTATION—cont'd

Nursing diagnosis 1: *Loss of energy and structural integrity in client (mother) related to anxiety.*
Goal: *Client will increase energy level through decreasing tension by 6/6/80.*

Objectives	Nursing orders	Scientific rationale
3. The client (mother) will use tension-release exercises on a regular basis, starting 5/13/80.	3a. On 5/13/80 the nurse will review with the client: The number of times she did the exercises the previous week. The sequence of doing the tension-release exercises. 3b. The client will verbalize any problems she may have had in regard to doing this activity and make necessary modifications. 3c. The client will set up times to do tension-release exercises on a regular basis: Mid-morning. Before dinner. (Joint family project.)	Evaluation is an integral part of learning.[10] Reinforcement by repetition is an important part of learning.[11] The client should be involved in all aspects of planning, and the plan must be tailored to specific individual needs.[2]
4. The client (entire family) will begin to use tension-release exercises by 5/27/80.	4a. All family members will learn and practice the tension-release exercises once a day, using the same techniques as described above with some modifications for the children in relation to appropriate developmental levels. (See plans 1a through 1d.)	Helping the family solve problems and develop coping abilities is essential to client participation.[2] Family-centered approach focuses on the family as a "unit of people" in which the health of one member affects the health of all others.[2]

Evaluation	Critique
The client did the T-R exercises only four times during the week.	
The client verbalized the sequence of tension-release exercises accurately.	
The client identified problems with the exercises:	
Felt "silly" doing them.	
Could not remember to do them at set times.	
The client did feel a little more relaxed after doing them.	
The nurse implemented plan 3a.	
The client set up alternate times to do exercises, such as midmorning and in the evening before dinner (with entire family) (5/13/80).	
The client is doing tension-release exercises at least once a day (5/28/80).	
Objective 3 met.	
Criteria statement:	*Objectives*
The family (client) will cite the following information:	Specific and family oriented.
1. The benefits of T-R exercises.	Appropriate to goal but not conclusive as to whether they will achieve it or are sufficient for it.
2. The sequencing of steps to achieve the T-R exercise.	Arranged in order of priority from individual to family.
3. The technique of T-R exercise.	*Nursing orders*
The nurse implemented plans as in objective 1 (1a through 1d).	4a is not as specific as it could be, especially in teaching T-R exercise to children.
The family members practiced the exercise with the nurse.	*Scientific rationale*
Family members demonstrated exercises with the nurse (5/13/80).	Family-centered support.
The family is doing T-R exercises (5/28/80).	*Evaluation*
Objective 4 met.	Criteria statement for plan 4a could be more specific for various age levels.
	Insufficient data as to family reactions to T-R exercises and plan implementation.
	Summative evaluation not clear; it is not known whether or not the goal is reached; could have checked BP after the T-R exercises for validation of reduction in BP.

Continued.

PLANS FOR IMPLEMENTATION—cont'd

Nursing diagnosis 3: *Alterations in nutrition related to mother's lack of knowledge.*
Goal: *Client will increase knowledge regarding therapeutic diet by 5/30/80.*

Objectives	Nursing orders	Scientific rationale
1. The client will verbalize the relationship and consequences of sodium and water balance in the body.	1a. The nurse will collaborate with the physician to reaffirm the client's need to decrease her sodium intake to below 3 g per day (5/20/80).	Collaboration Motivation: Individuals must be motivated to learn; the client must have high respect for the physician; support and encouragement from care givers is a motivating factor and a strength.[10,11]
	1b. The client will verbalize to the nurse what she presently knows about the significance of salt in the diet and its ultimate relationship to hypertension (5/24/80).	Teaching and learning; discussion: "Effective learning requires active participation and new learning must be based on previous knowledge and experience."[11]
	1c. The nurse will discuss with the client the importance of restricting salt in the diet on 5/24/80.	
	1d. The nurse will discuss with the client how salt is eliminated from the body system.	
	1e. The nurse will give written information to client regarding: Elimination of sodium from the body. High sodium foods to be avoided. Low sodium foods that are encouraged. Food preparation (including food likes and dislikes) for a low sodium diet.	Reinforcement (teaching and learning): The use of written information to reinforce the previous discussion may be used as a starting point in future teaching and discussion of this topic.[11] "The individual discovery of the meaning that the information holds for her will facilitate her learning process."[7]
	1f. The nurse will ask the client to read and study information for discussion at next visit on 5/30/80.	"Effective learning requires participation of the learner."[11]
	1g. The client will relate information to the nurse regarding salt, hypertension, and low and high salt foods in the diet (5/30/80).	"Evaluation is an integral part of learning."[11]

Evaluation	Critique

Criteria statement:
The client will verbalize:
  1. The importance of the balance of salt and fluid content to the body.
  2. The importance of restricting salt in the diet.
  3. The elimination of salt from the body.
  4. Foods that are to be avoided.
  5. Foods that are low in salt.
The nurse implemented plans 1a through 1g.
The client related the consequences of noncontrolled intake of salt: heart failure, stroke, kidney disease, retinal changes.
The client could name all foods with high salt content.
Objective 1 met.
	Goals
	Broad in scope.
	Appropriate to implement the nursing diagnosis.
	Realistic and attainable.
	Mutuality unknown.
	Objectives
	Stated in specific terms.
	Appropriate to goals.
	Lack of date-time measurement.
	Client focused.
	Nursing orders
	Appropriate to assessment data.
	Stated in terms of client and nurse behaviors.
	Incorporates collaboration activities (with physician).
	Sequentially placed.
	Scientific rationale
	Strategy and individuality are addressed.
	Insufficient information in regard to rationale for low sodium diet.
	Evaluation
	Criteria statement is appropriate.
	Formative evaluation describes nurse behaviors.
	Need to describe client's reactions to each point, especially her present knowledge, in 1b.

Continued.

PLANS FOR IMPLEMENTATION—cont'd

Nursing diagnosis 3: *Alterations in nutrition related to mother's lack of knowledge.*
Goal: *Client will increase knowledge regarding therapeutic diet by 5/30/80.*

Objectives	Nursing orders	Scientific rationale
2. The client will plan a daily diet that is a low-calorie hypoglycemic diet with a low sodium content (mutually agreed upon).	2a. The client will verbalize her own and the family's food preferences, by 5/30/80. 2b. The client will plan a menu using the prescribed hypoglycemic diet with a low-sodium modification for three meals by 5/30/80. 2c. The nurse will check the menu against prescribed regimen and norms. 2d. The client will prepare and eat planned therapeutic meals for 3 days during the week of 5/30/80 to 6/6/80. 2e. The nurse and client will discuss any problems (individual or family) that may have arisen from using this diet, such as food dislikes, poorly prepared food, or tasteless food.	The plan must be tailored to individual preferences and needs.[6] The care plan must be individualized to suit the client's needs and desires.[6] Active participation on the part of the client is necessary for learning. The client will choose which days she will implement the diet.[11] Evaluation is an integral part of learning.[14]

Evaluation	Critique

Criteria statement:
  1. The client will verbalize her likes and dislikes.
  2. The client will plan a menu for three meals and implement this menu for three meals sometime within the coming week.
Plans 2a through 2d were implemented and facilitated by the nurse and client.
The client discussed the problem of getting the family to eat certain foods on the diet.
Alternate plans will be addressed at a later date.
	Objectives
	Stated in specific terms.
	Mutually established.
	Insufficient data in regard to time and date.
	Nursing orders
	Appropriate to assessment data.
	Dated.
	Stated in specific terms for both nurse and client.
	Nursing action in 2d is not appropriate to objective 2; it goes beyond the scope of this objective; a new objective must be stated for this action.
	Scientific rationale
	Strategies are well supported and documented.
	Topic—content of low sodium diet—not supported by rationale.
	Evaluation
	Criteria statement lists behavioral outcomes.
	Insufficient data in regard to client reactions to nursing interventions.
	Insufficient data as to the foods that this family has problems with; should give an example.
	Include the individuality of the client (likes and dislikes).
	Reassess data.
	List specific concerns to be explored.
	Summative evaluation not present; attainment of goal not discussed.
	Insufficient data; evaluation incomplete (no alternate plan).

CONCLUSION

Members of the Davis family were subsequently seen over the next 6 months; Otto's and Levine's conceptual frameworks were used for continued assessment and implementation.

Other nursing diagnoses emerged (such as impaired communication in family members, potential pulmonary stress in the father related to hazardous working conditions, and decrease in intrafamily communication) as time went on. Goals and objectives were established, and many contracts were made and negotiated before the nurse closed the health records on this family. As each concern came into the awareness of both family and nurse, goals, objectives, and plans were mutually established, implemented, and eventually resolved in varying degrees.

Setting priorities for goal attainment and successfully resolving concerns as they arose, the family attained a higher level of functioning. Family strengths were present and identified throughout the difficulties, and potential strengths were pointed out in didactic sessions with the entire family. As a result of working through both their crises and their long-range concerns, this family now has greater strengths and resources.

REFERENCES

1 Bates, B.: A guide to physical examination, ed. 2, Philadelphia, 1978, J.B. Lippincott Co.
2 Clemen, S., Eigsti, S., and McGuire, S.: Comprehensive family and community health planning, New York, 1981, McGraw-Hill Book Co.
3 Hill, R., and Hansen, D.A.: Families Under Stress. In Christensen, H.T., editor: Handbook of marriage and family, Chicago, 1964, Rand McNally and Co.
4 Jacob, R.G., Kraemer, H.C., and Agras, W.S.: Relaxation therapy on the treatment of hypertension, Arch. Gen. Psychiatry **34:**1417, 1977.
5 Levine, M.E.: Introduction to clinical nursing, ed. 2, Philadelphia, 1973, F.A. Davis Co.
6 Little, D., and Carnevali, D.: Nursing care planning, ed. 2, Philadelphia, 1976, J.B. Lippincott Co.
7 Murray, M.: Fundamentals of nursing, Englewood Cliffs, N.J., 1976, Prentice-Hall, Inc.
8 Nicassio, P., and Bootzin, R.: A comparison of progressive relaxation and autogenic training as treatment for insomnia, J. Abnorm. Psychol. **83:** 253, 1974.
9 Orem, D.: Nursing: concepts of practice, ed. 2, New York, 1980, McGraw-Hill Book Co.
10 Otto, H.: A framework for assessing family strengths. In Reinhardt, A.M., and Quinn, M.D., editors: Family-centered community nursing, vol. 1, St. Louis, 1973, The C.V. Mosby Co.
11 Pohl, M.: The teaching function of the nursing practitioner, ed. 3, Dubuque, Iowa, 1978, Wm. C. Brown Co., Publishers.

BIBLIOGRAPHY

Bailey, J.T., and Claus, K.E.: Decision making in nursing, St. Louis, 1975, The C.V. Mosby Co.
Mahoney, E., Verdissa, L., and Shortridge, L.: How to collect and record a health history, New York, 1976, J.B. Lippincott Co.
Malasanos, L., and others: Health assessment, ed. 2, St. Louis, 1981, The C.V. Mosby Co.

NURSING PROCESS
of the community client

LINDA L. DELANEY
BONNIE L. SOMMERVILLE

This chapter examines the hypothetical community of Pleasant View. The nursing care plan is presented and critiqued. As in the previous chapters, the data here have references at the end of this chapter. References for this hypothetical community are, of course, fictitious but provide a sample format for documentation.

Data collection. Data have been collected using the tools of observation, interaction, and measurement, and categorized into structure and process. The critique column identifies the pattern of the data and data gaps, and provides a critique of the data presented. The data were all collected before the analysis and the implementation of plans.

Data analysis. During the analysis or the processing of the data, theories, models, and principles are used, data are compared with standards, and judgments are made as to whether the functioning of the community indicates a health concern or an asset. All aspects of the community are examined. However, the main focus is on data relating to health. Health resources are analyzed by looking at the direct services provided and the three categories of services recommended in *Healthy People: The Surgeon General's Report on Health Promotion and Disease Prevention.*[37] These categories are preventive health services, those services that can be delivered to individuals by health providers; health protection services, measures that can be used by governmental and other agencies to protect people from harm; and health promotion services, those activities that individuals and communities can use to promote health life-styles.

Goals, objectives, and plans. Knowledge regarding functioning of the community provides information as to what change strategies will be useful. The process of change, as conceptualized by Lewin, is used, and involves three steps: (1) unfreezing, (2) moving toward the new level, and (3) refreezing at the new level.[17]

Evaluation. Evaluation data are not collected, since this is a hypothetical process. Questions to indicate appropriate data are provided in the evaluation column. Criteria standards are also established.

DATA COLLECTION

Observations	Interactions

Category: *Structure*
Pattern: *Characteristics and uniqueness*

The sense of sight is used in the following:
1. West, south, and north boundaries are artificially construed with no visible geographic delineation.
   The east boundary is the Buckeye River.
   Boundaries exist mainly in rural areas.
   State route 24 divides area; it is the only four-lane road in the township.
   Topography gently sloping terrain.
   All residential areas bounded by farmland.
2. Area combination of residential housing and much farmland.
   Concentrated business zones with interspersed small businesses along one of the main arteries.

3. In housing development, lawns well maintained with healthy-looking shrubbery, perennials, lawns, and trees.
4. Housing relatively new—very few houses older than 20 years.
5. Farm dwellings older than housing developments.
   Over-all good condition of barns and farm houses.

6. Many brick houses in development. Two-car garages predominant with late-model automobiles in driveways.
   Garages filled with conglomeration of tools, bicycles, and lawn equipment. Lawn furniture evident in many back yards.
7. Only a few privacy fences.
8. Animals seen on leashes or in yards; no strays evident.
   Rabbits, birds, and squirrels observed in some of the developments.
9. No sidewalks.
   Two-way streets in minimum repair.
   Speed limits 35 mph in rural areas, 15 mph in neighborhoods.
   No centerline street markings except for main highway.

1. "The township border goes right through the northern section of my farm."[32]

2. "The area is characterized by well-drained soil underlain by sand and gravel."[6]

3. The value of houses in Pleasant View ranges from about $30,000 to $200,000. The average is $75,000.[8]

Measurements	Critique
	The data identified as "characteristics and uniqueness" are collected through conducting a windshield survey. (See p. 68, Chapter 6.) Although these are subjective data, they must be presented in an objective manner, as stated in Chapter 3. The inferences and hunches that are generated by the subjective data give clues about the community that can be further assessed using objective methods. During the collection of subjective data, the use of all the senses is helpful.
1. See Appendix A for map outlining boundaries. [*Editor's note:* Appendix A, map, not included here.]	Data regarding boundaries are objectively stated (O 1).
	"Much farmland" is a subjective statement. Would be more useful to have numbers of acres or percentage of farmland (O 2).
	Data gap: Ratio of farmland to developed land. Are crops growing in fields? What kinds? What kinds of animals are observed?
	"Healthy looking" shrubbery, perennials, lawns, and trees subjectively stated (O 3).
2. 51 square miles, estimated population 30,000.	Need documentation of source (M 2).
	Term "relatively" is subjective, but is clarified by the statement "older than 20 years" (O 4).
	Would be useful to know approximate age of farm dwellings. This would provide historical background information about the community. "Good" is an evaluative statement (O 5).
	"Many brick homes" is subjective term. An example of a more objective statement would be "approximately 85% of homes constructed of brick" (O 6).
	Data gap: Data state "many brick homes"—what are other construction materials—stone, wood, stucco?
	"Only a few privacy fences"—subjective term (O 7).
	Data objectively stated—concise and significant in that information is provided regarding uniqueness of community (O 8).
	"Streets in minimum repair" is subjective. Would be more useful to state actual conditions: "two way streets have large chuckholes and crumbling pavement" (O 9).

Continued.

DATA COLLECTION—cont'd

Observations	Interactions

Category: *Structure*
Pattern: *Characteristics and uniqueness —cont'd*

10. Children and adults seen on minibikes or bicycles riding on streets.
    Children observed in all areas roller-skating and skate-boarding on streets.

11. Neighborhood watch signs in all the four subdivisions.

12. People observed in neat but modest attire, appear clean, tanned, and sporting new cars, and riding 3-speed or 10-speed bikes.

The sense of hearing is predominant in collecting these data:
13. No heavy industry evident.

Taste is used while collecting these data:
14. Varied preference for food evident. Several fast-food restaurants featuring hamburgers, pizza, and chicken, plus Italian, Mexican, and "home-cooked" food establishments.

The sense of smell is used in the following:
15. Pleasant smells of honeysuckle and jasmine in residential areas. Air void of noxious odors, except near Highway 24. There, odor of gas fumes evident.

4. Angry residents gathered at City Commission meeting last night requesting stricter enforcement of speed limits or a ban on construction vehicles in Woodland Hills section. A petition with 200 signatures was presented along with verbal complaints.[25]
   Seven-year-old in "serious condition" in local hospital after being struck by truck while walking dog in street.[25]

5. "I'm the president of the north neighborhood organization. We have four of these organizations in this area. All are fairly active politically and all have organized neighborhood watch areas."[1]

6. Community free of noise except for sounds of traffic on two major N-S and two major E-W thoroughfares.

7. "When we want to raise money for a cause we have a pancake breakfast, steak fry, spaghetti supper, or ice cream social."[16]

8. People smiled and talked to one another in local business establishments. All people interviewed warm and friendly.

Measurements	Critique
	Objective presentation of datum with source stated. This datum may give information about unique characteristics of the community. For example, it provides information regarding citizens' participation (I 4).
	Data gap: Would be useful to know names of streets and buildings.
	Objective with documentation provided (I 5).
	Would be more useful to use term "late-model cars" rather than "new cars." "Sporting" as descriptive term suggests perceptual bias (O 12).
	Data gap: Who are the people observed in the community? Are they women with small children, teens, or older adults? What race are they?
	What evidence of politics is visible? Are there campaign posters or a party headquarters?
	Would be useful to know the names of these major thoroughfares (I 6).
	Objective, pertinent documentation provided. Taste is used while collecting these data. Objective data about the number and types of restaurants could be obtained from telephone book if more objective data needed (O 14, I 7).
	"All people interviewed warm and friendly" is a subjective phrase. More objective presentation would be to state, "All people approached were willing to talk, answer questions asked, and smiled throughout interview. No person that was approached refused an interview" (I 8).
3. Area lies in tornado belt, and precautionary measures in area include education in schools, tornado tips printed in local newspaper, and fire sirens signalling tornado warnings.[9]	*Data gap:* Number of tornadoes per year; amount of damage incurred (M 3).
4. Pollution index for Pleasant View: Suspended part. 56 mg/M³ Nitrogen oxide 58 mg/M³ Carbon monoxide 6 ppm[12]	"Pleasant smells" is subjective (O 15). Objective data, pertinent, provides documentation for data regarding observation of environment (M 4).
5. Average annual temperature: 52.2° F Average maximum temperature: 88° F Average minimum temperature: 4° F Average rainfall: 33" Average snowfall: 25" Average annual ppt.: 36"[19]	Objective relevant data, documented (M 5).

Continued.

Observations	Interactions

Category: *Structure*
Pattern: *Characteristics and uniqueness —cont'd*

Measurements	Critique

6. Total population

Year	Pleasant View	Poppulus
1970	26,555	233,239
1975	30,118	203,708

Strengths: Two separate years (1970, 1975) included, another area's statistics provided; these are useful statistics, as comparisons can be made (M 6).

Weaknesses: Age of statistics—not accurate representation of population at present time. No documentation as to source of 1975 population statistics.

Data gap: Need to have information regarding Poppulus—what relationship to Pleasant View? Useful for comparison data, but need explanation as to why this city was chosen.

7. Age distribution[36]

Objectively presented, documentation provided (M 7).

	Pleasant View		Poppulus	
	No.	%	No.	%
0-5	2,183	8.2	20,406	8.7
5-14	6,658	25.1	42,877	18.4
15-24	3,824	14.5	44,627	19.1
25-34	3,515	13.2	27,743	11.9
35-44	4,252	16.0	24,716	10.6
45-54	3,542	13.3	27,403	11.8
55-64	1,616	6.1	21,861	9.4
65-over	962	3.6	14,658	6.3
Nonwhite	21	.08	73,790	31.6
White	26,534	99.92	159,449	68.4

Age distribution of males and females in Pleasant View[35]

	Males		Females	
	No.	%	No.	%
0-5	1,098	8.5	1.085	8.6
5-9	1,605	12.4	1,569	12.4
10-14	1,823	14.1	1,661	13.1
15-19	1,381	10.7	1,274	10.1
20-24	563	4.4	606	4.8
25-34	1,631	12.6	1,884	14.9
35-44	2,097	16.2	2,155	17.0
45-54	1,863	14.4	1,674	13.2
55-59	513	4.0	462	3.6
60-64	338	2.6	303	2.4

Marital status

	Pleasant View		Poppulus	
	No.	%	No.	%
Married	13,257	49.9	103,897	44.5
Divorced	283	1.1	13,569	5.8

8. Birth rate

$$\frac{\text{No. live births in year} \times 1{,}000}{\text{Avg. (midyear) population}}$$

Strengths: Useful to present formulas used for calculation; comparative data useful (M 8).

	Number	Rate
Pleasant View	462	17.4
Poppulus	3,245	13.6

9. Death rate

$$\frac{\text{No. deaths in year} \times 1{,}000}{\text{Avg. (midyear) population}}$$

Would be useful to calculate rate so could compare with national statistics; statistics 1976—need to be consistent with year and statistical source (M 9).

Data gap: Are fetal death statistics for Pleasant View or Poppulus?

	Number	Rate
Pleasant View	148	5.6
Poppulus	2,886	12.3

	White	Nonwhite
Fetal deaths	5	0
Perinatal deaths	4	0
Neonatal deaths	3	0

Continued.

DATA COLLECTION—cont'd

Observations	Interactions

Category: *Structure*
Pattern: *Characteristics and uniqueness—cont'd*

Category: *Structure*
Pattern: *Community resources*

16. Few people at bus stops; busses approximately one third full.

9. Two bus lines serve area; one Mega City and one Local Runs, Inc. They travel a circuitous route (see map) connecting many traffic generators. Transportation available only on highly traveled thoroughfares.[10] [*Editor's note:* Map not included here.]

10. "We have one of the finest school systems in the area. Our children score well above average on standardized tests. Yet the district spends less per pupil to educate our children than do most areas around us."[22]

Measurements	Critique

10. Sex distribution

	Pleasant View	Poppulus
Males	50.3%	47.1%
Females	49.7%	52.9%

Comparison data provided, percentages calculated; would be useful to state numbers of males and females in Pleasant View and Poppulus so reader can check calculations (M 10).

11. Approximately 9,408 households in Pleasant View, 98% of which are in single dwellings.

Would be useful to have number of single households; what about the other 2%—apartments, condominiums, duplexes? (M 11).

12. Income of families

	Pleasant View	Poppulus
Under $3,000	—	6.2%
$3,000-$5,999	10.2%	14.1%
$6,000-$9,999	24.9%	33.9%
$10,000+	58.8%	51.7%
Median income	$13,197	$12,234

Data objectively presented, documentation provided; pertinent (M 12).

Data gap: Migration statistics, religion and nationality information.

Educational attainment of persons 25 years and older

	Pleasant View	Poppulus
No school	0.3%	0.8%
Graduated from high school	50.5%	69.6%
Attended college	24.5%	17.4%
Median school years completed	13.0%	12.2%

Leading causes of death

	Pleasant View	Poppulus
Heart disease	40.6%	37.0%
Malignant neoplasms	32.7%	18.8%
Cardiovascular disease	40.4%	9.2%
Accidents	13.7%	3.0%
Respiratory system	9.7%	2.7%
Suicide	1.7%	1.5%

Occupation

	Pleasant View	Poppulus
White collar workers	48.5%	49.4%
Manufacturing	35.4%	38.2%
Other	16.1%	12.4%

Data gap: Would be useful to know categories of "other."

13. 57 people per day ride Mega City bus line.[15]
    18 people per day ride Local Runs, Inc.

"Few" subjective: an example of an objective datum would be "three people observed at bus stop" (O 16).

The Mega City bus line would be considered a process datum, in the "obtain" category, because this is energy obtained from the environment (I 9). (See p. 70, Chapter 6, for further details.)

Data objectively reported, documentation provided (M 13).

Data gap: Total capacity of bus line.

14. 1.7% families: no car.
    28.4% families: 1 car.
    56.2% families: 2 cars.
    13.5% families: 3 cars.

Need documentation source (M 14).

Comparison of dollars per pupil spent with other general areas would be useful; also useful to have information regarding standardized tests (I 10).

Continued.

DATA COLLECTION—cont'd

Observations	Interactions
Category: *Structure* **Pattern:** *Community resources—cont'd*	11. "A problem I see in the high schools is the increase in reported cases of venereal disease. I've been here 3 years, and I've seen an increase each year. There are about 150 known cases of VD. These are only the reported ones—goodness knows how many other cases are untreated and unreported. Blue County doesn't have a VD clinic; students must go to Poppulus County Health Department or to their private physician for diagnosis and treatment. We don't have any formal sex education classes taught in high school—we give out brochures about birth control and VD in health class. But there is no guarantee they get read."[30]

Measurements	Critique
15. School system: 51 square miles; includes all of Pleasant View Township plus small portions of two adjacent townships. Public schools: one high school (grades 10-12), two junior high schools (grades 7-9), and six elementary schools (grades K-6). Students can attend Blue County Vocational School for specialized training. Two parochial schools, St. Mary's Grade School (2-8) and Bishop High School (9-12). Student enrollment in public schools 1979/80, 7,674. High school enrollment 1991. Enrollment in parochial schools 1,700 (400 St. Mary's and 1,300 Bishop High). Certified staff of Pleasant View schools includes 361 teachers, 4 registered nurses, and 24 administrators. Student-teacher ratio 24.75 to 1 at elementary level, 25.41 to 1 at junior high level, and 22.9 to 1 at senior high level. 260 classified employees including secretaries, clerks, teacher aides, lunchroom employees, bus drivers, maintenance workers and custodians. Board of education composed of five members. Elections held in each even-numbered year. Terms staggered with two seats 1 year and three seats following election. Four individual education classes for children identified as having slow learning rates. These classes consist of 12-16 students. Also learning disability program with six classrooms and six tutors. Within school district free bus service for all students living one mile or more from school and for all kindergarten students. Also 345 students transported who live within 1 mile, because of hazardous traffic conditions.[20]	Pertinent information; need more information as to what is being done in this area. Has there been a report of this to school officials and parents? Any plans for educational programs in adolescent health? (I 11). *Data gap:* Need statistics from health department on reported cases of veneral disease. Data regarding school system have both interactional and measurement data included. Measurement data consists of numbers: 51 square miles, 1 high school, 6 elementary schools. Documentation provided (M 15).
16. Resource identification: 5 parks in area 4 private swimming pools, each of which has at least 4 tennis courts 1 bowling alley 1 skating rink 1 private tennis club 1 private racquetball club 6 free tennis courts at high school Numerous ballfields.[15]	Pertinent data; "numerous" subjective term (M 16).

Continued.

DATA COLLECTION—cont'd

Observations	Interactions

Category: *Structure*
Pattern: *Community resources—cont'd*

17. Telephone and electric lines along roads and streets.

12. Resource identification: Fuel oil and electricity are major source of home heating. Natural gas has been opened to area in last 3 months. So far 100 homes have signed up. Two county systems and one private system provide water to the area. Approximately one third of the houses have wells. The county sewage system serves three fourths of the area.

18. Streets and yards clean, garbage cans sitting along curbs in front of approximately half the houses.

Category: *Structure*
Pattern: *Government*

19. Trustees' meetings open to public.

Category: *Process (Obtain)*
Pattern: *Health resources*

13. Pleasant View lies within Blue County. Blue County encompasses nine cities, including Mega (the county seat), Skyville, Oldtown, and Pleasant View; and 11 townships.

Measurements	Critique
	These are sources of energy obtained. They would be more appropriately recorded as process data in the category of "obtain." (See p. 70, Chapter 6.) Needs documentation (O 17, I 12).
	Data gap: Source of fuel oil and electricity.
	Need to separate measurement data from interaction data (I 12).
17. Fire department: five fulltime and one part-time firemen, 67 volunteers.	Objectively stated, documentation provided (M 17).
Equipment: five pumpers, one four-wheel drive vehicle, one rescue van, and one tanker.	"Streets and yards clean" is subjective statement; more objective way of stating this would be "streets and yards free of paper, trash, and garbage" (O 18).
Emergency squad: 23 paramedics and four ambulances. Paramedics are volunteers.[28]	
18. About one fourth of homes have septic tanks.[24]	
19. Three independent refuse companies serve the area.	*Data gap:* Information regarding snow and leaf removal would be useful (M 19).
20. Three church-operated nursing homes.	Objectively presented data, documentation provided (M 20).
Four pharmacies, nine dentists, nine physicians and surgeons, one medical laboratory, one emergency clinic open 6 PM to 9 AM nightly, equipped to handle most mild to moderate emergency situations.	"Mild to moderate" subjective term.
Pleasant View Rescue provides emergency medical treatment and transportation to any hospital in vicinity.	
Two church-sponsored nursery schools. Two day care centers: privately owned, providing day care from infancy to 12 years. After-school pickup and summer programs provided.	
Four movie theaters.	
Police Department consists of 16 full-time officers; one Police Chief, one lieutenant, two detectives, and 12 patrolmen.	
23 Protestant churches and one Catholic church; one Mormon Church.[3]	
21. Township trustee form of government designated by State Revised Code. Administered by three elected trustees and an elected clerk/treasurer. Two men and one woman now serving as trustees. Trustees elected for 4-year terms with elections held every 2 years.[24]	Data pertinent and objectively stated; documentation provided (M 21).
	Obtain refers to energy, information, and matter that are obtained from the suprasystem to help the system function. It is the same as "input."
22. Blue County population in 1975 132,321. Projected population 182,000 in the year 2000.	Need documentation of source (M 22).
	These are structural data (I 13).

Continued.

DATA COLLECTION—cont'd

Observations	Interactions
Category: *Process (Obtain)* **Pattern:** *Health resources —cont'd*	14. Blue County Health Department offers many health services to county residents: Immunization clinics: daily in mornings in Blue County Health Department offices in Mega. Prenatal classes: Mega, Skyville, and Oldtown once a week. TB screening: at schools as needed; at Mega Central Office three times a week. Well child clinics: once a month in Pleasant View. Once a month in Mega. Well baby clinics: three times a week in Skyville and Mega, ½ day a week in Oldtown and Pleasant View. Visiting nurse: as needed by physician referral. Home care. Environmental and inspectional services: as needed. Dental clinic (waiting list): one day a week in Mega. Heart clinic (for diagnoses and follow-up of heart defects on children): must be referred by physician and seen only by appointment; held twice a year. Pediatric otological diagnostic clinic: four times a year. Epilepsy clinic for diagnoses and management of patient with seizures: once a year.[3] 15. Anyone in Blue County is eligible to attend these clinics regardless of income. One well baby clinic held in Pleasant View.[5] 16. Blue County Board of Health and Relaxation provides services of five agencies: a. Children's Mental Health Program: Counseling for young people with mental health problems. Preventive services. Parenting classes. b. Blue County Residential Services for the Mentally Retarded: Housing, foster homes. c. Blue County Guidance Center: Outpatient service—group counseling and walk-in crisis center. Creative living service—day service and recreation. After-care—follow-up for clients. d. Emergency Supportive Service: Crisis intervention. One walk-in center in Mega. Telephone hot line and walk-in service run by volunteers. e. Commission on the Aging: Services to senior citizens.[4]

Measurements	Critique
	Data objectively presented; documentation of source provided (I 14).
	Data gap: Location of these services—in Mega only, or in other locations?
	Source documentation provided (I 15).
	Data gap: Would be useful to know information regarding fee for service; set fee? Sliding scale?
	Objectively presented, source documented (I 16).
	Data gap: Location of services?

Continued.

DATA COLLECTION—cont'd

Observations	Interactions

Category: *Process (Obtain)*
Pattern: *Health resources—cont'd*
	17. Blue County Educational Activities Training for developmentally disabled citizens of Blue County, in charge of:
	  a. Daytime School: preschool ages 3-6, school ages 6-21. Provides early infant stimulation; has training consultant, physical and speech therapy, and physical development specialist.
	  b. Daily Living Skills Lab: an adult activity program for continuation of development in skills of self-help, social and family living, basic academics, and prevocational training.
	  c. Blue County Sheltered Workshop: for handicapped and retarded men and women. Provides job training and placement, vocational rehabilitation, and long-term sheltered employment.[3]
	18. Blue County Speech and Hearing Program provides:
	Home care service to help rehabilitate patients with speech loss.
	Evaluation and rehabilitation service to the mentally retarded, patients in Blue Memorial Hospital, and those in extended care facilities.
	Summer clinic to prevent a lapse of service to Head Start teachers.[7]
	19. To receive any of the above services, residents must travel to Mega or Skyville. Services do not seem to be widely known in the Pleasant View area.
	Five hospitals are within 10 miles of Pleasant View: Blue Memorial Hospital in Blue County; other four in adjacent Poppulus County—Clark General, St. Mary's Hospital, Wright Memorial, and Children's Hospital.
	Main source of daily health care consists of private physicians within Pleasant View and surrounding communities.
	20. Six 4-year colleges, two junior colleges, two business schools, and one diploma nursing program within 20-mile radius. Two are state colleges and one is a county school.
	Within these schools one can attain a degree in medicine (MD), a baccalaureate in nursing (1); an associate degree in nursing (2); and a diploma in nursing (1). Also offered within these colleges are degrees in respiratory therapy (2), dental hygiene (1), and laboratory technology (2).[3]

Measurements	Critique
	Objectively presented, source documented (I 17). These data could have a dual heading of Health resources and education. *Data gap:* Location of services—is transportation to these facilities available?
	Objectively presented, source documented (I 18).
	Sources need documentation; "services do not seem to be widely known in Pleasant View area" is subjective statement made by community health care provider that should be investigated further with statistics (I 19). *Data gap:* Statistics to demonstrate use of these services by Pleasant View community residents.
	Source provided, objectively presented; pertinent data (I 20). Measurement data.

Continued.

DATA COLLECTION—cont'd

Observations	Interactions
Category: *Process (Obtain)* **Pattern:** *Recreation*	21. Blue County has approximately 60 recreational parks. Cultural activities within 20-mile radius include: Museum of Natural History. Art Institute. Local philharmonic orchestra. Local regional ballet company. Local modern dance company. Four local theater groups, three college theaters. A major league baseball team is within 1 hour's drive of Pleasant View. A major league hockey team is within a 15-minute drive. Five daily newspapers. Three local television stations. Several UHF and VHF radio stations.[3] 22. Legislative action initiated at township level must go through county and state levels before ratification can be made. Trustees are directly responsible for statutes concerning zoning. This is the only area in which trustees have authority to institute laws without state action.[9]
Category: *Process (Obtain)* **Pattern:** *Education*	23. Two laws affecting school district this coming year: a. Each child must show verification that he has received all immunizations within 20 days following beginning of school or child will be excluded until he receives them. b. PL 94-142 entitled "Education for All Handicapped Children" stipulates that handicapped students must be provided the best education in least restrictive environment. School district has set budget of $200,000 to upgrade and reconstruct schools to facilitate use by handicapped children. 24. One junior high and two elementary schools are barrier free. Students with cerebral palsy and muscular dystrophy are being mainstreamed.[23]
Category: *Process (Obtain)* **Pattern:** *Transportation*	25. Major commercial airport 14-25 miles from Pleasant View, serviced by several major airlines, with both nonstop and commuter flights available.
Category: *Process (Contain)* **Pattern:** *Development*	
20. Approximately 100 people at one township meeting discussing proposed mall.	26. Shopping mall proposed at intersection of state route 24 and Hanes Road.[25] Pleasant View task force formed to study impact of mall on area.[25]
21. Land surrounding proposed mall site gently sloping farmland with scattered crops and trees.	27. Conservation group claims proposed mall located on a flood plain and should not be developed.[25]

Measurements	Critique
	Objectively presented, documentation provided; pertinent (I 21).
	Objective data, documentation provided (I 22).
	Data gap: Would be useful to know statistics regarding numbers and types of handicapped students. These data would provide needed information for health planning (I 23).
	Datum unclear: what is meant by "barrier free"? Needs to be more specific so reader does not have to make inferences (I 24).
	Need documentation (I 25).
	Contain refers to matter, information, or energy that the community is trying to "contain" within the environment (keep out of the community system). See p. 70 of Chapter 6.
23. Three major Anchor stores have signed agreements.	Documentation provided (I 26).
	Data gap: Need more data regarding this topic.
	Pertinent datum (I 27). Need more information. Documentation provided.

Continued.

DATA COLLECTION—cont'd

Observations	Interactions
Category: *Process (Contain)* **Pattern:** *Development—cont'd*	
22. Roads on east and south of proposed mall area two-lane, no center line. Area is fairly flat plain with corn growing. River is across the road.	28. Southwest neighborhood organization submits petition with 200 names protesting proposed mall. Citizens state that area roads cannot handle increased traffic that would be generated.
23. Area of proposed landfill adjacent to area of high population density.	29. Residents in the northwest area are violently opposed to a proposed landfill in the area.[14] 30. One of the present landfills serves Skyville and one serves Pleasant View. The proposed landfill would serve part of Oldtown and the College Ridge housing area. 31. Residents fear that close proximity of the landfills would be environmentally undesirable and would result in lower property values.[24] 32. Residents who live in the landfill area have septic tanks and wells.[26]
24. Area of proposed housing bordered by two-lane county road and large housing developments. No sidewalks.	33. Sugar Valley Church donates land for low income apartment complex.[25] 34. Pleasant View residents opposed to changing zoning regulations to allow low income apartments.[25] "In reality, Pleasant View is not suitable for this type of dwelling. We have no mass transit systems, the area is not within walking distance of necessary services or schools. Children have to be transported to extracurricular events, so those kids would be left out of school activities. Also, housing prices would undoubtedly drop and that's not fair to the residents who have invested in this area!"[34]
Category: *Process (Contain)* **Pattern:** *Expansion*	35. Local citizens testify that proposed annexation of 30 acres of Pleasant View and Skyville is improper and illegal. The majority of residents in area choose to stay in Pleasant View. In addition, this annexation would be across county lines.[25]
Category: *Process (Retain)* **Pattern:** *Independent data (more than one datum needed to form a pattern)*	36. Each child must show verification that he has received all immunizations within 20 days following beginning of school year or he will be excluded until he receives them.

Measurements	Critique
	"Area is fairly flat" is subjective statement. "River is across the road" unclear datum; across the road from what? Needs more information to determine significance (O 22).
	Needs documentation (I 28).
	Data gap: Need more data regarding number of area roads and size of roads—traffic flow at present versus projected flow.
	"200 names" is measurement data.
	"High population density" is subjective or analysis statement (O 23).
	Data gap: Would be useful to provide statistical data as to density, such as number of houses in specific area.
	Residents "violently opposed" is judgmental statement (I 29). State data in terms of residents' quotations or direct observations.
	Need more data in this area (I 31).
	Data gap: How do residents perceive it would affect the environment—sights, odor, potential for rodent infestation?
	Potential health hazard; would be useful to collect more data regarding this (I 32).
	Objective presentation of residents' perception of proposed project; documentation provided (I 34).
	Documentation provided (I 35).
	Data gap: More data needed in this area.
	Retain refers to the matter, information, or energy the community is trying to retain, or keep in the system. For more information, refer to p. 70 of Chapter 6.
	Need documentation (I 36).
	Data gap: Would be useful to have statistical data as to number of children with current immunization statistics available through school health records.

Continued.

DATA COLLECTION—cont'd

Observations	Interactions
Category: *Process (Retain)* **Pattern:** *Independent data (more than one datum needed to form a pattern)—cont'd*	37. "One of the big reasons Pleasant View is working for incorporation is to keep our share of local taxes. Our return on tax dollars is much less than it would be if we were incorporated."[11] 38. "St. Paul Episcopal Church has just opened a coffee house located in the church basement. The hours are 7-10 PM Friday and Saturday nights. Bring your guitar and sing along or perform for the group. All Pleasant View teens ages 13-17 are invited."[33] 39. "School district has set aside monies to upgrade and reconstruct schools to facilitate usage by handicapped children."[23]
Category: *Process (Dispose)* **Pattern:** *Production*	40. Whirr Company manufactures small electric motors.[38] Tech, Inc. contracts with various manufacturers and the federal government to provide research and technical services.[35] 41. "Local merchants sponsor Pleasant View resident for Miss Ohio title."[25] "Local Barbershop Quartet travels nationally competing in contests."[25]
Category: *Process (Integration)* **Pattern:** *Communication* 25. Local newspaper, *Pleasant View News*, carries pictures and announcements of local events, such as society and 4-H news, school news, social events, and local meetings. 26. Posters on telephone poles advertise various candidates. Billboards and posters in local stores advertise local events (fund raisers, candidates, and school events). 27. Clear plastic bags being hung on door by woman. 28. Each swimming club prints monthly letter. (See Appendix B.) [*Editor's note:* Appendix B not included here.] School prints monthly newsletter. School calendar with events and statistics mailed to every home in Pleasant View. Fire Department and Police Department print annual reports. 29. Chamber of Commerce acts as information center for Pleasant View. Has pamphlet library available to citizens with much information (such as churches, businesses, and safety information in relation to tornadoes).	42. "Local merchants advertise through our services. We get housewives to deliver circulars each week."[31]

Measurements	Critique
	Data gap: Need more information in this area (I 37).
24. Five of the local churches have youth groups for the teens.	*Data gap:* More data needed. Data state that five church groups are providing activities for teens; would be useful to know number of teens attending, and how long this has been in effect (I 38).
25. $200,000 budget.	*Data gap:* More data needed; what kinds and number of handicapped students are in Pleasant View? Does this apply to all schools? What does "upgrading" mean? Specifically what will be done to facilitate mainstreaming handicapped children? (I 39)
	Dispose refers to what the community is trying to dispose of into the environment. These may be positive or negative aspects. For more information, see p. 73 of Chapter 6.
26. Employs approximately 300 people.	Objectively presented; documentation provided (I 40).
27. Employs approximately 1,500 people. 28. 850 seniors per year graduate from Pleasant View High School.[21]	*Data gap:* Number of Catholic high school graduates (M 28). Examples of energy disposed of into the environment (I 41).
	Integration refers to how the subsystems of the community interrelate to accomplish the system's functions. Pertinent data, objectively stated (O 25).
	Pertinent data, objectively stated (O 26).
	Unclear datum—more useful way of stating datum would be "woman hanging clear plastic bags, approximately 12″ × 18″, filled with printed advertisement material, on doorknobs of houses" (O 27). Objectively presented; provides examples of methods of communication within the community (O 28). *Data gap:* Quantity of distribution.
	Data gap: How do people know Chamber of Commerce exists? Number of people using center? (O 29).

Continued.

DATA COLLECTION—cont'd

Observations	Interactions

Category: *Process (Integration)*
Pattern: *Communication—cont'd*

30. School closings announced on three area radio stations.
31. Local telephone book distributed by advertising firm with Pleasant View private residences and businesses.

43. Reasons neighborhood councils came into being include: neighborhood watch groups being formed, protesting some proposed changes such as landfills and mall. Have evolved into neighborhood voice in township council meetings.[24]

Category: *Process (Integration)*
Pattern: *Sustenance*

44. Public services—Road Department provides snow removal and tree removal and trimming on the township's right-of-ways.
    Finance Department—finances governed by Board of Trustees and Clerk Treasurer. Tax rate $55.95 per $1,000.[24]
45. Many of the social services offered to Pleasant View residents are in coordination with the Jaycees and Jaycettes. A sampling of their various programs includes:
    a. Sports programs such as tee ball for children ages 6-10, shooters education program for ages 8-14, including gun safety, and Punt-Pass-Kick programs for ages 10-14 years.
    b. Fund-raising programs such as a Haunted House with money going to the Cancer Society, Multiple Sclerosis Society, and Cerebral Palsy Foundation; and a marathon scheduled for September 16, 1980, with proceeds going to a blood mobile used by nine area counties.
    c. Community health promotion through CPR instruction taught by 19 members of the Jaycees who are certified instructors; the Jaycettes perform puppet shows in the schools for grades 1-3, teaching the dangers of smoking, drinking, and drugs; meals on wheels for the elderly, and bike safety for motorists.
    The Jaycees have various goals for the community. This includes educating 60% of the adult population in CPR techniques. Also, a future program called The Vital Information Program is planned to provide medication cards of elderly Pleasant View residents to the Fire Department, Police Department, and the home. This will provide information at times of emergencies. Another goal is to initiate crime and drug abuse counseling within the school system beginning at the junior high level.[16]
46. Free bus service for all students living 1 mile or more from school and for all kindergarten students.

Measurements	Critique
	Objectively presented (O 30).
29. Four neighborhood organizations.	Objectively presented (O 31). Pertinent data, documentation provided (I 43). *Data gap:* Number of people participating in neighborhood group.
	Measurement data (I 44).
	Objectively presented, pertinent; documentation provided (I 45). *Data gap:* Need statistics regarding juvenile crime rate and drug abuse problem.
30. 345 students transported who live within 1 mile, because of hazardous traffic conditions.	Unclear datum, needs documentation. "Because of hazardous traffic conditions" needs further and statistical documentation (M 30).

Continued.

DATA COLLECTION—cont'd

Observations	Interactions
Category: *Process (Integration)* **Pattern:** *Governance*	47. Trustee form of government designated by Ohio Code. Any legislative action initiated at the township level must go through county and state levels before ratification can be made. The trustees are directly responsible for statutes concerning zoning. This is the only area in which the trustees have authority to institute laws without state action. 48. Trustees hold administrative responsibility for seven areas within township: zoning, fire department, police department, cemeteries, zoning commission, Board of Zoning Appeals, and roads. Zoning Commission appointed by trustees. Zoning Commission hears all zoning cases and makes recommendations to trustees. To overrule these recommendations a unanimous vote is needed by trustees. In all other areas, decisions are made by majority vote. Trustees responsible for all township personnel. Clerk/Treasurer's responsibility deals with financing and budgeting for township. No vote with trustees. 49. Six task force committees have been organized to study township issues: Intergovernmental: coordinates with two other local townships. Police Task Force: studies needs of department in relation to community and makes recommendations to trustees for proposed levy. Incorporation Study Group: studies effects that incorporation of Pleasant View would have on community. Library Committee: initiates plans for construction and maintenance of new library. Health Advisory Committee: studies health needs of Pleasant View community. Park Board: acquires, sets policies for, and maintains local parks.
Category: *Process (Integration)* **Pattern:** *Protection*	50. Services offered by Fire Department include blood pressure screening every Sunday, CPR training with nine certified instructors, and training programs for nursing home, restaurant, and school personnel. Assistant Fire Chief is fire inspector and conducts inspections regularly for nursing homes and other businesses. "Main problem is not having enough volunteers. This is a result of having extensive training program required of all volunteers."[28] 51. Levy to be proposed next election; if it passes, money will be used to hire additional policemen. Patrolling is divided by state route 24. One cruiser takes area south of state route 24 and the other north of state route 24.

Measurements	Critique
	Documentation needed. Data objectively stated (I 47).
31. Last year (1979) 904 runs made by emergency squad. Most of these runs to Wright Memorial. Second most used hospital was Clark General. Most emergencies involved auto accidents—4,766 men responded to the 904 runs in 1979.[27]	Objectively presented (M 31).
32. Four fire stations: response time to emergency and fire calls about 6 minutes.[27]	
33. 343 fire runs involving 3,657 firemen. Financial 500,000. Most fire calls for dwelling fires, grass, brush and trash fires, and auto and truck fires.	"Financial 500,000" is unclear datum. Relationship to other data not specified (M 33).
34. Crime rate has dropped in those areas that participate in neighborhood watches.[29] Two cruisers on patrol at all times throughout day. Department has five cruisers and one motorcycle.	*Data gap:* Need to include statistics to document that crime rate dropped (M 34).

Continued.

DATA COLLECTION—cont'd

Observations	Interactions
Category: *Process (Integration)* **Pattern:** *Protection—cont'd*	52. School health program services: Emergency first aid. Immunization records. Referral to appropriate agencies for needs of handicapped. Teacher in-service for health-related problems. Sex education classes for lower grades up to seventh grade. Notification of Lion's Club for purchase of eyeglasses and notification of Blue County Health Department to assist with health needs of those who cannot afford private medical care.[7] 53. Baccalaureate degree minimum educational requirement for school nurses, although no nurse in system has this degree. Nurses must begin work on a degree within a 4-year period or contracts will not be renewed. 54. Duties of school nurse: home visitation and eye and hearing screening. Nurses assisted by trained Red Cross volunteer aides. School psychologist conducts individual studies of students with learning or behavioral problems. 55. Tuberculosis tests mandatory in grades 1, 7, and 11, and are conducted by Blue County Health Department. 56. Free lunches offered in school to children whose family's incomes lies within the guidelines. 57. Guidelines not strictly enforced, and a family with large medical expenses or other financial burdens can usually qualify. 58. Senior citizens can eat lunch in Pleasant View lunchroom for $0.70.[22]

Measurements	Critique
	Listing of health services is objective datum that demonstrates relationship with other community components. Documentation provided (I 52).
	Data gap: How is program formulated? Group or individual effort? Who implements program? How many in-services? Topics of in-services? High school or grade school? Topics covered in sex education?
	Documentation needed (I 53).
35. Four school health nurses hired by School Board.	Documentation needed (M 35).
	Objective presentation of integration data (I 54). Documentation needed. Data superficial.
36. Four speech and hearing therapists provide services to elementary and junior high students.	*Data gap:* Number of students serviced. What children screened? What services?
	This datum belongs in the "obtain" category because it is a service obtained from the suprasystem (I 55).
37. $6,262 for a family of four through $12,800 for a family of twelve.[22]	
	Data gap: Number of senior citizens using this program (I 58).
	Documentation provided, qualifying data provided (I 56-58).

ANALYSIS/SYNTHESIS OF DATA

Analysis/synthesis	Critique

Structure

Pleasant View is a dynamic rural and suburban community,[a] consisting of an estimated population of approximately 30,000.[b] It is a rural and suburban community interspersed with farmland, housing developments, and business. Statistics indicate that Pleasant View is a spacious, upper middle class, well-kept community.[c]

The population has increased since the 1970 census; there is an average of three persons per household. According to Klein, adequate space is imperative for physiological and psychological integrity.[17]

The physical environment of Pleasant View is overall a positive one. Community residents have an adequate supply of pure water[d] for drinking, bathing, and recreational needs. The area is adequately supplied with telephone services and energy for power and light.[e] Although there is a concentration of gasoline odors in the primary intersection of Pleasant View, the pollution index is well within normal limits as determined by the National Weather Bureau.[f] The positive environmental aspects of adequate water and pure air is congruent with Nightingale's environmental concepts.[g]

The primary mode of transportation of the approximately 30,000 Pleasant View residents is private car. The 51 square miles of the community are divided by state route 24, the area's only four-lane highway. Other streets and roads that provide access to the residents are narrow two lane roads.[h] This results in traffic congestion on primary roads.

Statistics show that the greatest number of residents are in the 35-44 age group. The median age is 26.9 years, with 40.3% under 18 years and only 3.6% over 65 years of age.[i]

According to the U.S. Census statistics the median income of Pleasant View families was approximately $13,197, which is well above the national median of $9,867.[j] Analysis of statistics shows a possible correlation between the family income and educational level.[k] Both the educational level and median income are higher in Pleasant View than in a nearby city.

Pleasant View's birth rate is higher than that of the city of Poppulus, and the death rate is lower. This is consistent with the age distribution of both areas. The sex ratio of males and females is about equal in Pleasant View; this correlates with the small divorce percentage in this community. According to statistics, 98.3% of all families in Pleasant View have at least one car, and almost 70% have two or more. The average value of the homes in Pleasant View is about $70,000; in comparison the national average value is approximately $45,000, according to the Board of Realtors President.[l]

These statistics reveal that Pleasant View[m] is a young, growing, affluent yet stable community where families enjoy an income well above the national median. The age distribution statistics and knowledge of Erikson's developmental tasks[13] provide documentation for the needs for specific health care facilities. Such facilities would include children's health facilities, child care facilities, and women's health facilities.[n]

[a]*Data gap:* Need information as to what is considered rural and suburban.
Sanders, Irwin T, *Rural Society*, Prentice-Hall, 1977, provides useful discussion regarding rural society.

[b]"Population of approximately 30,000": is this 1975 population statistic as reported in data collection? Need to be consistent with statistics and document year used.
Data gap: Need reference.

[c]No theory to support statement of "spacious, upper middle class, well-kept community."

[d]Data state that approximately one third of the houses have wells. No statistics are available concerning purity of water in these wells. Need data to support analysis statement.
Data gap: Statistics regarding water purity and pollution.

[e]No documentation in data to support statement of "adequately supplied."
Data gap: Statistics about telephone service and energy for power and light.

[f]"Pollution index within normal limits" is supported by documentation.

[g]Need source for theorist.

[h]This information would be available through the Department of Highways; might also be useful to talk with task force committee studying the potential impact of proposed mall.
Data gap: Number of cars on community roads.

[i]What conclusions or inferences from this data? Could compare data with that of Poppulus or with national statistics.

[j]Need documentation of source.
Data gap: Theoretical basis for correlating income and education.

[k]Data support statement. Inference.

[l]Need to cite primary source. No documentation as to Board of Realtors source.[8] Data not in data bank.

[m]These inferences are supported by data:
"Growing": statistics indicating population increase.
"Affluent": median family income above national median.
"Stable": divorce rate low.
"Young" is inference.
Data gap: Need to establish a frame of reference for this statement. Is age distribution same as, younger than, or older than Poppulus or national average?

[n]Unclear correlation between Erikson and health care facilities.
Data gap: Are these facilities available?

ANALYSIS/SYNTHESIS OF DATA—cont'd

Analysis/synthesis	Critique

The leading causes of death in Pleasant View are in the same rank and order as the nation's, as indicated in the Surgeon General's report on Health Prevention.[o]

There are a total of eleven schools in the school system that provide education for kindergarten through twelfth grade. Special provisions are made for slow learners and handicapped students. Free bus service is provided to all students living within 1 mile of schools.

Numberous recreational facilities, including parks, swim clubs, tennis courts, bowling alleys, skating rinks, racquetball courts, ball fields, and movie theaters are available to community residents.

Protective services are provided by Fire and Police Departments. There is a shortage in both these departments within the Pleasant View area.[p] The Police Department is understaffed, and has a need to double its staff. The department hopes that a pending levy will alleviate the problem.[q] The Fire Department also lacks manpower because of its voluntary status.

Process

Klein contends that communications are imperative for a community to exist. Without communications there would be no interplay between components.[17] A strength in the Pleasant View community is the open communications. There are a variety of modes used to transmit information to community residents. Citizens are informed about issues and concerns. Community meetings are well attended, and much input is provided by Pleasant View residents.[r] The predominant method of communication is the *Pleasant View News.* The newspaper is published locally, 6 days a week, and is received by approximately three fourths of the households.[s] The editor is a resident in the community and is a major power holder in the system. The Pleasant View citizens also have much impact on the functioning of the community.[t]

Decision making refers to the way the community goes about getting and using resources in order to carry out the processes of adaptation and integration.

The community is governed by a Board of three elected trustees.[u] Any legislative action initiated at the township level must go through county and state levels before ratification can be made. The only area in which the trustees have authority to institute laws without state action is in the area of zoning. Decision-making power is dispersed among a number of Pleasant View citizens, in that the trustees organize task force committees to study township issues. Presently there are six such committees.[v]

The most evidenced transactional modes, as described by Bridemeier (Smoyak, pp. 407-409) are those of team cooperative and Gemeinschaft. Many residents and store owners give time, energy, and support to community activities and projects because of common interests and loyalty to the community system.[w]

---

[o]Documentation provided for standard.

[p]No data to support shortage of police and fire department staff.

Data gap: Would be useful to compare response time of fire department with national standards.

[q]No mention of proposed levy in data collection.

Note: Would be useful to know how the health services are communicated to residents or if they are. Would also be useful to have statistics regarding Pleasant View residents using Blue County health facilities.

[r]What is the criterion for "well attended"?

[s]No data to support statement in data collection.

[t]Need data to support statement.

[u]The number of elected trustees not in data collection.

Data gap: Would be useful to have more information regarding selection of task force committee members. How is this selection made? Are the same people on the committees or are all committees different?

[v]Information present in data bank.

[w]Need to show relationship between theory and data used to make this judgment.

Data gap: Theoretical basis for this judgment.

Continued.

ANALYSIS/SYNTHESIS OF DATA—cont'd

Analysis/synthesis	Critique

Preventive health services

There are 5,919 (46.8%) women of childbearing age in the Pleasant View community.[x] The birth rate is 17.4/1,000.[y]

Childbearing during adolescence is a high-risk experience for mother and child alike. A major concern that urgently needs addressing is inadequate knowledge of and access to information on sexual behavior and family planning services.[37,z] Family planning services available in Pleasant View are through private physicians.[aa] Planned Parenthood provides birth control devices and abortion counseling. However, this agency is located in Poppulus, approximately 15 miles from Pleasant View.[bb] Direct transportation other than by automobile is not available.

In Pleasant View, 14.5% of the population is between the ages of 15-24.[cc] A health concern was expressed by the high school nurse regarding the incidence of veneral disease in the school. The nurse stated that there are about 150 reported cases. Statistics show that that is approximately 7.5% of the high school population. However, there is no organized program to inform this population of signs, symptoms, prevention, or treatment of venereal disease. Treatment and education are available only through private physician and the Poppulus Health Department.[dd]

Comprehensive prenatal care is one of the leading ways to reduce infant and maternal mortality.[37,ee] Prenatal care is available in Pleasant View through private physicians and public health clinics.[ff] Only one public health prenatal clinic per month is available in the Pleasant View community.[gg] Public transportation to this clinic is not available. Infant care is available through private physicians, public health clinics, and federally sponsored children and youth projects (C & Y). One Public Health Well Child Clinic per month is held in Pleasant View. No C & Y sites are in the local community. In fact, few of the residents surveyed were aware of the services.[hh] Supplemental food supplies can be obtained through the Special Supplemental Food Program for Women, Infants, and Children (WIC). Few Pleasant View residents would qualify for the program because of income qualifications. Last year state law decreed that any child in school had to show proof of immunizations before November 1, or would not be allowed to attend school until proof was shown.[ii] Approximately 25% of the students were unable to show such proof. The Blue County Health Department held immunization clinics in the various schools, and students whose parents had signed consent forms could obtain their immunizations for a nominal[jj] fee or free; 125 students used this service.[kk]

Blood pressure screening is provided weekly at the fire stations in Pleasant View.[ll] Nursing students from a local university hold blood pressure screenings in two local grocery stores four times per year.[mm,nn]

[x]This datum not present in data bank.
[y]Need to cite method of calculating women of childbearing age.

[z]Theoretical basis of need for access to information regarding sexual behavior and family planning services established.
[aa]*Data gap:* Have any programs been formulated? By whom have they been implemented?
[bb]Number of women from Pleasant View using Planned Parenthood services.
[cc]Need community data to compare with theory base.
Data gap: Number of adolescents bearing children.

[dd]Theoretical basis of need for information and service regarding venereal disease established.
[ee]Theoretical basis for prenatal care established.

[ff]*Data gap:* Number of women attending public health clinic in Pleasant View.
[gg]*Data gap:* Number of women attending public health clinic in other Blue County areas.

[hh]Not in data bank.

[ii]*Data gap:* What immunizations were required?
[jj]"Nominal" is subjective term.
Data gap: Which immunizations were offered?
[kk]Data indicate further investigation of child health practices necessary. Unclear whether child health services not being sought or whether parents do not keep good records.
[ll]Need to establish why blood pressure screening is important (leading cause of death in Pleasant View, cardiovascular disease; relationship between it and blood pressure).
Data gap: Number of people screened.
[mm]*Data gap:* Is health teaching part of screening?
[nn]No conclusions drawn from data; so what?

ANALYSIS/SYNTHESIS OF DATA—cont'd

Analysis/synthesis	Critique

Health promotion services

Health promotion programs are held on a sporadic basis in Pleasant View. The high school and junior high have a film once a year on the effects of tobacco on the body. They also have a film on drug abuse.[oo] Teens[pp] can also be seen standing outside the high school smoking, and at extracurricular school functions many of the students can be seen smoking.

Exercise and physical fitness programs are abundant during the elementary and high school years through organized sports programs.[qq] Murray and Zentner state that this is an age when exercise is essential for muscular development, refinement of coordination and balance, and the enhancing of other body functions such as circulation, aeration, and waste elimination.[rr] Soccer and baseball organized by the Jaycees are quite well attended.[ss] The four swimming clubs have swimming teams. Physical education programs in the schools are mandated by state law, but the schools meet them only minimally (once a week). In addition the junior high and high schools have intramural teams in basketball and interscholastic teams in gymnastics, baseball, softball, track, football, basketball, and soccer.

Benefits of these programs are low cost, open participation, promotion of community spirit, and family involvement.[tt] Constraints are that private transportation is required for all but physical education classes, and time and energy are required for organization and execution of programs.

Regular exercise is also beneficial for adults. People who exercise regularly report they feel better, have more energy, lose excess weight, and improve muscular strength and flexibility. Cardiovascular fitness and a sense of well-being are also associated with regular exercise.[37,uu]

Statistics indicate that most working residents in Pleasant View have occupations that do not require physical exertion.[vv] Although there are many resources available for achieving physical fitness and exercise in Pleasant View (aerobic dance, men's softball and baseball teams, swimming clubs, tennis and racquetball clubs, and adult soccer league),[ww] these programs are not as well attended[xx] as children's physical fitness programs.[yy]

In addition, there has been no community effort to educate the public on the benefits of regular physical exercise.[zz,ab,ac]

[oo]Need to establish relationship between smoking, drug abuse, and health. No conclusions drawn from data.
[pp]"Teens" inferential data.

[qq]*Data gaps:*
  Number of participants.
  Number of female participants.
  Number of male participants.
[rr]Relationship between exercise and health established.
[ss]Inference made that team sports meet physical fitness requirements. "Well attended" is subjective term.

[tt]No data to suggest promotion of community spirit and family involvement.

[uu]Relationship between exercise and health established.

[vv]How do statistics indicate this?

[ww]Inference that physical fitness can be achieved through mentioned sports.
[xx]"Not as well attended" is subjective term.
[yy]Not documented.
Data gap: How many participants?
[zz]*Data gap:* Programs available.
[ab]*Data gap:* Theoretical framework documenting relationship to health.
[ac]Many other documented health risks or prevention promotion activities not addressed: substance abuse, nutrition, mental health and stress support systems, dental care.

Continued.

ANALYSIS/SYNTHESIS OF DATA—cont'd

Analysis/synthesis	Critique

Health preventive services

Environmental protection services are provided by the Blue County Health Department; included in these services are housing inspection, water inspection, restaurant inspection, pollution monitoring, and rodent control.[ad]

Data indicate that Pleasant View residents have available the human and environmental resources to meet Maslow's primary physiological needs.[ae]

[ad] No theoretical data presented. Adequacy of services not addressed.

Data gap: How often are these services provided? Voluntary or mandatory controls for these services?

[ae] No definition of Maslow's needs. No data to support that human and environmental resources meet Maslow's physical needs.

NURSING DIAGNOSIS

Diagnoses	Critique
Three nursing diagnoses have been identified and arranged in order of priority. Plans have been formulated for only the first diagnosis.	*Data gap:* Theoretical basis for arrangement of nursing diagnosis. Even though the theoretical basis for arranging the diagnoses is not provided, the order does follow a logical sequence.
1. Potential for increasing incidence of sexually transmitted disease (STD)* in the high school population, related to absence of health teaching.	Data provide more statistical documentation to warrant intervention in the area of STD than unwanted pregnancy. Health promotion activities are lower priority than prevention services.[37]
2. Potential for increasing incidence of unwanted pregnancy because of inaccessibility of low-cost family-planning services.	Statistics do not support strong need for diagnosis 2. However, *Healthy People* addresses this concern.
3. Potential for decreased health potential of residents related to lack of regular health promotion programs.	Data document the existence of sporadic health promotion activities in Pleasant View. *Healthy People* emphasizes the need for a regularly scheduled health promotion program.

*The high school nurse talked about cases of venereal disease. However, *Healthy People* uses the broader term of STD.

PLANS FOR IMPLEMENTATION

Nursing diagnosis: *Potential for increasing incidence of sexually transmitted disease (STD) in the high school population related to absence of health teaching.*
Goal: *The Pleasant View High School population will have decreased incidence of STD by June 1982.*

Objectives	Plans	Scientific rationale
1. The community will have access to information regarding STD by October 1981.		Unfreezing: for change to take place, community has to become dissatisfied with status quo.[17]
	1a. Interview local physicians regarding incidence of STD in community.	Important to identify and gather support from community gatekeepers; community tends to listen to those with informal power.[39] Empirical rational mode of change. Men are rational; if they hear the facts they will make reasonable decisions based on them.[2]
	1b. Contact local newspapers regarding incidence of STD in community. Offer to write series of three articles reporting: Incidence and specific diseases involved. Signs and symptoms of specific diseases. Interview with local leaders, physicians, teachers, clergy, school board members, and public health officials regarding the problem.	Essential elements for controlling STD include education of public to understand early signs of disease and the kinds of sexual behavior that increase risk.[37]
	1c. Have several people write to newspapers commenting on problem and suggesting measures to decrease incidence of STD.	Quoting local leaders lends credence to concern necessary for social action.[39]
	1d. Have several people call local talk radio station and comment on articles.	Keep issue before public; raise consciousness.[17]

Evaluation	Critique
Evaluation criteria Outcome criteria: 1. Newspaper articles will appear describing incidence, mode of transmission, manifestation, complications, prevention, and treatment of STD. 2. Community groups will discuss above information. 3. Community groups will request a program to inform the at-risk population of danger of STD. Formative: 1. Who was contacted? What was response?	How was time frame selected? *Data gap:* Plans need to be more specific; who, when, and what? Scientific rationale: Are there data to support the fact that these are community gatekeepers? Plan: Is some response expected?
Was newspaper contacted? Were articles written and printed?	Plan: A written teaching plan on the articles would be useful in an appendix. Scientific rationale: Why was local newspaper chosen as vehicle for transmission? *Data gap:* Who will contact newspaper? When? Who will write article? Copies of planned articles?
Were letters to newspapers written and printed? Was local talk show called? What type of response was elicited?	Scientific rationale specifies local leaders; the plan refers to having several people write, not specifically community leaders. *Data gap:* Be more specific: how will people to write be chosen? What do you want them to say? Important to have alternate plan here. Calling talk show risky for positive acceptance; is listening audience liberal or conservative? How do you know? What is the scientific rationale for calling local talk show? *Data gap:* How will people to call be chosen? What do you want them to say?

Continued.

PLANS FOR IMPLEMENTATION—cont'd

Nursing diagnosis: *Potential for increasing incidence of sexually transmitted disease (STD) in the high school population related to absence of health teaching.*

Goal: *The Pleasant View High School population will have decreased incidence of STD by June 1982.*

Objectives	Plans	Scientific rationale
2. The community will take action to inform the at-risk population of the hazards and prevention of STD by December 1981.		Moving to the new level. Community norms and values have to integrate. Community involvement will in part determine whether or not changes will be accepted.[17]
	2a. Suggest to school board formation of task force to plan program on STD to be offered in high school: Task force to be composed of parents, teachers, clergy, physician, and nurse. Task force to look at specific content and the way the course is to be taught: Elective. With parental permission. As required assembly. During school hours. After school hours. 2b. Implement program.	Middle-class people like to be involved in decision making.[17] Important to establish trust and a climate for collaboration between groups.[17] Allowing community to make decisions regarding content and course planning facilitates community acceptance.[17]
3. The community will provide access to screening and treatment for STD by March 1982.		Refreeze new level (since change has been brought about by community forces, it should persist).[17] Essential elements of controlling STD are screening procedures, medical treatment, and follow-up procedures.[37]
	3a. Contact health department, local physicians, and local service organizations regarding facilities available, cost, and community acceptance of this type of service.	Other communities have used these groups to provide screening and treatment for STD.
	3b. Suggest to trustees formation of citizen's task force to look further into the concern.	Pleasant View has demonstrated active participation in community decisions; acceptability of services is more likely when community is involved in decision making.[17] One key to successful program planning is determining what consumer believes he needs and what he wants to do about it.[18]

Evaluation	Critique
Outcome criteria: 1. School board will have STD as an agenda item at a monthly meeting. 2. A task force will be formed to plan a formal program. 3. The program will include information on incidence, mode of transmission, manifestation, complications, prevention, and treatment. 4. The program will be offered to all students 13-18 years.	Outcome criteria sound as if writer has predetermined idea of program in mind.
Formative: Was a task force formed? When? Who was on the task force? What content will be taught? Where and when will course be taught? Who will teach it? Who will attend?	Plan too vague. If you are going to establish credibility you must have specific goals and objectives for contacts. Know what you're going after and how to get the information. How were these professions chosen as being on the task force? Scientific rationale: Need to establish reasons community would be involved with this specific content; for example, issues involving moral conduct or sexually sensitive issues. Evaluation: Data complete. Plan: The task force doing the planning may demonstrate favorable acceptance, but further planning would be necessary to facilitate acceptance by community at large. *Data gap:* What content will be examined? When?
Was program implemented as planned? If not, why not? What modifications?	
Outcome criteria: 1. There will be a local screening program for STD. 2. Everyone in the community will have access to the program. 3. Confidentiality will be ensured. 4. Treatment will be available for cases of STD.	Objective 3 appears to be inconsistent with 2; it addresses at risk population (13-18), but 3 addresses community. Need to be consistent, or provide rationale for altering population. Evaluation 3 same concern; not consistent with evaluation 4 of objective 2. Scientific rationale: Need documentation.
Formative: Who was contacted? By whom? When? What facilities available? What was cost? Community acceptance?	Plan: Not complete for objective achievement. These two steps seem to be reversed. The task force should be doing the contacting, since they will have authority and power. Also, it is doubtful that these two steps would lead to objective achievement. *Data gap:* Need to be specific: who will contact? When, and what will be said?
Summative evaluation Were evaluation criteria met? Formative: Did meeting evaluation criteria lead to goal achievement?	

REFERENCES

1 Becker, A.: Community resident, interview.
2 Bennis, W.G., and others: The planning of change, ed. 3, New York, 1976, Holt, Rinehart & Winston.
3 Blue County: Blue County Resource Directory.
4 Blue County Bureau of Social Services: Social services directory, 1979.
5 Blue County Health Department: Blue County annual health report, 1976.
6 Blue County Health Department environmentalist: Interview.
7 Blue County Health Department nurse: Interview.
8 Board of Realtors President: Interview.
9 Board of Trustees: Interview.
10 *City Bus Schedule*, 1979.
11 Committee for Incorporation Chairperson: Interview.
12 Environmental Protection Agency: Pollution index, 1979.
13 Erikson, E.: Childhood and society, ed. 2, New York, 1963, W.W. Norton & Co., Inc.
14 Holcomb, Sarah, community resident: Interview.
15 Jaycees: Know your community.
16 Jaycees President: Interview.
17 Klein, D.C.: Community dynamics and mental health, New York, 1968, John Wiley & Sons, Inc.
18 Lancaster, J.: Community mental health nursing: an ecological perspective, St. Louis, 1980, The C.V. Mosby Co.
19 National Weather Service: National weather service bulletin.
20 Pleasant View Board of Education: Annual report, 1979.
21 Pleasant View Board of Education: School calendar, 1979.
22 Pleasant View Board of Education, School Board member: Interview.
23 Pleasant View Board of Education, School Principal: Interview.
24 Pleasant View Board of Trustees, trustee: Interview.
25 Pleasant View Daily News, April 8, 1980, June 5, 1980, June 24, 1980, June 28, 1980, August 13, 1980, and September 16, 1980.
26 Pleasant View Department of Sanitation, sanitarian: Interview.
27 Pleasant View Fire Department: *Annual Report*, 1979.
28 Pleasant View Fire Department Fire Chief: Interview.
29 Pleasant View Police Department Police Chief: Interview.
30 Pleasant View School Nurse: Interview.
31 Quik Ad: Interview with manager.
32 Sites, T.: Interview.
33 St. Paul Episcopal Church: Flyer.
34 Task Force to Study Proposed Housing Development Chairman: Interview.
35 Tech, Inc.: Annual report, 1979.
36 U.S. Census Bureau: Population of the United States, 1970.
37 U.S. Department of Health, Education, and Welfare: Healthy people: the Surgeon General's report on health promotion and disease prevention, Washington, D.C., 1979, The Department.
38 Whirr Co.: Annual report, 1979.
39 Wigley, R., and Cook, J.R.: Community health: concepts and issues, New York, 1975, D. Van Nostrand Co.
40 Zoning Commissioner: Interview.

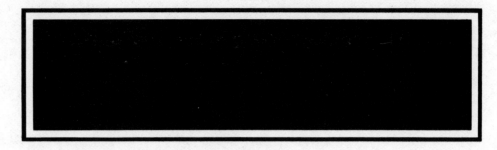

APPENDIXES

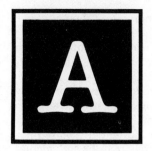 Glossary

accountability Ability to explain rationale for actions taken that is consistent with the responsibility for which the nurse contracted.

advocate One who acts in the interest of the health care consumer.

autonomy Having the freedom to develop and control oneself.

behavioral objective A statement describing a specific expected observable behavior of the client that is relatively short-term in nature.

caring Concerned with or interested in another.

catalyst A person who promotes actions and reactions and enables them to proceed under optimum conditions.

client Individual, family, group, or community.

collaboration A joint effort for the purpose of creating change toward a mutually desired goal.

colleague A peer functioning in a group in which each member openly shares knowledge and has equal opportunity to exercise power and authority.

community A specific population living within a defined perimeter or a group that has common values, interests, or needs.

community process The way the components of a community system function.

community structure The arrangement of animate or inanimate properties or parts of a community at a given moment.

communication techniques (facilitative) Methods used to promote open dialogue between people.

    clarifying Asking the client what was meant by a particular statement or question.

    consensual validation Asking the client the meaning of a particular word that was used in the conversation.

    focus Restrict discussion to obtain specific information.

    open-ended statements and questions Statements and questions that cannot be answered with a "yes" or "no" answer.

    reflect feelings or content Share with the client your (interviewer's) thoughts or feelings of the content spoken.

    related questions Questions that are relevant to previous statements for the purpose of obtaining more information about the topic.

    restate, repeat main idea Restate what the client said verbatim or pull together the main idea of what the client said and state it. This is used to promote elaboration on the topic or validation of what was said.

    sharing perceptions Telling the client what your (interviewer's) impressions are of a given statement or situation.

    summarize Share with the client succinct impressions or conclusions drawn from data.

    verbalize the implied State what the client implied to validate the interviewer's impressions.

comprehensive Reflecting the totality or wholeness of the client's life experiences.

concept A complex mental formulation of objects, events, or ideas that can be symbolized by a word label.

conceptual model A matrix of concepts, theories, or ideas that are interrelated, but in which the precise interrelationships among the concepts are not clearly defined.

concurrent evaluation Ongoing examination of activities as they are occurring.

coordination Regulation and combination of effort for harmonious performance.

criteria statement A statement reflecting the expected qualities, attributes, or characteristics that measure a client's performance.

consultation Invited communication with an expert who serves in an advisory capacity for the purpose of information exchange or analysis.

continuum A continuous whole whose fundamental common character is discernible amid a series of variations.

data Units of information obtained through the use of the senses and the designated tools of observation, interaction, and measurement.

dependent Relying on or requiring the support of others for the authority to perform activities.

depleted health Alteration in the dynamic pattern of functioning whereby there is an inability to interact with internal and external forces as the result of a temporary or permanent loss of necessary resources.

developmental needs Any requirement arising from the natural process of situational concerns of growth and differentiation.

family Dynamic system of two or more individuals who consider themselves a family and share a history, common goals, obligations, instrumental and affectional bonds and ties, and a high degree of intimacy.

family process Functions and group interactions by which the family operates; the salient features that differentiate it from another collection of individuals.

family structure Names, ages, health states, and occupations of family members.

formative evaluation Ongoing process for determining the completion of the steps of plans for implementation and objectives.

goal A broad or abstract statement of client performance that is relatively long-term in nature.

health care system The organized distribution of services and personnel to meet the health needs of others.

health care team An organized group of health care workers who have common goals, cooperative relationships, and coordinated activities related to the health care needs of the client or group of clients.

health concern An actual or potential health problem, disability, deficit, or limitation.

health maintenance The act of protecting and preserving patterns of maximum potential for health.

health promotion The advancement of patterns of functioning that foster and encourage health.

health restoration The advancement of patterns of functioning from depleted or impaired health to health maintenance.

health status The state of health.

holistic The view that an integrated whole has a reality independent of and greater than the sum of its parts.

impaired health Alteration in the dynamic pattern of functioning whereby there is a diminished ability to interact with internal and external forces as the result of a reduction in necessary resources.

independent Assuming autonomous authority to perform activities.

inference A judgment made from data obtained compared with health norms, concepts, principles, or standards.

interdependent A mutually collaborative effort in performing health care activities with other health care professionals and the client.

interpretation (personal) An individually biased perception of a given event that may be judgmental.

interviews Transitory relationships or exchanges of information that are goal directed.

   directive-interrogative Discussion between the client and nurse for the purpose of obtaining information.

   open-ended Discussion between the client and nurse for the purposes of obtaining information and building rapport.

   rapport building Discussion between the client and nurse for the purpose of establishing a relationship.

leader A person with foresight who is able to influence others in a positive direction, who is accountable for his own beliefs, who is willing and able to take risks, and who accepts power and uses it judiciously.

leadership A complex relationship between individuals whereby interpersonal influence is exercised through the process of communication toward the achievement of specific goals.

maximum potential for health The client's ability to achieve or develop the highest pattern of functioning possible within the client's health perimeter.

measurable Able to be determined in terms of extent, dimension, rate, rhythm, quantity, or size; used for a given behavior, performance, or characteristic.

multifocal The view that clients are composed of multiple foci, such as biophysical, spiritual, psychological, developmental, and sociocultural.

nonjudgmental Free from personal interpretation and bias.

norm The generally accepted range of behavior, performance, or characteristics.

nursing orders Actions chosen by the nurse and client to achieve the goals and objectives.

nursing prescription See nursing order.

nursing process A deliberate intellectual activity whereby the practice of nursing is approached in an orderly, systematic manner.

   assessment The ongoing process of data collection and analysis/synthesis of data that results in conclusions about the client's health concerns and strengths.

   diagnosis A clear, concise, definitive statement of the client's health status that can be affected by nursing intervention.

   evaluation A systematic, continuous process of comparing the client's response or observable behavior with the established goals and objectives.

implementation The nurse and client executing the plans.

plans for implementation Interventions determined to assist the client in resolving concerns related to the restoration, maintenance, and promotion of health.

objective See behavioral objective.

objective data Data free from personal interpretations and bias.

objective domains Categories on which to base objectives.

affective domain Reflects interests, attitudes, values, or feelings.

cognitive domain Reflects knowledge or intellectual abilities and skills.

psychomotor domain Reflects ability to perform a manipulative or motor skill.

outcome or performance evaluation Examination of the result of nursing actions according to the client's change in behavior and health status compared with objectives and goals.

pattern A composite sample of traits or behaviors that is characterized by rhythm, rate, intensity, duration, and amount.

perception An individual's idea of an event or situation that is based on the use of all senses and past experience.

performance Any behavior of a client that can be directly or indirectly assessed.

principles Guiding rules or laws that have been supported over time through research.

process The interaction of the components of a given system.

process evaluation Examining the actions and interactions of the nurse.

reliable Stable, dependable, accurate, consistent, and relatively predictable.

research A systematic inquiry to discover facts or test theories to obtain valid answers to questions raised or solutions for concerns identified.

resource External or internal source of strength or assistance.

responsibility Obligation to fulfill the terms of implied or explicit contractual agreement in accord with professional and legal nursing standards.

retrospective evaluation Examining the nurse's actions for effectiveness after the client is discharged from care.

role A dyadic relationship that is an actual or expected behavior pattern determined by socialization, including the interaction and interpretation of given norms, status, or position.

spiritual An internal essence or quality that gives meaning to a client's existence.

standard Acceptable, expected level of performance that is established by authority, custom, or general consent.

structure The arrangement of animate or inanimate properties or parts of a given system at a given moment.

structure evaluation Examining the physical facilities, types and availability of equipment, and the organizational components.

strategy (nursing) An overall plan or tactic that serves as a guide for individual nursing orders (prescriptions).

subjective data Data that may be biased by the observer's life experiences.

summative evaluation A description of whether and to what extent or degree the goals have been met.

systematic An organized and planned method of completing a given project.

synthesis The integration of theories and concepts into varied patterns.

theoretical framework A collection of concepts whose interrelationship describes or explains phenomena, which has not been proven.

theory An internally consistent body of relational statements and concepts that describes, explains, or predicts phenomena.

tools for data collection Methods by which the nurse obtains data from the client.

interaction Mutual or reciprocal exchange of verbal information.

measurement The use of all the senses as well as instruments to allow quantitative value of observations.

observation The use of all the senses to obtain information about a client.

unique The way clients differ from each other by virtue of heredity, environment, particular experiences, perception of such experiences, and the manner in which they react to such experiences.

valid The quality of data or data collection method to accurately reflect what was intended to be reflected.

validation The process of determining the accuracy of data.

vulnerability State of being at risk or susceptible.

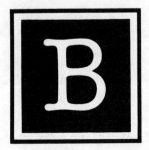

Guidelines for the NURSING PROCESS

A. Nursing assessment: data collection
   1. Data collected are comprehensive and multifocal.
   2. A variety of sources are used for data collection.
   3. Appropriate tools are used for data collection.
   4. The data collected are objective and nonjudgmental.
   5. A systematic format is used for data collection.
   6. The data collected reflect updating of information.
   7. The data collected are recorded and communicated appropriately.
B. Nursing analysis/synthesis
   1. The data are categorized and comprehensive.
   2. Data gaps and incongruencies are identified.
   3. Patterns of behavior are identified.
   4. Appropriate theories, models, concepts, principles, norms, and standards are compared with patterns.
   5. Health concerns and strengths are identified.
C. Nursing diagnosis
   1. The nursing diagnosis is concise and clear.
   2. The nursing diagnosis is client centered, specific, and accurate.
   3. The nursing diagnosis is stated as a descriptive or etiological statement.
   4. The nursing diagnosis provides direction for nursing intervention.
   5. The nursing diagnosis can be treated by nursing interventions.
   6. The list of nursing diagnoses reflects the client's current health status.
D. Goals and objectives
   1. Goals
      a. Goals are client focused and reflect mutuality with the client.
      b. Goals are appropriate to their respective diagnosis.
      c. Goals are realistic, reflecting the capabilities and limitations of the client.
      d. Goals include broad or abstract indicators of performance.
   2. Objectives
      a. Objectives are client focused and reflect mutuality with the client.
      b. Objectives are appropriate to their respective goals.

      c. Objectives are realistic, reflecting the capabilities and limitations of the client.

      d. Objectives include specific indicators of performance.

      e. Objectives are numbered in the appropriate sequence to achieve the goal.

E. Plans, implementation, and scientific rationale

  1. Plans (nursing orders)

      a. The plans are dated and contain the signatures of the responsible nurses.

      b. The plans (implementation strategies and nursing orders) are appropriate to their respective objectives.

      c. Plans are written in terms of client and nursing behaviors sufficient to achieve goals and objectives.

      d. The nursing plans are stated in specific terms.

      e. The plans include preventive, promotional, and rehabilitative aspects of care.

      f. The nursing plans include collaborating and coordinating aspects of care.

      g. The plans are placed in an appropriate sequential order according to priority.

      h. The plans incorporate the autonomy and individuality of the client.

      i. Plans are kept current and revised and include alternate plans when indicated.

      j. Plans for the client's future are included.

  2. Scientific rationale

      a. The scientific rationale addresses the identified topic and strategy and the individuality of the client.

      b. The scientific rationale incorporates appropriate supportive research findings and current literature.

F. Nursing evaluation

  1. The criteria for measuring client objectives are determined if appropriate.

  2. The formative evaluation describes whether and to what extent the nurse and client have implemented the stated plans and objectives.

  3. The summative evaluation describes progress or lack of progress toward the goal.

  4. The care plans indicate revisions if the goals and objectives are not adequately met.

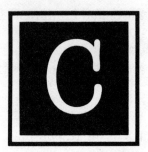

Other frameworks and models

JANET W. GRIFFITH

HALL'S CONCEPTUAL MODEL

Lydia Hall's model of nursing[4] began appearing in the nursing literature in the late 1950s. She describes nursing as consisting of three major components: care, core, and cure. These components are interrelated and depicted as three interlocking circles. Although these components are interactive, one component may be predominant, according to the client's level of health. The components may change predominance as the client progresses toward optimum health. Hall's model of nursing[5] has been used at the Loeb Center for Nursing and Rehabilitation at Montefiore Hospital and Medical Center.

The *care component* relates to maintaining the client's body functions and basic physical needs and promoting comfort. The nurse assists the client with activities of daily living that the client may require to promote the client's physical well-being and comfort.

The *core component* refers to the client as a person who needs to examine both the change in health status and the effect of these changes on his life-style. The nurse's role consists of the therapeutic use of self. The nurse assists the client in explorations concerning behavioral reactions, difficulties, and the future. The nurse facilitates the client's sharing of feelings in these areas. This promotes self-awareness and growth to handle changing self-concepts and life-style resulting from alterations in health.

The *cure component* reflects an interdisciplinary approach to the client, involving all members of the health team as well as the client, family, and significant others in the medical aspects of care. The nurse's role is as an active client advocate to bring together and facilitate the assistance of those health team members involved with the client.

In summary, Hall's care, core, and cure components address the physical, emotional, and interactive needs of the client. The nurse functions independently to meet the care and core aspects and works interdependently with other health team members in the cure component. This model is useful for assessment, analysis/synthesis, and especially planning of the nursing process for individual and family clients.

274

JOHNSON'S BEHAVIORAL SYSTEM MODEL

Dorothy Johnson's model[7] is a synthesis of theories and concepts from the behavioral and biological sciences that is integrated into a systems framework. Theories of stress and adaptation are also applied in this model. Man is viewed as a behavioral system, composed of seven subsystems. The subsystems interact and are interdependent. They strive to achieve balance and stability both internally and externally. Man strives to maintain balance and to function effectively by adapting to environmental forces through learned patterns of response. When these forces are too great, or when man is unable to adapt, behavioral instability develops in one or more of the subsystems. This reduces functional capacity and efficiency and depletes energy.

Nurses help clients maintain efficient and effective behavioral functioning by preventing illness and promoting health. They regulate the external forces to preserve the client's behavioral (biopsychosocial) system at an optimum level by imposing external regulations or controls, changing structural units in desirable directions, or fulfilling functional requirements of the subsystems.

Johnson's model is based on the interaction of the behavioral system and the subsystems and on their patterns.

Behavioral system. In systems theory, a system is a whole with interdependent parts. The parts have a structure and a process, or pattern of behavior. Systems are characterized by organization, interaction, interdependence, and integration of the parts. Through interaction both within the subsystems and with the external forces acting on it, the system strives to maintain balance and stability by adjusting and adapting.

Subsystems. There are seven interdependent subsystems. A disturbance in one may affect the others. Each subsystem has a unique function or special task necessary for an integrated performance of all the subsystems, and each has both structure and function. Four structural elements influence each subsystem. First is the *goal* or *drive*, defined as the purpose of the behavior and the consequences achieved. In general, the goal of each subsystem is universal for all people, but individual variations exist. Second, an individual's subsystem *set* reflects the "person's predisposition to act with reference to the goal."[7] Set distinguishes the range of behaviors available to the individual to achieve a particular goal. Preferred behaviors are developed through learning, maturation, and experience. Third, each subsystem has a *choice* of alternative behaviors to achieve specific goals. The goal is achieved by the individual's subsystem *behavior*, which is the only observable aspect of each subsystem. This behavior is examined for its efficiency in achieving the goal.

Each subsystem has an established set of behavioral responses or tendencies toward a common goal or drive. These responses are developed through maturation, experience, and learning. They are influenced by biopsychosocial factors. Over time, responses may be modified; but an observable recurrent pattern of responses continues.

There are seven subsystems, each with a unique goal:

1. Attachment or affiliative: This subsystem's goal is to relate to or belong to something or someone. Its purpose is to achieve social inclusion, intimacy, and strong social bonds for security and ultimately survival.

2. Ingestive: The goal is to take in from the environment needed resources to maintain integrity, achieve pleasure, or internalize the external environment.[3]
3. Eliminative: This subsystem expels biological waste from the system.
4. Dependency: The goal is to obtain resources needed for assistance, attention, reassurance, and security. This aids in gaining approval, attention, trust, and reliance.
5. Sexual: This subsystem's goal is procreation and gratification at feeling attractive to and cared about by others.
6. Aggressive: The goal is protection of oneself and others from potentially threatening objects, persons, or ideas. It serves as a self-preservation mechanism.
7. Achievement: This subsystem's goal is to master or control oneself or one's environment through seeking some standard of excellence, such as physical, social, or creative skills.

System requirements. Each subsystem requires that functional needs be met and regulating mechanisms be intact to maintain stability and balance. Functional requirements are met through the individual's own efforts or through assistance from the environment. These requirements include protection, nurturance, and stimulation. *Protection* refers to safeguarding the individual from noxious influences with which the system cannot cope, defending the individual from unnecessary threats, and coping with a threat on the individual's behalf.[3] *Nurturance* means supporting the individual's adequate adaptive behaviors through nourishment, training, and conditions that support appropriate behaviors. *Stimulation* promotes continued growth and development. Different forms of stimulation are used for different purposes to maintain or enhance behavioral stability.

Individuals use a variety of *regulating and controlling mechanisms* to evaluate and choose desirable behavior. These mechanisms are learned through experience in childhood and are usually internalized by adulthood. The three major types of regulating and controlling mechanisms that individuals use are biophysiological, psychological, and sociocultural.[3] These mechanisms provide a monitor and feedback to the system. They guide behavioral alterations and coordination among the subsystems.

Behavioral patterns. Each system and subsystem develops patterned, repetitive, and purposeful responses to form an organized and integrated functional unit. These patterned responses determine the interaction between the subsystems, the system, and the environment. The behavioral patterns establish the relationship of the system or person to objects, events, and situations in the environment. These patterns are orderly, purposeful, and predictable. They maintain efficient functioning of the system.

Summary. In Johnson's model man is viewed as a behavioral system, interacting with the environment and composed of seven subsystems. These subsystems develop distinct behavioral patterns through maturation, experience, and learning. Each subsystem functions according to goals, a predisposed set, choices of alternatives, and observable behaviors. The subsystems receive input from the environment through sensory modes. They act upon the input through behavioral responses and provide output through verbal, motor, or physical exchanges with the environment. Regulating and controlling mechanisms provide feedback to alter or maintain the system.

When the system cannot cope with environmental forces, the n̶
individual adjust and adapt by meeting or guiding functional
to restore stability. Johnson's behavioral system model is ₴
individual clients in the nursing process. It is a comprehensiv̶
includes biopsychosocial aspects, but additional approaches ̶
mental aspects may be required for nursing assessment and analysis.

BETTY NEUMAN'S HEALTH-CARE SYSTEMS MODEL

Betty Neuman's model[11] is based on systems theory, Selye's theory of stress, adaptation theories, and holistic approaches to individuals and health care. This open systems model views the individual as composed of interrelated physiological, psychological, sociocultural, and developmental variables. As the individual interacts with the environment, stressors—intrapersonal, interpersonal, and extrapersonal factors—affect the individual and generate varying responses. Nursing aims to attain and maintain maximum wellness by reducing the stressors or strengthening the individual's line of defense.

The aim of Neuman's model is to "provide a unifying focus for approaching varied nursing problems and for understanding the basic phenomenon: man and his environment. The model is based upon an individual's relationship to stress—his reaction to stress and factors of reconstitution—and is thought of as dynamic in nature."[11] The model considers three factors: the occurrence of stressors, the reaction of the client to the stressors, and the client's physiological, psychological, sociocultural, and developmental status.

Neuman's concepts defined

Individuals. Man is an open system interacting with the environment through interpersonal and extrapersonal factors. Each individual is unique with characteristic responses within a normal range, which provide an internal set of resistance to stressors. Individuals are open systems with physiological, psychological, sociocultural, and developmental variables that dynamically influence the state of wellness or illness. Individuals are continuously exposed to various stressors in the environment and respond by adjusting to the environment or adjusting the environment. Through interactions and adjustment, the individual attempts to maintain harmony and balance both internally and externally.

Stressors. There are a variety of stressors, which may be categorized as: intrapersonal—forces operating within the individual; interpersonal—forces operating between the individual and others; and extrapersonal—forces outside the individual. Stressors are considered to be any situation, condition, force, or potential source that is capable of creating instability within the individual or reducing the individual's effective lines of defense or resistance.

Lines of defense and resistance. These consist of everything the individual possesses internally that assist in dealing with stressors. An individual's line of defense is flexible and dynamic, and varies according to such influencing factors as physiological structure, condition, and functioning, age, sex, sociocultural background, developmental state, and cognitive skills.

The individual's lines of resistance vary with the interrelationship of these factors and the number and degree of stressors experienced at any time. The lines of defense serve as a buffer to reduce stressors and prevent them from disrupting the system.

Nursing interventions. Nursing intervention is directed at all the individual's variables that respond to the stressors, and help the individual attain or maintain maximum health. Nurses assist the individual toward reconstitution, the "resolution of the stressor from the deepest degree of reaction back toward the normal line of defense."[15] Nursing intervention may be initiated when a stressor is suspected or identified and is based on four factors: degree of reaction, resources, goals, and anticipated outcome.[11]

Intervention strategies are developed in three levels of prevention, namely primary, secondary, and tertiary, as defined by Venable.[15]

Primary prevention consists of interventions initiated before or after an encounter with a stressor; it includes decreasing the possibility of encounter with stressors and strengthening the flexible lines of defense in the presence of stressors.

Secondary prevention consists of interventions initiated after encounter with a stressor; it includes early case finding and treatment of symptoms following a reaction to a stressor.

Tertiary prevention consists of interventions generally initiated after treatment; it focuses on readaptation, reeducation to prevent future occurrences, and maintenance of stability.

Summary. Neuman's model is applicable in all components of the nursing process. It is especially useful for individual and family clients with stress and for guiding nursing implementation strategies. It is a broad model that can be used across all clinical areas.

ROGERS' FRAMEWORK OF NURSING

Martha Rogers' framework[12] is based on a synthesis of the behavioral and social sciences. She views the focus of nursing as "a science of unitary man." The education and practice of nursing are "directed toward the maintenance and promotion of health, prevention of illness, and care and rehabilitation of the sick and disabled."[13]

The basic assumptions underlying Rogers' framework are important. She believes that individuals are unique, unified wholes possessing individual integrity. This wholeness results from living in a dynamic environmental interaction that is continuous, creative, evolutionary, and uncertain. Rogers views individuals as open systems in continuous interchange of energy with the environment. The life process of individuals evolves in one direction along an irreversible space-time continuum. The individual is the totality of all life events experienced at a given time. Pattern and organization identify individuals and reflect their innovative wholeness. An individual's pattern and organization provide for self-regulation, rhythmicity, and dynamism. Last, the fundamental characteristics of humans are attributable to their ability for abstraction and the use of imagery, language, thought, sensation, and emotion.

From these assumptions Rogers defines four concepts essential to her framework.

Energy fields represent a unifying concept of the changing nature and infinity of the universe. Rogers views man and environment as energy fields that are more than the sum of their parts, each having its own integrity. The fundamental unit of unitary man and environment is an energy field.

Openness refers to the infinity and unboundedness of the energy fields, which are continuously open.

Pattern and organization explain the identity of the energy field. This is a universe of open systems with creative and innovative change. "Human and environmental fields are continuously characterized by wave pattern and organization, but the nature of the pattern and organization is always novel, always emerging, always more diverse."[13]

Four-dimensionality means synthesizing the dimension of time with the three dimensions of space; thereby "reality [is] perceived as a synthesis of non-linear coordinates from which innovative change continuously and evolutionally emerges."[13]

In Rogers' humanistic framework, each human field and each person's environmental field are unique but coexist within the universe as integral to each other. Man has the ability to reason and feel, and possibly the capacity to participate knowingly in the process of change. Rogers defines man and environment in the following ways.

Unitary man is a four-dimensional, negentropic energy field identified by pattern and organization and manifesting characteristics and behaviors that are different from those of the parts. They cannot be predicted from knowledge of the parts.

Environment is a four-dimensional, negentropic energy field identified by pattern and organization. It encompasses all that is outside a given human field.

From the above framework, Rogers developed three principles of homeodynamics, which are "broad generalizations that postulate the nature and direction of unitary human development."[13]

1. Principle of helicy: "The nature and direction of human and environmental change [are] continuously innovative, probabilistic, and characterized by increasing diversity of human field and environmental field pattern and organization emerging out of the continuous, mutual, simultaneous interaction between the human and environmental fields and manifesting nonrepeating rhythmicities."[13]
2. Principle of resonancy: The human field and the environmental field are identified by wave patterns and organization manifesting continuous change from lower-frequency, longer wave patterns to higher-frequency, shorter wave patterns.
3. Principle of complementarity: The interaction between human and environmental fields is continuous, mutual, and simultaneous.

These principles only apply to Rogers' framework of unitary man. The principle of complementarity is really subsumed within the principle of helicy. To bring this framework together, Rogers[13] states, "Unitary man and his environment are in continuous, mutual, and simultaneous interaction, evolving toward increased differentiation and diversity of field pattern and organization. Change is always innovative. There is no going back, no repetition. Causality is contradicted."[13] To use Rogers' framework in the nursing process requires greater knowledge of these concepts.

AGUILERA AND MESSICK'S THEORY OF CRISIS INTERVENTION

Donna Aguilera and Janice Messick[1] synthesized the views of several behaviorists in their crisis intervention theory. They consider crisis a stressful event or change in the individual's life. It involves a loss or threat of loss that disrupts the individual's equilibrium. Crises are categorized as maturational or situational. Maturational crises are those events that occur routinely. They include marriage, pregnancy, going away to school, and the death of a friend or spouse. Situational crises are unexpected events, such as failing an exam, losing a job, receiving a promotion, or sustaining an injury.

These authors describe three balancing factors. Each factor must be present in a threatening situation to avert a crisis. These factors reduce the risk of a crisis and help the individual maintain equilibrium. The three factors are realistic perception of the event, adequate situational supports, and adequate coping mechanisms.

Realistic perception of the event. The meaning an individual attaches to an event influences the perception of it. Sometimes past experiences evoke feelings unrelated to the event; these feelings may distort the individual's perception and magnify the consequences of the event. When an individual attaches great significance to an event, a distorted perception is likely. The individual's feelings and emotions may create an unrealistic picture of the present and future, which hinders effective decision making and may lead to crisis. Those individuals with a realistic perception of the event are able to view the situation in perspective. This reduces the chance that their emotions will cloud decision making. A realistic perception of the event may avert a crisis.

Situational supports. Individuals rely on others to assist them in times of need. Significant others reflect an appraisal of the individual's self-worth and the meaning of the event. When faced with a loss or threat of loss, individuals share the meaning of the event with significant others. This sharing helps the individual place the event in perspective. Situational supports are considered adequate when the individual feels he can share the concern with and receive support from significant others. Sometimes an individual cannot share the concern with others for fear of losing their respect or esteem. When an individual lacks others with whom to share events or concerns, his situational supports are inadequate. This may cause disequilibrium and lead to a crisis.

Coping mechanisms. From life experiences, individuals learn a repertoire of coping responses or patterns. These patterns assist individuals in reducing tension, in adapting to daily stressful events, and in maintaining equilibrium. Occasionally, a stressful event occurs that overwhelms the individual. It may be an unfamiliar situation, the magnitude of the concern, or several concerns occurring simultaneously. Usual coping responses are ineffective, resulting in disequilibrium and crisis.

Summary. This theory of crisis intervention describes three balancing factors: realistic perception of the event, situational supports, and coping mechanisms. Each factor must be adequately present to maintain equilibrium and avoid a crisis. In crisis intervention, each factor is assessed and if one is missing or inadequate, means are sought to enhance or develop that factor. Crisis theory is an excellent one to use in the nursing process with individuals or families experiencing situational or maturational crises. This theory guides all components of the nursing process and is applicable in planning nursing implementation strategies.

BEAVERS' HEALTHY FAMILY FRAMEWORK

W. Robert Beavers[9] identified five components representative of healthy families. These components address the interrelationships among family members. This framework can be used to determine family strengths and weaknesses.

Family power structure. In the healthy family, power is shared and based on competence from experience. There is a clear hierarchy of power, with leadership in the parent's coalition. The children exert an influence on family decisions. The power is flexible without marked dominance and is experienced as benign leadership.

Degree of family individuation. Family members are able to express themselves freely, assuming responsibility for their own thoughts and actions. Members respect each other and recognize their unique experiences and differences; their receptiveness to each other is shown by open communication and empathy. There is a closeness among the members; yet distinct boundaries of separateness exist. Individuals clearly express their feelings and thoughts but feel accepted in spite of their mistakes or limitations.

Acceptance of separation and loss. The healthy family with a strong parental coalition is able to accept loss as part of life. There is evidence of strong relationships outside the family. Parents accept their own aging as part of reality and operate on the basis of a functional transcendent value system that incorporates loss as a natural phenomenon.

Perception of reality. The family unit perceives itself as a group with specific functions congruent with reality. There is a sense of time-binding experiences that bind the members together during the passage of time. This provides a matrix of shared meaning of the family as it acknowledges and accepts the passage of time and growth of its members. There is a sense of future and timelessness for the achievement of growth and change in the family and its members.

Affect. The healthy family is able to express a sense of humor and hopefulness directly, with an optimistic mood of warmth and caring prevailing. Family members are sensitive to and understand each other's feelings, conveying openness, trust, love, and respect for each other. They feel comfortable reaching out to other members to express their needs and are receptive to the needs of others.

Summary. Beavers' framework identifies components of a healthy family, which is depicted as sharing power according to competence. There is a healthy respect for each member's uniqueness, and members are able to share their feelings comfortably and reach out to others. The healthy family share meaningful experiences that bind them together, and are able to accept aging and loss as part of life.

Beavers' framework is a useful guide for all the family nursing process components. Since it mainly addresses interpersonal relationships, it may be necessary to supplement the assessment and analysis with a physiological approach.

ERIKSON'S DEVELOPMENTAL MODEL

Erik Erikson[2] is a lay psychoanalyst who extended Freud's theories on man. He emphasized the influence of sociocultural and biophysical dimensions on the individual's development. In Erikson's model, human development is interrelated with cultural and physical growth over eight distinctive stages. Each stage represents a developmental task: a foundation for the next stage. Each task is never fully resolved, and it may resurface in later years. The critical task at each stage holds a zenith position at that period of development; it becomes less dominant later but may arise again. If the specific task is not accomplished during the critical period, Erikson notes the consequences in the development of undesirable behaviors.

Erikson's eight stages of man

Trust versus mistrust. In infancy, the central task is to develop a sense of trust that basic needs will be adequately met. As these needs are met, the infant learns that the world is a safe place to live in. There is a predictable pattern that can be trusted. Mistrust in the safety and predictability of life occurs when the infant's needs are not satisfactorily met.

Autonomy versus shame and doubt. The toddler who has learned to trust begins to test the environment, determining the extent to which the environment can be manipulated. Autonomy develops as the toddler explores and learns control of self and the environment. If independent actions are thwarted or are unacceptable to others, the toddler experiences shame. When attempts made to manipulate the world are ineffectual, the toddler may develop doubt.

Initiative versus guilt. As the preschooler tries to be assertive during interactions with others and the environment, approval from others fosters initiative. When the preschooler's actions are not permitted or are disapproved of by others, the child has a sense of guilt.

Industry versus inferiority. The school-age child directs energy toward learning knowledge and skills applicable in the real world. The child who receives satisfaction from those efforts will continue to be industrious. The child who has difficulty and whose unsatisfying efforts go unrewarded may feel inferior and inadequate.

Identity versus role diffusion. During adolescence the individual searches for current and future identities. This is an attempt to integrate life experiences into a sense of self. To master identity the adolescent must feel an internally consistent self-image. It must agree with others' views. The adolescent who is unable to integrate life experiences and self-image into a consistent identity experiences role diffusion. Feelings of being lost or confused may occur.

Intimacy versus isolation. The young adult seeks relationships with others to acquire a sense of sharing, caring, and intimacy. An individual who is unable to share close relationships and feel comfortable in intimate relationships may have a sense of isolation from friends or family members.

Generativity versus stagnation. In adulthood the primary task is satisfaction with productivity. This includes work, family, home, and citizenship. These activities and a sense of accomplishment provide the individual with intrinsic rewards, but the adult who is dissatisfied in these areas may feel stagnation. With lack of productivity, the adult may indulge in self-absorption and develop derogatory attitudes toward others.

Integrity versus despair. The older adult, satisfied with life and its meaning, who believes that life is fulfilling and successful, has integrity. A sense of despair develops when the older adult fears death and finds failure with oneself and others.

Summary. Erikson's developmental model depicts eight psychosocial stages in the life cycle. It identifies critical developmental tasks at each stage and the consequences when a critical task remains unaccomplished. Although each task is age appropriate, the tasks are never completely resolved and may arise at any time in the life cycle. This developmental model has limited use in the nursing process. Each client should be assessed and analyzed according to the age-appropriate developmental level. The model is used in conjunction with other, broader frameworks that include biopsychosocial concepts.

HILL AND HANSEN'S FAMILY CRISIS MODEL

From the study of families in crisis, Reuben Hill and Donald A. Hansen[6] identified major factors that influence a family's ability to cope with or adapt to a crisis. These factors were categorized in four groups that are interrelated but conceptually distinct. This analytical model provides an excellent base for assessing both the meaning of the crisis to the family and their ability, as individuals and as a unit, to adapt to the situation. Family strengths and deficits can be identified from the model, and nursing intervention strategies generated from it.

Characteristics of the event. A major concern of the entire family is the change in the biological system of the affected family member. The type of disability, prognosis, and potential for rehabilitation affect both the individual member and the family unit. The significance and perception of the concern in relation to the pathophysiological factors, knowledge of the condition, including potential limitations, and the response of others need to be explored by each family member and the family as a whole.

Perceived threat to family relationships, status, and goals. When a crisis or illness occurs in a family, members may assume different roles temporarily or permanently. The family needs to identify what roles will change, which roles are given up by whom, and what new roles will be taken on by others. This has implications for all members, as roles are reciprocal and the changes may affect future family interactions. Family members need to identify past family roles, relations, and communication patterns, along with the changes necessitated by the crisis or illness. With role changes, decision-making patterns will also change, and this may alter family relationships. With a family crisis, both individual and family goals may change. The family members' feelings about the new roles, decisions, and goals need to be expressed openly to alleviate anger, hostility, and resentment, and prevent them from developing with the changing family situation in a crisis.

Resources available to the family. Resources may be considered as the abilities and skills of family members and friends or relatives, facilities in the community, financial means (such as income and insurance), and transportation. Both the quantity and quality of each resource must be considered so that deficient areas may be supported. Information about the household composition, including the age, sex, and educational background of the members, is important. Marital status, ethnicity, religion, occupation, and income are also important factors that influence the family's adaptation to a crisis.

Past experience with crises. Families who have dealt with previous crises may draw on these experiences in new crises to assist them in solving problems. In crises, new decision-making patterns may emerge in the family. Also, the family may turn to supportive individuals in the community whom they believe they can "count on," as they have in the past. Past experiences may strengthen or weaken the family's ability to cope.

Summary. This family crisis model is sufficiently broad and comprehensive to serve as a guide to each component of a family nursing process. It incorporates the basic approaches to crisis management and can guide the nursing assessment, analysis, and planning components.

KOHLBERG'S STAGES OF MORAL DEVELOPMENT

Lawrence Kohlberg's interest in moral development was stimulated by the work of Piaget, and he explored the responses of young adolescents to moral dilemmas in his dissertation study. From his research and his own beliefs, Kohlberg identified six levels of moral reasoning.[8] Kohlberg views moral development in children as moving gradually to higher stages based on the child's capacity for increasingly complex logical "operations," combined with an increasing empathy for others through social interactions. These stages emerge in an invariant sequence in response to both internal presssure and social interaction with others.

Level I: Premoral

Stage 1: Punishment-obedience orientation. The child defers to the superior power and position of authority figures, usually parents. The physical consequences of the child's behaviors, in term of goodness or badness, are determined by others, without regard for the meaning or value of the behavior. The punishment and power or authority of others determine for the child what is right or appropriate behavior.

Stage 2: Instrumental-relativist orientation. The child's behavior is based on meeting one's own needs. The child seeks immediate or future gratification from actions. When the child interacts with others, there is a sense of fairness, reciprocity, and equal sharing, not a sense of loyalty, gratitude, or justice. Action is based on getting something in return.

Level II: Convenience morality

Stage 3: Interpersonal concordance or "good boy–nice girl" orientation. The child's behavior reflects approval seeking and conformity to appease others. Good behavior receives the approval of others as it pleases them or shows that the child helps others. There is conformity to stereotyped expectations of appropriate behavior or concern for others.

Stage 4: Law and order orientation. The child's behavior is oriented toward adherence to authority, rules, and the maintenance of social order. Acceptable behavior consists of performing one's duty, respecting authority, and abiding by the social rules for their own goodness.

Level III: Principled morality

Stage 5: Social contract, legalistic orientation. The individual acts on the belief that justice flows from a contract between those in authority and those under authority that assures equality for all. Appropriate behavior is based on the general individual rights and societal standards. Rules for reaching contracts or consensus are considered with behavior geared toward the "legal point of view," but the possibility of changing this view is weighed in terms of individual values.

Stage 6: Universal ethical principles orientation. An individual's behavior is based on personally chosen moral principles that are universal to society, consistent, and logically comprehensive. These principles are abstract and ethical and form the basis of justice in reciprocity and equality of humans.

Summary

Kohlberg's stages of moral development are a useful supplementary or supportive approach in the nursing process. They can be applied to the individual or family client, specifically for nursing assessment and analysis. Since they consider only moral development, they have limited utility.

MASLOW'S HIERARCHY OF NEEDS

Advocates of human needs theory view individuals as integrated, whole beings who are motivated by internal and external needs that create tension. To reduce this tension, an individual seeks to meet specific needs through goal-directed behavior. Abraham Maslow[10] classified human needs into five categories of predominance and placed them in a hierarchy. This hierarchy of human needs begins with basic fundamental needs of the individual that must be satisfied before proceeding to the next higher level. Throughout life the individual strives to satisfy needs at each level, but at different periods needs within one or more categories may be predominant. The desire to gratify human needs at each level motivates the individual and strengthens goal-directed behaviors. Generally, the basic physiological needs and safety needs must be relatively satisfied in the individual before striving for higher level needs.

Physiological needs. There are a variety of fundamental physical needs that have been identified, including air, food, sleep, sex, fluids, exercise, elimination, and stimulation. For survival and satisfactory function, every individual must have these basic physiological needs met. The extent or degree to which each of these needs is met varies with the individual. Some people require more sleep or food than others, but individuals must satisfy these needs at their own specific levels.

Safety. When basic physical needs are relatively satisfied, safety needs emerge; these include security, stability, order, physical safety, freedom from fear, protection, and sometimes dependency. These needs reflect self-protection through the establishment of structure, law, order, and limits.

Needs for safety and protection from harm may become more prominent when the individual is threatened by body harm as in physical illness or potential injury. Safety needs involve both imminent danger or concerns and potential loss, such as loss of the security of a spouse or occupational position.

Love and belonging. As physical and safety needs are reasonably satisfied, the need for love and belonging emerges. Within this category are needs for affectionate relationships, identification within various groups (family, church, and work), and companionship. These needs may be expressed through contact with significant others, tenderness, affection, and intimacy in sharing time spent together. Love and belonging needs may include contact with and affection for family members, friends, and associates of all age groups and both sexes. When love and belonging needs remain unsatisfied, the individual may feel alone, alienated, estranged, and distant from friends and relatives. The need for love encompasses both giving and receiving mutually.

Esteem and recognition. When the above needs have been gratified, the individual's need for esteem and recognition arise. These needs include self-respect, self-esteem, prestige, respect, and esteem from others. An individual may be motivated by the desire to achieve fame, recognition, strength, competency, independence, or an outstanding reputation. This desire for esteem and recognition motivates each individual toward goal-directed behaviors to achieve or gratify these needs in his own unique way. As this need is relatively satisfied, the individual experiences a sense of adequacy, self-worth, self-fulfillment, and contentment.

Self-actualization. When the lower needs in the hierarchy have been relatively satisfied, an individual strives toward self-actualization. Young people may grow toward self-actualization, but the individual must usually reach maturity before he has a sense of self-actualization. Self-actualization means that the individual is relatively satisfied with most aspects of life. This includes what the individual thinks of himself and the level of achievement reached or the ability to fulfill that designated purpose in life. Some adults continue working toward self-actualization all their lives, while others arrive at a sense of fulfillment or accomplishment in midlife. The individual feels a sense of having achieved his purpose in life and used his capabilities to the fullest.

Summary. Maslow's hierarchy is a broad approach that can be used in all components of the nursing process. It is applicable to both individual and family clients. It is most useful in arranging nursing diagnoses in order of priority, but can also serve as a guide in assessing and analyzing data and in planning nursing implementation.

STEVENSON'S FAMILY DEVELOPMENTAL MODEL

Joanne Stevenson[14] describes the basic tasks and responsibilities of families in four stages. She views family tasks as maintaining a common household, rearing children, and finding satisfying work and leisure. These tasks also include sustaining appropriate health patterns and providing mutual support and acculturation of family members. The four stages are delineated by the number of years the couple are married and their approximate age. The tasks for each stage are described below.

The emerging family. There are two major family tasks in the first 7 to 10 years of marriage. First, the couple strive for independence from their parents. Second, they develop a sense of responsibility for family life. This includes economic, emotional, and sociocultural responsibilities. Independence and responsibility are accomplished in the following ways:

Advancing self-development and the enactment of appropriate roles and
   positions in society.

Initiating the development of a personal style of life.

Adjusting to a heterosexual marital relationship or to a variant companionship style.

Developing parenting behaviors for biological offspring or in the broader
   framework of social parenting.

Integrating personal values with career development and socioeconomic
   constraints.[14]

The crystalizing family. When families reach the early middle years with
teenage children, different responsibilities emerge. The family assumes responsibility for growth and development of individual members and outside
organizations. The parents provide assistance to both the younger and older
generations without exerting control over them. These tasks are accomplished by:

Developing socioeconomic consolidation.

Evaluating one's occupation or career in light of a personal value system.

Helping younger persons become integrated human beings.

Enhancing or redeveloping intimacy with spouse or significant other.

Assuming responsible positions in occupational, social, and civic activities, organizations, and communities.

Maintaining and improving the home or other forms of property.

Using leisure time in satisfying and creative ways.

Adjusting to biological or personal system changes that occur.[14]

The interacting family. In the later middle years, most of the children
leave the home but return periodically with grandchildren. The older family
members absorb the small children into the home. Relationships between
work and leisure change. The older family now assumes responsibility for
"continued survival and enhancement of the nation."[14] To accomplish these
responsibilities, the adult members are involved in:

Maintaining flexible views in occupational, civic, political, religious, and
   social positions.

Keeping current on relevant scientific, political, and cultural changes.

Developing mutually supportive (interdependent) relationships with
   grown offspring and other members of the younger generations.

Reevaluating and enhancing the relationship with spouse or most significant other or adjusting to their loss.

Helping aged parents or other relatives progress through the last stage
   of life.

Deriving satisfaction from increased availability of leisure time.

Preparing for retirement and planning another career when feasible.

Adapting self and behavior to signals of accelerated aging processes.[14]

The actualizing family. In late adulthood the aging couple are engaged in
discovering meaning in their lives. They accept the process of grief and
dying. They "assume responsibility for sharing the wisdom of age, reviewing
life, and putting [their] affairs in order."[14] This task is accomplished by:

Pursuing a second or third career, new interests, hobbies, or community
   activities.

Learning new skills that are well removed from previous learnings.

Sharing wisdom accrued from the past with individuals, groups, communities, and nations.

Evaluating the totality of past life and putting successes and failures into perspective.

Progressing through the stages of grief, death, and dying with significant others and with oneself.[14]

Summary. Stevenson's model describes family tasks and responsibilities over four stages. The stages encompass child rearing, spouse relationships, and interaction with community organizations. They also include sharing wisdom and knowledge with other generations and organizations, changing the focus of work and leisure, and the grief process. This model is useful in examining family psychosocial patterns at a specific developmental stage. The biological health of family members needs to be added to this model for the nursing process.

REFERENCES

1 Aguilera, D.C., and Messick, J.M.: Crisis intervention: theory and methodology, ed. 4, St. Louis, 1981, The C.V. Mosby Co.

2 Erikson, E.: Childhood and society, ed. 2, New York, 1963, W.W. Norton and Co., Inc.

3 Grubbs, J.: An interpretation of the Johnson behavioral systems model for nursing practice. In Reihl, J.P., and Roy, Sr. C., editors: Conceptual models for nursing practice, ed. 2, New York, 1980, Appleton-Century-Crofts.

4 Hall, L.: "Nursing: what is it? Virginia State Nurses Association publication, 1959.

5 Hall, L.: The Loeb Center for Nursing and Rehabilitation at Montefiore Hospital and Medical Center, Int. J. Nurs. Stud. **6**:81, 1969.

6 Hill, R., and Hansen, D.A.: Families under stress. In Christensen, H.T., editor: Handbook of marriage and family, Chicago, 1964, Rand McNally and Co.

7 Johnson, D.E.: The behavioral systems model for nursing. In Reihl, J.P., and Roy, Sr. C., editors: Conceptual models for nursing practice, ed. 2, New York, 1980, Appleton-Century-Crofts.

8 Kohlberg, L.: Collected papers on moral development and moral education, Cambridge, Mass., 1973, Moral Education and Research Foundation.

9 Lewis, J.M., and others: No single thread: psychological health in family systems, New York, 1976, Brunner/Mazel, Inc.

10 Maslow, A.: Motivation and personality, ed. 2, New York, 1970, Harper & Row, Publishers, Inc.

11 Neuman, B.: The Betty Neuman health-care systems model: a total person approach to patient problems. In Reihl, J.P., and Roy, Sr. C., editors: Conceptual models for nursing practice, ed. 2, New York, 1980, Appleton-Century-Crofts.

12 Rogers, M.E.: The theoretical basis of nursing, Philadelphia, 1970, F.A. Davis Co.

13 Rogers, M.E.: Nursing: a science of unitary man. In Reihl, J.P., and Roy, Sr. C., editors: Conceptual models for nursing practice, ed. 2, New York, 1980, Appleton-Century-Crofts.

14 Stevenson, J.S.: Issues and crises during middlescence, New York, 1977, Appleton-Century-Crofts.

15 Venable, J.F.: The Neuman health-care systems model: an analysis. In Reihl, J.P., and Roy, Sr. C., editors: Conceptual models for nursing practice, New York, 1980, Appleton-Century-Crofts.

INDEX